About the Author

ARTHUR C. KLEIN is the au
(Robinson, 1994), an evalua
based on an unprecedented
1,000 people in the USA with
result was described in the *Sunday Telegraph* as 'a truly excellent
book' and sold nearly half a million copies in the USA alone.
Klein's finding that exercise was the most powerful treatment for
many forms of arthritis led to a follow-up book, *Arthritis: What
Exercises Really Work*, which was published in the UK in 1996.

Note

This book is intended as a reference volume only, not a manual for self-treatment.

Every effort has been made to ensure the contents of this book are accurate and current. Medical and pharmaceutical knowledge is constantly changing and the application of it to particular circumstances depends on many factors. Therefore readers are urged always to consult a qualified medical specialist for individual advice. The writers, researchers and publishers of this book cannot be held liable for any errors or omissions, or action that may be taken as a consequence of using it.

Note from the author

Many of the 1,051 participants in the US nationwide Arthritis Survey performed the exercises in this book to good advantage. The program as a whole has been reviewed and approved by several US physicians who are considered experts on the topic of exercise. Nevertheless, your own physical condition may require special modifications and precautions. We encourage you to show this book to your doctor before beginning to practise this program.

The Daily Telegraph

ARTHRITIS

The complete guide to relief using methods that *really work*

Arthur C. Klein

ROBINSON
London

Constable & Robinson Ltd
3 The Lanchesters
162 Fulham Palace Road
London W6 9ER
www.constablerobinson.com

This revised edition published in the UK by Robinson,
an imprint of Constable & Robinson Ltd 2005

A combined edition first published in the UK by Robinson Publishing Ltd 1998.
Arthritis: What Really Works first published in the UK by Robinson Publishing Ltd
1994; first published in the USA as
Arthritis: What Works by St Martin's Press 1989.
Arthritis: What Exercises Really Work first published in the UK by Robinson
Publishing Ltd 1996; first published in the USA in 1993.

A copy of the British Library Cataloguing in Publication data
is available from the British Library

ISBN 1-84529-073-9
ISBN 978-1-84529-073-3

Printed and bound in the EU

3 5 7 9 10 8 6 4 2

Contents

Acknowledgments

Thanks to Regina Gload, most of all, and also to Bridget MacSweeney and Eva Collins, for handling all the clerical work involved in conducting the Arthritis Survey™;

To Kathleen Pratt, M.S., R.D., for turning the dietary suggestions of survey participants and researchers into the Arthritis Survey™ Diet and Thirty-Day Meal Plan;

To Anthony F. Hitchcock and Jean Lindgren, for their help with the on-line searches of the medical literature;

To rheumatologists Barry L. Gruber, M.D., and Michael V. Sobel, M.D., for their expert opinions and advice;

To Willibald Nagler, M.D., and Irene von Estorff, M.D., of the Department of Rehabilitation Medicine at The New York Hospital-Cornell Medical Center, for their careful review of the exercise recommendations;

To Jared Kieling of St. Martin's Press, for pursuing and endorsing this project; and

To the 1,051 Arthritis Survey™ participants, for sharing their knowledge and experiences.

Introduction

The treatment of arthritis can at times seem both complex and confusing. The range of remedies is certainly diverse, with orthodox doctors placing their trust in drugs and surgery while complementary practitioners tend to advocate more physical forms of therapy and dietary manipulation.

The great virtue of this book is that it makes sense of this confusion by allowing the real experts – arthritis sufferers themselves – to express their opinion on the relative merits of these two approaches.

The main reason for the multiplicity of different treatments is that, regrettably, no single cause for arthritis has been discovered. Genetic inheritance certainly plays a role in some variants such as osteoarthritis, and there is no doubt the main symptoms of pain and stiffness can become more severe with ageing. Yet the precise trigger that starts off the inflammation in the joints – and there must be one – has still to be identified. When the cause of arthritis is found – as undoubtedly it will be at some point in the future – then it might be possible to develop some new treatment that will stop the disease in its tracks. In the meantime, the only alternative for the individual is to find those treatments that suit them best by either palliating or minimizing their symptoms, or by slowing down the progress of the disease. But where to start?

The difference in approach between the mainstream and alternative therapies goes back to the 1950s when steroids and other anti-inflammatory drugs were found to have a dramatic effect in alleviating the symptoms of arthritis. Many doctors at the time thought these were the answer to combat arthritis, and became heavily committed to drugs as the only scientifically respectable mode of treatment, dismissing any other therapy. Regrettably, drugs – and particularly steroids in the treatment of rheumatoid arthritis – did not fulfil early expectations and their usefulness was soon found to be severely compromised by the serious side effects they caused.

The surge in popularity of complementary medicine, starting in the 1970s, led to the rediscovery of more traditional approaches to treatment that had been neglected by mainstream medicine, and nowhere was this more obvious that over the vexed issue of diet. In medical textbook terms arthritis was perceived as being the result of an aggressive attack by the body's immune system, causing severe inflammation of the joints and for which the obvious cure was through drugs that depressed the result of the inflammatory response – anti-inflammatory drugs. Doctors dismissed any suggestion that diet might be important because it was impossible to see how it might have fitted into this traditional mode of thought. Nonetheless many patients have since discovered that dietary changes such as cutting down on fatty foods or increasing the amount of fish consumed could on occasion be quite dramatically beneficial in easing their arthritis, and often much more so than the drugs they had been prescribed.

It is in this context where individual responses to any treatment – whether mainstream or alternative – is highly variable, that a dispassionate view is at a premium, and who better to provide it than the real experts: the patients themselves. The crucial message to emerge is that there is no 'right' or 'wrong' treatment in this matter but rather that people must test out remedies for themselves and should trust their own judgement.

This is exemplified by the comments of a 29-year-old teacher from Texas who is quoted in the section on nutrition: 'Most of the rheumatologists I have seen dismiss nutrition, other than to say it is important to eat balanced meals and not to become overweight. But, personally, I find that whenever I eat a lot of sugar products I will feel pains in one or more joints so I try not to indulge my sweet tooth too often and although I believe it is important to follow a doctor's advice, ultimately I am the judge of what is best for my body, because I know my body better than anyone else.' Exactly.

There is no doubt that the treatment of arthritis can predispose to entrenched views and that those disillusioned with the orthodox approach might be too readily scornful of what it can

genuinely offer while accepting uncritically every type of alternative therapy. Nowhere is this more revealing than in the question
of the value of copper bracelets. Many people with arthritis have
worn a bracelet at one time or another, perhaps because being
such a widespread practice it must be presumed to be of help.
But do copper bracelets make a difference? By an overwhelming
majority the participants in the survey conducted for this book
agreed it did nothing other than, as one pointed out, 'turn your
arms green. They jingle and get caught in things too. I wore one
on each wrist for approximately two months with no relief.'

Both these examples, first of diet and then of copper bracelets, illustrate how those with arthritis are prepared to explore
any avenue that might possibly be of benefit to them. Here in
this unique book they can learn from the experiences of others –
both positive and negative. In addition this book contains a complete volume of exercises which, carried out on a regular basis,
really can alleviate the stiffness and pain of arthritis. Again, these
exercises are ones which have been tried out and have worked
for sufferers, and I can think of no higher recommendation.

How good it is to have these two books published together in
one clear, comprehensive volume. *Arthritis: The Complete Guide to
Relief* really is a mine of invaluable information and help to
arthritis sufferers everywhere.

James Le Fanu

Foreword

When Arthur Klein first asked me to write a foreword to *Arthritis: What Exercises Work*, I was a little less than enthusiastic. I wondered whether I should accept the invitation, for I suspected the book might be 'just another patient care book,' whereas I have been deeply involved in rheumatology (the subspecialty of medicine that concentrates on all forms of arthritis) for forty years. As it turned out, I was honoured, delighted, and educated in reading – indeed *studying* – the manuscript. I believe that this book and its predecessor, *Arthritis: What Works*, are practical, scientifically sound, well written, and instantly comprehensible. Together, they offer the best advice available today in overall management of the two most widespread forms of arthritis, rheumatoid arthritis and osteoarthritis.

Arthritis: What Exercises Work deals with one of the most important and significant aspects of the management of these two diseases. Exercise is very commonly prescribed for arthritis, but that's about as far as it all too frequently goes. In other words, doctors give patients too little detail or instruction, with few illustrations, and no precise direction. Yet many of the most troublesome and disabling aspects of both rheumatoid arthritis and osteoarthritis are due to lack of exercise!

A joint that is immobilized initiates a series of changes that result in total destruction of the joint within about four months. This occurs even in the absence of disease – by dint of immobilization alone. Adhesions begin to appear in the joint, a strange tissue grows over the surface of the cartilage, and tears occur where tendons are inserted in bone. New planes of motion contrary to normal anatomical planes appear, followed by enzymatic degradation of the tissues. Ligaments become lax, losing their tensile strength. The cartilage that caps the ends of bones, and which is normally four times more slippery than Teflon, loses that slipperiness and becomes perforated by ulcers.

Many of the changes that occur in the joints of people with rheumatoid arthritis and osteoarthritis are assumed to be caused by a disease process, when in fact they are often a consequence of relative immobility. These findings underscore the enormous importance of exercise in the fight against arthritis. I always counsel my patients to exercise to their point of tolerance.

My advice to you, the reader, is the same. You should realize that immobility will set off the destructive set of events I outlined above in just a few weeks. After four or five months, such degeneration may be quite well along, so that even if you initiate a program of vigorous exercise, you may have to wait up to a year for the joint's normal motion to return. Therefore, I say, prevention is the order of the day.

Exercise exerts a very favourable influence on the immunological system, affecting the production of white blood cells, lymphocytes and leukocytes, as well as the whole spectrum of antibodies against various viruses and bacteria. A protective agent called interferon is induced by brisk exercise. There is even evidence that people who are exercising significantly lower their risk of cancer. Exercising also reduces obesity.

Actively exercising to the best of your ability helps you discover your own fountain of youth. Do not heed the warning that because you have a disease you should rest more and more, and not stretch yourself at all. That would be the worst thing you could do.

Stretching, described in the book, is of major importance as a prelude to walking and as a regular habit to maintain healthy ligaments, muscles, bones, joints, and tendons. A complete stretching program would require approximately ten to fifteen minutes a day. It is wise to stretch before and after a walk, to help you maintain optimum balance, and avoid stumbling and falls.

Warm up before you exercise, and cool down afterward with some postexercise stretching.

Walking, which almost everyone with rheumatoid arthritis or osteoarthritis can do to some degree, is of extreme importance as an integral, essential part of a program of disease management. I've come to use the term 'walk the walk' when urging my patients to carry themselves proudly, and to remember that self-confidence is the most important mental ingredient for success in arthritis management. The way you walk and move can strongly influence the way you think and feel. If your body is down, your thoughts and feeling will be down. If your body is up, your thoughts and feelings will be up, too.

Walking the walk means holding your head high and your chin up, while keeping your eyes forward, shoulders back, and arms swinging to the bounce in your step. It is difficult to walk the walk and say things like 'I'm awful,' 'I hurt,' or 'I can't do this.' Rather, a person who walks the walk says, 'I am confident in my ability,' 'I know how to handle pressure,' and 'I'm going to practice walking the walk by being aware of how I carry myself.'

When you focus on making positive physical changes, as this book shows you, you'll feel more positive and energetic.

To exercise, and especially to walk, is to induce the synthesis and release of a set of hormones called endorphins produced in the brain and the spinal cord. These normal, morphinelike substances actually diminish the perception of pain. Equally, or perhaps more important, is the fact that walking generates a sense of self-esteem, with increased optimism and decreased anxiety. Thus, walking confers both a physical and an intellectual appreciation of self-worth.

Increasing self-confidence not only makes you feel better physically and psychologically, but also improves sexual appetite and performance. You will look better and feel younger. You will grow tougher and more content. Best of all, you can say to yourself, 'I set out to do it, and I did it.'

Until recently, the question of how intensely one must exercise was unresolved. Taking a hint from a well-known fable, we can see that although the tortoise and the hare travel at different paces, the tortoise is the less anxious. You don't have to work up to a sweat to experience the stress-relieving and tissue-saving benefits of exercise. The evidence now is that walking, even at a slow pace, can induce the mechanisms in the body (arthritis or no arthritis!) that elevate mood, relieve anxiety, and improve one's overall self-esteem. Joint stiffness is reduced. Swelling tends to gradually disappear with regular walking. The prevention of bone loss is another benefit of walking.

As the author of this book points out, walking is one of the few exercises to which age and physical condition usually pose no barriers.

I also consider it of great importance to exercise your brain. By that, I mean I encourage you to practise memory methods, remain with the times, read, study, and be all you can be. I know I still see myself as an underachiever. I haven't run as fast as I can, I haven't walked as fast as I can, I haven't written as well as I can. Not yet! I can still strive to do better. And so can you. Regardless of the presence of a chronic disease – or anything else – you are capable of improved physical and intellectual performance. This book will help you achieve them.

John H. Bland, M.D.
Professor of Medicine, University of Vermont College of Medicine

Foreword to the First UK Edition

By Dr L. E. Glyn, MD (London), FRCP (London), Fellow of the Royal College of Pathology (London)

This unique book on arthritis was originally published in the USA and is based on the experiences of 1,051 people in that country suffering from osteoarthritis (564), rheumatoid arthritis (416) or both (71). The information it contains derives from these individuals' responses to a detailed questionnaire, which covered not only the type(s) of treatment, the type(s) of practitioner providing that treatment, and the respondents' assessment of the results, but also such additional treatments and coping mechanisms as the patients themselves found useful. Among these latter factors, modifications of diet feature strongly, and the author include some detailed suggestions for eating patterns based on what the respondents found helpful.

Readers in the UK may find it interesting to compare the provision of care for people with arthritis available in the USA with that available in Britain. Perhaps the most striking feature of this comparison is the relatively small number of consultant rheumatologists in the USA – that is, those who have passed the Board examinations corresponding to the similar specialist qualifications in Britain. In 1989, when this book was first published, there were only about 2,000 such rheumatologists in the USA, but 40 million people with arthritis: a ratio of one consultant to 20,000 patients. No wonder Americans may find it hard to track down a rheumatologist or to get an appointment to see one. In Britain, by contrast, almost every large district hospital has its rheumatological department with one or more consultants attached to it.

One consequence of this disparity in medical provision is that

US patients make far more use of non-medical practitioners, especially chiropractors and osteopaths. It is noteworthy that the results achieved by non-medical practitioners – at least as reported by the survey respondents – were far inferior to those achieved by rheumatologists.

Another feature of US medical practice which will strike the British reader as unfamiliar is the question of cost: the patients surveyed frequently refer to the high cost not only of consultation but also of drugs and other forms of treatment, even when these are partly covered by medical insurance. In Britain, patients have access to the appropriate specialist care on the National Health Service, though this may not automatically include access to non-medical practitioners such as chiropractors and osteopaths (see the Note on Health Care in the UK on p. xxvi).

The most important question facing the intending purchaser of this book is to what extent a person with arthritis in the USA resembles his or her counterpart in the UK. From my own experience dating back to 1947, and from much intercourse with American rheumatologists, I can assure readers that there are virtually no differences of note between the two groups or the treatments they undergo. Not only is orthodox treatment essentially the same, but the same unorthodox treatments also have their adherents. Even the copper bracelet will be found on about the same proportion of people.

The reader will find that most of the drugs used to treat arthritis bear the same names in Britain as they do in the USA. In the Note on Drugs (p. xxviii) a list is given of those drugs that are known under a different name or names in the two countries. A very few drugs mentioned in the text do not appear in the Data Sheet Compendium published by the Association of the British Pharmaceutical Industry and are therefore not available in these forms in the UK. A list of these is also given in the Note on Drugs.

About one-quarter of the book is devoted to nutrition and diet, and the role of these factors in influencing the manifestations of arthritis. There is no doubt that this area is exciting interest among British rheumatologists, and the subject is well reviewed in an article in a recent issue of the *British Journal of Rheumatology* (vol. 32, 1993, p. 507). Another article in the same volume (p. 982) discusses the beneficial effects of fish oils in reducing the need for non-steroidal anti-inflammatory drugs. It is highly improbable that any of the common rheumatic diseases is the result of malnutrition, but it is nevertheless highly probable that the condition of many patients would improve if some attention were paid to nutritional and dietary factors. British rheumatologists today are much less likely to take up the dogmatically antagonistic stance to this approach described by the respondents as characteristic of many of their American doctors.

Arthritis can be a serious, sometimes a disabling, disease. It comes in many forms, of which the two commonest – rheumatoid arthritis and osteoarthritis – are covered in this book, and it cannot be stressed too strongly that accurate diagnosis requires medical expertise, usually at the highest level. The proper supervision of treatment is best provided by that patient's own general practitioner, and no form of self-medication should be undertaken without your GP's knowledge and support. With this one caveat I can warmly recommend *Arthritis: What Really Works* to all those in the UK who suffer from this disease.

Dr Glyn was formerly Deputy Director of the Medical Research Council Rheumatology Unit, Taplow, and Director of the Kennedy Institute of Rheumatology, London.

Foreword to the Second UK Edition

By Professor Howard A. Bird, MD FRCP, Professor of Pharmacological Rheumatology, University of Leeds

This intriguing book, which is to be published in parallel in the USA, now reaches its second UK edition. It is a privilege to be invited to provide this foreword.

The first edition was based on the results of a United States postal questionnaire sent to individuals with arthritis, particularly those suffering from either osteoarthritis or rheumatoid arthritis. The results were re-fashioned into a style that might be of broad interest to the general public by two distinguished medical authors. This new edition has been updated with the results of a web-based survey conducted in the United Kingdom in January 2005. Nearly 500 osteoarthritis and rheumatoid arthritis sufferers responded to the survey questions and provided new insights into the conventional and complementary treatments they found helpful. A number of changes were noticeable from the earlier survey – perhaps the most significant being the widespread use of supplements such as glucosamine by arthritis sufferers. This new edition has expanded the coverage of these supplements and looks at the scientific evidence for their effectiveness.

First, there are a few notes of caution, particularly applicable to readers in the UK. Before a drug can be marketed, a licence has to be granted by the appropriate regulatory authority for the country concerned. Some are stricter than others and for this reason, in general, the number of drugs available in the USA, where the original questionnaire was circulated, is less than in the UK. For this reason your favourite drug that you take at present may not have been included in the survey. It has also been necessary to translate the different proprietary names under which the same drug may be sold in different countries. A reminder about important differences in the style of health care between the two countries is also provided.

A questionnaire study of this type, although of much interest, will not necessarily be an accurate chronicle of up to 150 different sorts of arthritis that can affect joints. Some of these types of arthritis have quite specific treatments and if you have one of the rarer sorts of arthritis, you may be disappointed to find the particular remedy you need is not covered. However, the questionnaire was circulated to patients with the two most common types of arthritis (osteoarthritis and rheumatoid arthritis) so it is probable that for most the general advice covered in responses will still be applicable to you.

Inevitably, it takes time to analyse a questionnaire and then to compile a book based upon the findings. As a result, some quite important drugs that have been introduced in the last five years are also not mentioned within these pages. Examples of treatments you will not find are leflunomide, a disease modifying drug for rheumatoid arthritis, consideration of the multiple use of several drugs at the same time for the better management of rheumatoid arthritis and the new and expensive 'biologic' agents such as the TNFα blockers and the blockers of other cytokines such as IL-1.

In addition, it should be remembered that the recent controversy about the benefits of a highly specific type of NSAID called a COX-2 inhibitor and the associated cardiovascular side effects that might occur with such drugs was barely dreamt of when this book was revised. Indeed, this is an area that just at present is changing almost by the week rather than by the year.

Against that background, the greater part of this book has and will stand the test of time and the patient perceptions of all the treatments they have tried, both conventional and unconventional, provide a unique resource of information that is not always gleaned through the more formal scientific or medical studies conducted by doctors. Many health professionals who play a significant role in the management of arthritis, not always with the full support of the medical profession, also receive honourable mention with realistic assessment of the advantages and disadvantages of each of the treatments they offer.

So, this book should provide a useful source reference and practical information based on the experience of the people that really count, the patients who suffer from arthritis. The author is to be congratulated on his achievement and it is hoped that this book will do much to explain many questions that the medical profession is often unable or disinclined to answer. I hope you enjoy reading it.

A Note on Health Care in the UK

While the kinds of practitioners and treatments described in this book are very similar in both the UK and USA, the structure of health care in the two countries is very different. Access to free health care for individuals in the UK is provided through the National Health Service, and your first port of call as a person with arthritis should always be your GP. He or she will then refer you to your local hospital or other specialist practice for the appropriate consultancy and treatment. Rheumatology units offer specialist facilities to people with arthritis. Many employ rheumatology nurse practitioners who work with the rheumatologists. Some units have their own rheumatology physiotherapists and occupational therapists. Both these health professionals work closely with the rheumatologist to offer specific support and treatment. Since the introduction of the 'internal market' in the NHS, the facilities your doctor will be able to offer you and the details of the necessary arrangements may vary from one practice and health authority to another, but in all cases it will be necessary to obtain referral from your GP before you see a specialist.

Your GP may also be willing to refer you to a chiropractor, osteopath or acupuncturist if you wish; alternatively, you may consult any of these practitioners privately, in which case of course you will have to bear the full cost. He or she may also be able to arrange for you to see an occupational therapist, who can be particularly helpful in advising on aids and adaptations to make many aspects of daily life easier and thus to help you retain as much independence as possible. Most large hospitals have an occupational therapy department; an alternative route is through your local social services department, which may well employ one or more occupational therapists.

One or two differences in terminology should be noted. Physiatry in the USA has much in common with physiotherapy as practised in the UK, although there are some differences. Access to physiotherapy is via the referral from your GP or hospital consultant. Some GP practices employ their own physiotherapist. Others employ counsellors to whom you can be referred. Podiatry is simply the American term for chiropody. Osteopaths in the USA are classified as medical doctors and may prescribe drugs, whereas their counterparts in the UK are classified as non-medical practitioners and therefore may not issue prescription-only drugs.

A Note on Drugs in the UK

In both the USA and the UK there is a strict division between 'over-the-counter' drugs, which anyone may buy from a pharmacy or chemist, and 'prescription-only' drugs, which may be obtained only on the authority of a doctor. In the USA, a licence to market drugs, whether through the medical profession or directly to consumers, is given by the Food and Drug Administration; in the UK the corresponding role is played by the Committee on the Safety of Medicines, a body responsible to the Secretary of State for Health which advises on the issue of clinical trial certificates and product licences. Without a product licence, a drug or other medical product cannot be marketed in the UK.

Most of the drugs mentioned in this book are available in both the UK and the USA under the same names. Some, however, are known by different names in the two countries, and these are listed below. Where a name is the 'generic' or 'approved' title by which a drug is known, it appears in roman (normal) type; where it is the brand or trade name by which it is sold by a particular manufacturer, it appears in bold type.

Name in USA	Name in UK
acetaminophen	paracetamol, **Panadol**
Advil	ibuprofen
Ansaid	**Froben**, flurbiprofen
Datril	paracetamol
etodolac	**Lodine**
ketorolac	**Toradol**
Meclomen	**Ponstan**, meclofenamate sodium
Mono-Gesic	**Disalcid**, salsalate
Nalfon	**Fenopron, Progesic**
Nuprin	ibuprofen
Relifen	**Relifex**

Rheumatrex	methotrexate, **Matrex**
Tylenol	**Tylex***
Voltaren	**Voltarol**

*Although Tylenol is a very popular over-the-counter drug in the USA, in Britain Tylex is available only on prescription because in addition to paracetamol, each tablet contains a smaller amount of codeine.

The nearest equivalent of the fish oils available in the USA under names such as **Promega** and **Proto-chol** is MaxEPA. Equivalents of the various liniments mentioned are **Aspellin** and **Sloan's**.

Drugs Not Available In the UK
The following drugs are not available in the UK, although most are variants of similar drugs that are prescribed in Britain.

Anacin, Excedrin (multi-ingredient products containing aspirin)
Anaprox (naproxen)
carprofen/**Rimadyl**
isoxicam
oxaprozin
Parafon Forte (a multi-ingredient product containing paracetamol)
Proquazone
Oraflex (benovaprofen) is not now available in Britain. It was formerly prescribed under the brand name **Opren**, but was withdrawn owing to a high incidence of serious side-effects. Butazolidin (phenylbutazone) is available under the brand name of **Butacote**, but is licensed only for the treatment of ankylosing spondylitis, a form of inflammatory arthritis primarily affecting the spine.

A Note on the Recipes for the UK

The recipes in chapter 13 use the American version of the imperial system of measurement – that is to say, pounds (lb) and ounces (oz) rather than grams (g) and kilos (kg) for weights, and pints (pt) and fluid ounces (fl oz) for volumes.

There are two particular points that British readers will need to note. First, the American pint contains only 16½ fluid ounces, whereas the imperial pint contains 20 fluid ounces. Second, Americans measure volumes in 'cups': one cup is half an American pint, that is to say 8⅓ fl oz.

If you prefer using the metric system of weights and measurements, any cookery book will contain a conversion table.

The abbreviation *T* in the recipes means (level) tablespoonful; *t* means level teaspoonful.

Part 1
Arthritis: What Really Works

Section 1
New Findings and a New Source of Help

To move freely without restriction due to pain, disability, or weakness is among the most basic of human rights. Any disorder that impairs mobility; limits the capacity to touch, embrace, or protect; and interferes with personal hygiene, physical labour, or recreation threatens a person's sense of dignity and self worth.

Stephen R. Kaplan, M.D., and Edward V. Lally, M.D., from an article on arthritis treatments in *The Journal of Musculoskeletal Medicine* (September 1986)

May the work you do to help the suffering and educate the public be blessed by God.

Survey Participant #440, a Canadian psychologist, minister, and mother of four

Chapter 1
You Have Good Reasons to be Hopeful

• A new kind of knowledge about helpful treatments for arthritis • Startling findings from an unprecedented nationwide survey • Questions you dare not ask your doctor — answered here

If you've read only this far, you already know something about arthritis. Maybe you know how it feels to lie imprisoned in bed each morning by knees and hips that have hardened to cement during the night. Or maybe you know the ringing noise that aspirin blares in your ears after you've swallowed your tenth or twelfth tablet of the day, or the fatigue that knocks you down in mid-morning, before you've had a chance to do half the things you used to accomplish with ease, or the anger that flares up when television commercials describe your ailment as 'minor aches and pains.'

No doubt you would like a *different* sort of knowledge about arthritis. What would help most to kill the pain? Would a change in diet help? Which experimental treatments hold real promise? Is surgery worth the risk? Can exercise slow the deterioration of the joints? Who gives the best care for arthritis? Which drugs fight inflammation best? Is there any harm in wearing a copper bracelet or drinking cod liver oil? How does one carry on — homemaking, making a living, making love — in spite of arthritis?

Your doctor may lack the time or the information to address these questions as fully as you might wish. Indeed, you dare not even ask some of the questions, for fear your doctor will laugh at you. And so you are left to ferret out the answers on your own.

This is a book of answers — a guide to the practitioners, treatments, and self-help strategies that can change your life for the better. It is based on the collective experience of more than one thousand people with osteoarthritis or rheumatoid arthritis* who took part in a US nationwide Arthritis Survey and over 450 people who took part in the 2005 UK Survey, and who have, among them, tried literally everything.

This is *not* a book of anecdotes, although as you read it, you will hear people telling their stories in their own words. Instead, it is a detailed report of *what's out there*, with a painstaking analysis of *what works*.

Because this book draws heavily on people's actual experiences, it covers everything from the orthodox to the outlandish. Rather than dismiss alternative approaches and so-called 'quack' remedies with a sneer, we explore them in detail, since some of our participants tried them – and since you may be tempted to try them, too.

Because this book *also* draws on the rich store of information in the current medical literature, it introduces you to a few of the experimental therapies that are too new to be widely available yet, and some of the revolutionary developments in nutrition research that suggest how changes in diet may benefit people with arthritis.

In fact, so many treatments work to relieve arthritis pain that the real challenge is to discover *which* ones will work best for you. You can use the information in this book to help you:

- Find the kind of doctor best qualified to treat your arthritis
- Get extra help from nonmedical practitioners who can significantly improve the quality of your care
- Discover which practitioners are best avoided
- Put together a new diet plan that may relieve pain and control inflammation
- Minimize the risks of the prescription medications and over-the-counter drugs you take
- Replace the vitamins and minerals that medications may rob from your body

---

* Osteo- and rheumatoid are the two most common forms of arthritis. Osteoarthritis is the 'wear and tear' disease – the breakdown of cartilage inside one or more joints. Rheumatoid arthritis is a whole-body disease that inflames many different tissues, but especially the membranes that line the joints.

- Enjoy pain relief from simple techniques you can use at home or at work
- Learn how to exercise safely and effectively to preserve the natural motion of your joints
- Prepare for joint surgery so as to improve the likelihood of a successful outcome
- Manage your emotional reactions to arthritis and control pain-aggravating stress
- Explore the value of some unorthodox approaches, such as acupuncture and Yoga
- Continue to carry on your everyday activities with the help of a wealth of practical tips

You may want to go through the material from start to finish, or turn immediately to the topics that intrigue you the most. The text is full of cross-references, so you can be sure to find all the information on any given subject, even if you don't read the chapters in order.

The voice that speaks to you from this book is a far cry from the entreaties of those around you who *insist* that you try what they tried or go to the foreign clinic where Aunt So-and-So was cured.

It isn't the voice, or rather the countless disparate voices, of alternative health-care providers who have a cause to promote, or product manufacturers with a gimmick to sell.

The voice that speaks to you from these pages is broadly informed and charged with the encouragement, support, and advice of a thousand other people who have at least one thing in common with you – arthritis. But what makes this book a voice of authority?

Arthritis: What Works is based on a nationwide US survey conducted of 1,051 people with arthritis, updated with the results of a UK survey of over 450 people with arthritis, *and* on a rigorous search of the medical literature that pertains to arthritis. It is at once people-centered and scientifically supported. The individuals who took part in the survey shape the book by virtue of their interests and experiences. *The medical literature validates their views in most cases*, helps explain why they reacted as they did to various kinds of treatment, and shows you the surprising new directions that arthritis research is taking today.

The participants in the US survey were a microcosm of the 37 million Americans with arthritis. As a group, they match the national arthritis picture in terms of their age, sex, and the kinds of treatment they've received. What's more, the pooled experiences of the participants repeatedly mirror the results of medical studies on some of the topics covered here. For example, forty-eight survey-group members have tried methotrexate, a treatment borrowed from cancer therapy for use against particularly destructive cases of rheumatoid arthritis. Fifty percent of these participants (twenty-four individuals) said they enjoyed dramatic improvement on the methotrexate therapy – virtually the same rate of significant relief reported in a 1984 study of 189 patients at the University of Utah. In the UK survey twenty-six participants had tried methotrexate and 42 percent had experienced dramatic long-term relief.

In telling us their honest opinions of prescription anti-inflammatories for arthritis, to cite another example, participants suffered headaches from Indocin (indomethacin) and diarrhoea from Meclomen (meclofenamate) with precisely the same frequency as subjects in clinical trials of these drugs. The difference here, of course, is that participants also tell what *else* happened – how they resolved the difficulties, what other things they tried, and with what success. The survey participants can function as your national self-help group in print. You can compare your experiences with theirs and use their collective advice to guide your next choices.

Nor is their advice limited to the kinds of things your doctor might tell you. It has a broader range, addressing the whole gamut of arthritis care, from over-the-counter to under-the-counter and everything in between. Anything hyped on television or claimed in catalogues to be an arthritis 'cure' is subject to scrutiny here – because all treatments offered and all promises made about arthritis are of potential interest to people who have arthritis. As a result of the survey, we can use participants' assessments of chiropractic care, for example, to rate and compare what these doctors achieve to what medical doctors and other health-care practitioners have to offer you. We can take a serious look at the likes of copper bracelets, DMSO, been venom, honey, and apple-cider vinegar, and appraise their relative risks and benefits. In some of these areas, where respectable research has not been done, participants' advice may be the *only* source of unbiased information available to you.

On the question of nutrition many participants say there *is* a connection between nutrition and arthritis, having found that a change in diet amounts to a measure of pain relief or a reduction of inflammation. Many researchers agree and are busying themselves with landmark studies that show how certain foods can aggravate arthritis, while others apparently ameliorate the symptoms. Fascinating findings about fasting, about vitamins, and about specific food intolerances are spelled out here, both from the perspective of the individual survey participant, who has perhaps replaced red meat with fish, and the researcher in the hospital setting, who has watched patients with severe chronic rheumatoid arthritis *respond* to dietary therapy.

Many participants volunteered extra information not asked for – the probable *cause* of their arthritis, for example, the history of arthritis in their families, or the effects of the weather (dampness, cold, changes in humidity) on their pain. A few even took us to task for not probing these topics. But we intentionally avoided such questions in order to focus on purely practical matters, being after the tools and strategies that worked to make participants feel better – not the root cause of their problems. It was beyond the scope of the project to consider the influence of genetic or environmental factors in causing arthritis, and surely the weather is beyond anyone's control.

Our aim – and we achieved it – was to learn what works best for the most people: what stops pain, what reduces inflammation, what gets stiff joints moving in the morning, what practitioners offer the most help, what diet makes the most sense, what exercises can improve joint function, what techniques allow people to do what they must in spite of disability. If this is the kind of information you've been looking for, please read on.

Chapter 2
These People can Help You

• How early proper treatment changed a family history of arthritis • How gold reclaimed one woman's life • Surgery banished this man's pain • Experimental drug to the rescue • Diet makes a difference after all • Stories of people who helped themselves with exercise, grit, and guts

You are about to read a few case histories selected from the 1,051 stories in the US Arthritis Survey. These particular vignettes were chosen because each one of them recounts an experience shared by tens, scores, or hundreds of other individuals in the group. The accounts present some of the most important elements of arthritis care – and they introduce the people who help make this book a message of hope and encouragement.

When M.W. was a little girl, she saw her father stricken and then crippled by arthritis before his thirty-fifth birthday. He walked on crutches for the rest of his life, she recalls. 'I knew I didn't want to go through what I saw him go through.' And so, three years ago, when M.W. began to feel pain herself in her knees, elbows, and fingers, she suspected arthritis and sought treatment immediately, even though she was just twenty-eight at the time.

'When I began seeing the rheumatologist, I was naturally concerned and more worried than some people might have been. The rheumatologist was a real help to me. He was a good listener and took the time to talk to me, so I could get through that rough period and become determined to do what I needed to. He stressed the importance of a doctor and a patient working together for the patient's benefit. He helped me to believe that medications would help me resume a normal life, and I have found that to be so.'

M.W.'s father never saw a rheumatologist, nor did he know that there was such a thing as an arthritis specialist. These doctors were extremely helpful to participants, as you can see in Chapter 3 by the way they compare to other kinds of medical practitioners. Chapter 4 describes the non-medical practitioners, such as physiotherapists, who offer the best help for arthritis.

'I took aspirin in the beginning,' M.W. continues, 'and it helped a little, but I am doing much better with my arthritis since I have been using a prescription anti-inflammatory drug called Feldene. The arthritis no longer interferes with my shopping and cooking and taking care of my three children.'

Feldene and most other drugs like it did not exist when M.W.'s father was a young man. Today they are a mainstay of treatment, and drug companies keep coming out with new ones. You can read a full account of their pain-killing and anti-inflammatory effects in Chapter 5. Non-prescription drugs, including aspirin, are covered in Chapter 6.

H.L. was also young – thirty-five – when rheumatoid arthritis came on suddenly, invading all her joints with pain so intense she could barely function. And although her doctor tried to help her with several of the new anti-inflammatory drugs, including Feldene, she got no relief from any of them.

'When he saw that the arthritis was not getting better, he sent me to a rheumatologist who started me on gold injections and physiotherapy,' she writes. 'Then I began to get better in a hurry.' She felt her first moment of pain relief while soaking in the warm water of a hospital's whirlpool bath. She used the whirlpool every day for the next two weeks, and got hot-wax wraps for her hands from the physiotherapist, as well as hand splints to wear while resting or sleeping. These things all helped her feel better while she waited for the gold salts, called Solganal, to build up in her body with each weekly injection.

'The rheumatologist told me the gold shots would take at least three months to work, maybe six months, but I felt about 100 percent better in *six weeks*. After only two months on gold, I found I could do almost anything I had been able to do before I got sick. I have little discomfort at all, now. When I do, I take two aspirin a day. A warm bath helps a lot, too. Other times I might get that drained feeling and need to lie down for a few minutes. But the gold injections work so well I can do whatever I want.'

H.L. no longer sees the rheumatologist who helped her so much. Her family doctor has taken over her care again and gives her the necessary injection of Solganal twice each month.

Gold injections, which have been used as rheumatoid arthritis treatment on and off for the last sixty years, have also been joined by gold in pill form, to be swallowed instead of injected. You can see how the two compare in the second half of Chapter 5, and size them up against other specialized treatments that come into play when anti-inflammatory drugs fail to help.

L.F., an English professor, talks about his arthritis in the past tense, thanks to two total hip replacements he had six years ago, at the age of sixty-five. 'I do have a little arthritis in my thumbs,' he concedes, 'and I can't turn my neck very far, but I have *no* constant aches anymore, and I take *no* pain medications.'

After discovering he had osteoarthritis, L.F. relied on aspirin, then switched to the newer anti-inflammatory drugs. He also joined a health club, where he found '*great* relief and help' from swimming and using the Jacuzzi about three times a week. But his rheumatologist and orthopaedist agreed at the end of seven years that he could be dramatically improved with surgery.

L.F.'s two operations were scheduled six months apart, and he had the benefit of physiotherapy twice a day, including exercise instruction, during each hospital stay. The result? 'I have no pain! I suppose it took months to *fully* recover from the surgery, but I remember that I drove to the health club after two weeks. Now that I've retired, I work in the yard and do all my own housework. I can only have praise for my doctors and my therapist because I am pain-free. If my hips come "unglued" in the future, I'll go back to my surgeon.'

Because his artificial hips were cemented in place, there is a chance that they may loosen sometime in the next ten years, or 'come unglued,' as L.F. aptly describes the possibility. However, other surgical techniques, described in Chapter 7, make use of 'cementless' joints that encourage your own bone to grow into the replacement parts and form a living, lasting fusion. In Chapter 8, you can find out about a dozen 'extra' measures, including many forms of physical therapy, that can ensure the best possible outcome from surgery – or from any other treatment, for that matter.

'Two years ago I could hardly move my wrists, elbows, shoulders, ankles, or knees,' writes C.E., a forty-five-year-old high school guidance counsellor. 'Just walking from the chair to the kitchen was a *major*, painful chore. I cried every day because it all seemed so futile. I was getting no sleep, I couldn't make love, and I was about to give up and just "sit."' The drug treatment that brought C.E. out of this terrible state was considered experimental at the time. It is called methotrexate and was first used in the treatment of cancer.

Every Monday, at 8 A.M., 3 P.M., and 10 P.M., C.E. swallows one small yellow tablet of methotrexate, in addition to the anti-inflammatory drug she takes every day. 'Now, three and a half years after my rheumatoid arthritis began, I am in semi remission with the methotrexate therapy.'

We look at methotrexate and other drugs in detail in Chapter 5.

As though he hasn't had enough to do, helping to care for his thirty-one-year-old brain-damaged son and managing his own rheumatoid arthritis for the past twenty-six years, P.D. has had three episodes of cardiac arrest and lives with a constant reminder of his years as a coal miner – the respiratory disease called black lung. For his arthritis, P.D. has taken aspirin, anti-inflammatory drugs, and prednisone. He's had steroid injections, physiotherapy, and surgery to replace his left hip and knee. And while he speaks well of the help he's received in all these avenues, the thing that makes the biggest difference to him now is the dietary change he prescribed for himself. 'I eat a lot less meat, bread, and sweets, and drink less coffee and cola. I eat more raw fruits and vegetables. I don't know how this diet would affect others, but I've found, beyond a doubt, that the closer I stick to it, the better I feel.'

The internist who first diagnosed P.D.'s arthritis didn't say anything about nutrition, beyond the standard advice to eat a balanced diet, but P.D. says, 'I believe that a diet without animal products, wheat products, sugar, salt, and cola can be of great benefit to the arthritic. To eat fresh raw fruit and vegetables will cause even further improvement.'

Several mainstream specialists have been seriously exploring the role of nutrition in arthritis prevention and treatment – *and* calling for an intensified research effort in this area, as you will see in Chapter 11. P.D.'s diet specifics are spelled out in Chapter 12, with other advice from the more than one hundred participants who say they have reduced their pain by changing the way they eat. Their suggestions, together with findings from new medical research on nutrition's role in arthritis, form the basis for the thirty-day meal plan that comprises Chapter 13. The vitamins and minerals that you may be missing, either because of your arthritis or the drugs you take to treat it, are discussed in Chapter 14, with specific recommendations.

R.D. had shrugged off minor arthritis pain in his knees for nearly thirty years, but when the arthritis settled in his spine, the pain became agonizing and relentless. Although he had only recently retired at age sixty-six, the pain was beginning to make R.D. think that he had perhaps lived long enough. He certainly didn't feel he had anything good to look forward to, and he still vividly remembers the night the pain sent him to the local hospital emergency room, begging for a strong painkiller or anything else that might help him find relief. Then his doctor encouraged him to lose weight and got him started on an exercise program with a phsyiotherapist. Today, forty pounds lighter and the veteran of eight years of regular exercise, R.D. controls his arthritis pain with nothing more than an occasional tablet of **Advil** (ibuprofen).

'I do two sets of exercises for my back – one for the upper spine and shoulders, and another for the lower back and legs. These are standard exercises recommended by doctors and registered physiotherapists. They take, on average, not over fifteen minutes each day. And yet I am confident that the exercises did *more than anything else* to relieve the terrible pain I was having.'

Exercise has proven to be so beneficial for treating arthritis that no one questions its value any longer. If you don't already have an exercise regimen, you can turn to Chapter 17 for a rundown of the best overall fitness activities, as described and rated by our participants, as well as specific exercises for specific joints.

For all the help she has received from doctors – and there's been a lot for which she's thankful – G.N. has boosted herself over some of the worst times by her own grit. Other survey participants also find that a positive outlook and some well-chosen strategies for reducing stress, controlling pain, and working around their limitations, as described in Chapters 15, 16, 18, and 19, make them feel in control of their lives again.

'My vanity has been very helpful to me,' G.N. writes. 'At the onset of the disease, when I couldn't comb my hair until two o'clock in the afternoon, I steadfastly refused to cut it off, and decided that I must learn to look good. I've continued to do this, and although people's comments imply that I can't have a chronic disease when I look so well, it's a source of pride to know that the "outside" looks good even when the "inside" is a mess.

'One of the most annoying aspects of living with arthritis is people's attitudes toward it. I, for one, look perfectly normal (except for the splint I wear), and I find that most people either do not understand the physical limitations that I have, or don't really believe they exist. I feel it is of the greatest importance to admit what one cannot do and learn to adapt or ask for help. My attitude is that there are many people who enjoy helping others, so why deprive them? I've also found that asking for help (when it's needed) helps others understand the limitations that the disease imposes.

'Another thing I've had to learn to do is express *feelings* to those who are close, so they can understand my mood shifts. This was so difficult for me at one time that I started out by putting notes on the refrigerator. Gradually, I was able to *say*, "I'm having a **** day." (Put in any four-letter word you like.)

'I've also learned that love doesn't stop because I have a chronic disease, and that I can be a valuable person despite my physical limitations. Ironically, it was my rheumatoid arthritis that taught my older son the sensitivity to cope successfully with his wife's disease when she learned she had multiple sclerosis. And it has taught me that people can continue to have intimate relationships and be needed by the able-bodied.'

Section 2
How to get Significantly Better Results from Professional Care

May I never forget that the patient is a fellow creature in pain. May I never consider the patient merely a vessel of disease.

> – from the Code of Maimonides, an oath taken by graduates of Mount Sinai Medical School

I will remember that there is art to medicine as well as science, and that warmth, sympathy and understanding may outweigh the surgeon's knife or the chemist's drug.

> – from 'A Modern Hippocratic Oath,' by Dr. Louis Lasagna, taken by graduates of Tufts University School of Medicine

Anyone with arthritis needs many warm fuzzies and insights that are not available in doctors' offices.

> – Survey Participant #238, a freelance writer from New Mexico

Chapter 3
Medical Doctors:

Which Ones to See, Which Ones to Avoid

• *Why rheumatologists and orthopaedists are so effective* • *How to find an arthritis specialist* • *The advantages of a family doctor* • *Where to get medical advice on exercise* • *How to talk to your doctor*

Getting the correct professional help right away is extremely important. Unfortunately for them, a number of the participants accepted what they called the 'inevitability' of arthritis and ignored the pain and stiffness as long as possible before seeking medical attention. Now they look back at the time they spent being stoical or philosophical and curse themselves for the delay. 'I self-doctored myself until about two years ago,' wrote a disabled printer from California. 'I feel now that this has been much to my downfall, and I would *not* recommend it to anyone. What helped me the most was finally admitting that I could not handle the arthritis by myself. Now I am seeing a specialist in this field, and I have full confidence in him, so I follow his instructions to the letter. And I am no longer bedridden, thanks to his treatments and advice.'

Other participants *tried* to get help right away, but got nowhere because the doctors they saw had some serious misconceptions about arthritis. For example, the myth that arthritis is a disease of old age persists in the minds of some medical professionals. As a result, a few of our participants in their twenties or thirties weren't taken seriously, because they were 'too young' to have arthritis. Now they have one or more artificial joints, even though they're 'too young' for those, too.

This chapter names and rates the various types of doctors who treat arthritis. As you will see, there are a few kinds of specialists who far outstrip the others in achieving dramatic success. If you haven't been examined by one of these practitioners and you are not satisfied with your present care, you owe yourself a trial visit. Also, check the tips at the end of the chapter for suggestions on how to make *any* visit to the doctor more productive.

Participants rated their doctors by judging the kind of help they'd received from each one, whether it was dramatic long-term relief, for example, moderate long-term relief, temporary relief, or no relief, which meant that the practitioner was ineffective. As you'll see, some practitioners only succeeded in making participants feel *worse*, either because of the treatment they provided or the negative attitude with which they offered their advice. Some survey participants did not rate this or that practitioner because they had started treatment too recently to make a judgment, or because they'd seen the doctor only for diagnostic tests or a second opinion about surgery.

First on the list are the rheumatologists, who in both the US and UK Survey turned out to be the most effective practitioners for providing long-term help.

Rheumatologists

- These arthritis specialists got praise for providing long-term relief, especially for rheumatoid arthritis.
- Aside from being the most knowledgeable about arthritis treatments, including experimental approaches, they may teach you a lot about self-care.

Rheumatologists, together with orthopaedists (see pages 28–30), are the popular heroes in the battle against arthritis. Rheumatologists are medical doctors who have gone on for at least two years of special training in the many different types of arthritis and related conditions. This extra measure of education and experience makes them the reigning experts on the disease and most aspects of its treatment. 'I am sure that if my GP had not been so good and referred me to rheumatologist in Christchuch Hospital I would not still be working,' wrote a sixty-year-old woman from Bournemouth. 'I have so much support from the team, which includes practitioners and occupational therapists. I have a demanding job but adjustments are regularly made so that I came continue to work.'

A fifty-eight-year-old woman from Clacton-on-Sea reported, 'The best therapy is acceptance of the complaint and doing your best to overcome the disabilities along with specialist advice and medication from a rheumatologist.'

'My rheumatologist is top-drawer,' wrote a housewife from Maryland. 'He's up on the latest data, sees more actual cases of arthritis, and thus he inspires more confidence. He listens more, cares more, due to his very choice of rheumatology as a specialty. He advises correctly and adds caution where necessary.'

In cold, hard statistics, rheumatologists top the charts. Nearly half of those rated in the US survey and over half of those rated in the UK survey were credited with helping participants attain *dramatic* long-term relief. Here are the figures.

	US Survey	US Survey Percentage	UK Survey	UK Survey Percentage
Total number of rheumatologists seen	482		179	
Number rated by participants	456*	(95%)	100	
Outcome of treatment:				
Dramatic long-term relief	217	(48%)	98	(55%)
Moderate long-term relief	77	(17%)	39	(22%)
Temporary relief	97	(21%)	24	(13%)
No relief (ineffective)	49	(11%)	16	(9%)
Made participant feel worse	16	(3%)	2	(1%)

* Although we list the total number of practitioners seen in each specialty, we use the number *rated* to calculate the outcome of care. In other words, the 217 rheumatologists who provided dramatic long-term relief account for 48 percent of the 456 who were rated. (And these 456 rheumatologists account for 95 percent of the total 482 who were seen by our participants.)

What do these numbers mean? They mean that your chances of finding help with a rheumatologist are better than four out of five, since in both surveys over 85 percent of those rated were able to provide *at least* temporary relief or better. Much of this relief comes in the form of drugs, including aspirin and other anti-inflammatory pills and shots that *could* be dispensed by any doctor or osteopath. But rheumatologists are probably better acquainted with these drugs than other practitioners because they use them all the time, observing their good effects and their not-so-good side effects in hundreds or thousands of patients every year. It follows that rheumatologists are also more conversant with the less familiar treatments for arthritis, such as gold injections and penicillamine (see Chapter 5). And, if you have a particularly painful, disabling case of rheumatoid arthritis, for example, that defies all of these approaches, then the rheumatologist is the one who will try to attack the disease with more potent, possibly experimental, therapies.

More than Medicine

The best rheumatologists, however, don't limit their advice to what they can write on a prescription pad. They are firm believers in patient education. They explain what they're going to do and why, enlisting you as a partner in your own care. They teach exercise, or refer you to someone who can, such as a physiotherapist. They offer advice about ways to protect your joints and perform your day-to-day activities, or recommend an occupational therapist or self-help course teaching these strategies. If you need joint replacement or other surgery for arthritis, the rheumatologist will help you find an orthopaedic surgeon to perform those operations. And if you are overweight, the rheumatologist will no doubt tell you that losing a few pounds will minimize the stress on your joints. 'The rheumatologist was the most helpful,' said a New York actress, 'since he advised exercise and weight loss as being the best treatment. He instructed me on daily exercises that would strengthen my muscles and reduce the stress on my joints, and these have given me excellent help.'

The good rheumatologist is also a crackerjack diagnostician. Over and over, we heard our participants tell of months or years spent wondering what their problem was – until they either were referred to a rheumatologist or wound up in one's office through sheer persistence. 'The acceleration of my osteoarthritis is the result of an inherited blood disease,' reported a fifty-year-old chemist from California. 'Before this was diagnosed, my advanced arthritis condition puzzled the following practitioners: internist, acupuncturist, body worker, podiatrist, and orthopaedic surgeon. Finally, a rheumatologist identified the primary cause and much of the picture fell into place.'

'It took going to four different doctors before finally getting to this rheumatologist and getting proper treatment,' recalled a thirty-seven-year-old radio disc jockey from Louisiana. 'In that six-month searching period, I became totally disabled. Despite continued misdiagnosis, I kept trying different doctors until I got to this specialist.'

Ideally, the rheumatologist not only recognizes the problem but also understands the other problems arthritis can cause, from the stress of living with pain to the fear of not being able to continue working or caring for a family 'My present rheumatologist,' wrote a clinical laboratory supervisor from Ohio, 'knows the pain is real, not imaginary. He is compassionate, encouraging, and sympathetic, while also reassuring me that I will be able to cope and adapt.' A retired teacher from South Carolina thanked her rheumatologist for being 'not only extremely helpful, but a great morale booster, too.'

A Slight Advantage in Treating Rheumatoid Arthritis

Although rheumatologists are highly regarded by our whole survey group, the fact is they do better treating people with rheumatoid arthritis than those with osteoarthritis. This is because of the so-called 'second-line' or 'remittive therapies' – Plaquenil is one example – that they can offer to their patients with rheumatoid arthritis, but which are generally considered useless in treating osteoarthritis. Looking just at the reports from US survey participants with rheumatoid arthritis, we find that 57 percent of rheumatologists treating them are able to give dramatic long-term help. The comments from these participants are likewise more glowing: 'I can honestly say my rheumatologist was a godsend,' wrote a nursing-home administrator from Pennsylvania, whose rheumatologist is treating her with an experimental drug. 'I was in so much pain, and he knew exactly what to try and what to do to help. If I'd found him sooner, I would never have lost any joints.'

For those US survey participants with osteoarthritis, on the other hand, 'only' 34 percent of rheumatologists achieved dramatic long-term results. This is still an extremely good track record. What's more, when we add on the figures for moderate long-term improvement and temporary help, it turns out that fully 79 percent of our US survey participants with osteoarthritis who saw a rheumatologist also saw some improvement.

The Trouble with Some Rheumatologists

As you can see from the ratings, 11 percent of the rheumatologists in the US survey and 9 percent in the UK survey were ineffective, and 3 percent in the US survey and 1 percent in the UK survey made their patients – our participants – feel worse. The problems had to do with bad reactions to certain drugs, insensitivity, and personality mismatches between doctors and participants.

'My rheumatologist has always been very supportive,' explained a computer operator from Missouri. 'But I had to fault him when I was having problems with allergic reactions and unusual side effects to medications, because I couldn't convince him these were serious problems. I remember that Methotrexate caused nausea, hair loss, severe swelling of my lower legs and feet, and red quarter-sized lesions with white centres of pus on my legs. Yet it took six weeks of suffering on my part to convince him that this wasn't working. On one other occasion, I finally refused to continue my medication, despite his objections, because of its side effects.'

There's no question that most rheumatologists rely on drug treatments. 'The rheumatologist prescribed many drugs,' a New Jersey homemaker recalled, 'which gave me severe rashes, nausea, and diarrhoea, and I also found myself becoming depressed. But the doctor was not very concerned about depression, and told me there was another new drug I could try. After that visit, I decided not to expose my system to further side effects. I asked the doctor whether a change in diet would help, but he said there was no connection between nutrition and arthritis.'

Asking some rheumatologists about nutrition can be as inflammatory as anything going on in your joints. Many of them are rigidly opposed to the concept of dietary help for arthritis because it smacks of quackery. Some have watched patients follow fad diets that turned out to be useless, or harmful, and that left them feeling duped. What's more, rheumatologists, like most doctors, receive little or no formal training in nutrition and may not know what counsel to offer – other than the casual advice to eat a balanced diet and keep the weight down. A few rheumatologists, however, are involved in exciting new research showing that certain foods and supplements can indeed have a positive effect, while other foods can aggravate arthritis in allergic or sensitive individuals. (See Section 5 for a full discussion of nutrition and arthritis, including the Arthritis Survey Diet and Thirty-Day Meal Plan in Chapter 13.)

Every rheumatologist is a human being first, and some doctors' personal skills just don't measure up to their technical expertise. This is a no-win situation for someone treating people with a chronic disease, patients who may require regular, even frequent, doctor visits over a period of years. A writer from North Carolina expressed the sentiments of many participants when she said, 'It has been important to me to be treated as an intelligent human being of worth, and to be included as a thinking participant in my treatment. I have left doctors who did not inform me or consult me.'

'As with any profession,' concluded a twenty-nine-year-old Texas teacher, 'I have seen some great rheumatologists and some quacks. The doctors who truly helped me spent time with me, made me feel good about myself. The doctors who did the most damage belittled my self-confidence, spent zero time with me, and were impatient in answering my questions. One doctor told me I'd probably become a quadriplegic and that I might as well accept the fact that I could never have what normal people have due to my arthritis.' This woman, we are pleased to report, has since improved tremendously through a combination of physical therapy and drug treatment from her present rheumatologist.

General Practitioners and Family Doctors

- When these doctors know you well, they often know best how to care for your arthritis.
- GPs can work effectively with rheumatologists to take over your continuing care, even if you require specialized treatments.

If you have a good relationship with a nonspecialist who cares for 'the whole you,' consider yourself truly fortunate. 'My GP has known me and my medical history for thirty-four years,' wrote a forty-one-year-old homemaker from New York. 'He sent me to a rheumatologist, and I went for the tests, but I didn't think that doctor was taking my other ailments into consideration. I have diabetes, glaucoma, anemia, and asthma. So I'm sticking with my GP. He read the rheumatologist's report, and prescribed medications and treatments that fit me, the total person, in terms of what I can afford, what I can manage with my other conditions, my lifestyle, and my emotional needs.'

Many of our participants enjoyed the best of both practitioners. Having seen a rheumatologist one or more times for an expert assessment of their state, they went regularly to their family doctor for medical treatment – such as periodic gold injections, if necessary – and moral support. Arthritis, after all, is a chronic condition that waxes and wanes. There are times that it demands the ultimate from modern medicine, whether in the form of a bold drug combination, a high-tech diagnostic procedure, or a feat of surgical derring-do. There are also times when nothing is more important than the sympathetic ear of a doctor who knows you well.

General practitioners or family doctors often work very effectively *with* the specialists their patients have consulted. The rheumatologist who is too far away or too busy to take you on as a patient, may be only too happy to suggest a plan of action for your regular doctor to pursue with you. 'My family doctor always treats me when I have a bad flare-up,' said a plant engineer from Iowa, 'since the rheumatologist is at the university, quite a ways away from here.'

As the ratings from our US and UK survey participants show, general practitioners and family doctors are reasonably effective in providing temporary to long-term relief.

	US Survey	US Percentage	UK Survey	UK Percentage
Total number of GPs and family doctors seen	418		302	
Number rated by participants	397	(95%)	302	(100%)

Outcome of treatment:

Dramatic long-term relief	117	(29%)	82	(27%)
Moderate long-term relief	99	(25%)	72	(24%)
Temporary relief	121	(30%)	96	(32%)
No relief (ineffective)	46	(12%)	46	(15%)
Made participant feel worse	14	(4%)	6	(2%)

Many of the benefits offered by GPs seem due partly to the long-standing nature of the doctor-patient relationship in many cases, and partly to plain old-fashioned good appropriate care. 'My family doctor has treated me from the beginning, and I credit him for my not being laid up permanently at this stage of my life,' wrote a fifty-four-year-old Pennsylvania salesman who has had rheumatoid arthritis since age thirty-two. 'I have been on gold for many years, plus anti-inflammatory drugs, exercise, good nutrition, and vitamins and minerals.' Other survey participants raved about the practical advice they got from their family doctor, or the diet that launched their successful weight loss efforts.

A fifty-three-year-old office manager from California told this story: 'When I first went to a rheumatologist, he gave me no relief, but just kept saying, "Wait and see." I also saw a chiropractor, a physical therapist, and a Yoga instructor, who were helpful so long as I wasn't in intense pain. My family doctor is the *only* one who started me on various anti-inflammatory drugs, and we experimented until I found the right combinations. He also had me using splints to rest my hands, and when I could no longer walk, I had wonderful results from arthroscopic surgery done on both knees by an orthopaedic surgeon he recommended.'

However participants who were *dis*pleased with their general practitioners or family doctors made comments such as the following: 'Most GPs just don't have knowledge about arthritis,' said a banker from New Hampshire. 'They really don't seem to care about how one feels fighting stiffness, pain, and the inability to get around and do things.'

At their worst, general and family practitioners may prescribe the wrong drugs. 'My regular doctor,' noted a beautician from Alaska, 'was the one who just gave me codeine. I kept telling him that there must be a better answer, and he said that was all he could do. That's when I decided to go to an orthopaedic surgeon – someone who knew about joints and could tell me what to do for my problem without turning me into a drug addict.' The orthopaedist switched her from painkillers to anti-inflammatory agents, gave her exercises to do, and taught her how to combine ice and heat for her knee pain.

Orthopaedic Surgeons

- Their surgery, when needed, may greatly improve the quality of life.
- Orthopaedic surgeons can give nonsurgical advice that equals that of any other practitioner.

Earlier in this chapter, we called these doctors heroes. They enter their specialty as the veterans of five years of post-medical school training in diseases and injuries that affect the bones and joints, as well as the muscles, ligaments, tendons, and the nerves that power them. Orthopaedic surgeons do some of their most glorious battle in the operating room, where they have transformed a ravaged painful knee, for example, into a smoothly functioning joint that can bend readily, straighten painlessly, and do its part in helping you walk well without a crutch or a cane.

Surgery, when it works, works wonders. (See Chapter 7 for a detailed examination of surgery for arthritis.) 'My orthopaedic surgeon has helped me more than anyone,' wrote a retired teacher from Kansas. 'He has performed eight operations on me – replaced both my knees, several joints in both hands, my left shoulder, and my right elbow – and the surgery has kept me out of a wheelchair. He has prescribed physical therapy and exercise as follow-up care, and he watches me carefully with periodic checkups.'

Outside the operating room, orthopaedic surgeons can and do provide many other kinds of treatment for arthritis, from prescription drugs and cortisone shots to braces and exercise advice. 'The orthopaedic surgeon took X rays and told me I was not ready for surgery,' said a Wisconsin homemaker. 'Instead, he talked to me about the right way to bend and sit, and how to make hot packs out of towels.'

'My orthopaedic surgeon prescribed a TENS unit [see Chapter 8] for me to use at home,' a Florida pharmacist reported, 'and it really helped.'

A forty-nine-year-old secretary from Missouri, who had seen just one doctor in the twenty years she's had osteoarthritis, said of her orthopaedist, 'He is very sympathetic and encouraging. He's willing to listen to me, and he adjusts my medication for the most benefit to me.' In short, there's nothing to stop an accomplished surgeon from being a good doctor in the best sense of the term.

	US Survey	US Percentage	UK Survey	UK Percentage
Total number of orthopaedic surgeons seen	350		128	
Number rated by participants	334	(95%)	128	(100%)
Outcome of treatment:				
Dramatic long-term relief	160	(48%)	56	(44%)
Moderate long-term relief	57	(17%)	23	(18%)
Temporary relief	68	(20%)	20	(16%)
No relief (ineffective)	30	(9%)	22	(17%)
Made participant feel worse	19	(6%)	7	(5%)

Orthopaedists' ratings were not far below those of rheumatologists for providing dramatic and moderate long-term relief. The ratings match closely in the other categories too, except that orthopaedic surgeons were nearly twice as likely (in the US Survey 6 percent versus 3 percent) to make their patients feel worse after treatment – because of the wrong advice, a poor surgery outcome, or a bad attitude. Here are some examples:

The wrong advice. 'My orthopaedic surgeon caused me the most harm by advising me to rest, instead of exercise,' said a forty-three-year-old tennis instructor from New York.

Poor surgery outcome. 'It's probably my own fault for going to the local hospital in the small town where I live,' conceded a retired factory worker from Michigan, 'but the orthopaedic surgeon was incompetent and he hurt me. I walked with a cane before my foot surgery. Now I have to use crutches.'

Bad attitude. A thirty-five-year-old vocational counsellor from Texas reported that her orthopaedist used scare tactics, actually 'threatening' surgery if she didn't do her exercises. In California, a thirty-seven-year-old home health aide found an orthopaedic surgeon who told her, 'There's nothing you can do for it, and it's just going to get worse as years go on.' 'I believed him,' she recalled, 'but I found out through trial and error that exercise relieves my arthritis pain. The experience with the doctor led me to seek my own solutions – since he presented none.'

Neurosurgeons

- Neurosurgeons may be able to provide dramatic relief if you need surgery on your back or neck.
- If you don't need surgery, you may receive no help at all.

While an orthopaedic surgeon is usually willing to treat people with arthritis *whether or not* they require surgery, a neurosurgeon is strictly a surgeon who operates on the brain, the spinal cord, and the other nerves. If your problem requires their special expertise, you're likely to get relief. But if not, don't expect other help to be forthcoming. This situation accounts for the very high percentage of neurosurgeons rated as ineffective in the survey.

	US Survey	US Percentage	UK Survey	UK Percentage
Total number of neurosurgeons seen	22		22	
Number rated by participants	22	(100%)	22	(100%)
Outcome of treatment:				
Dramatic long-term relief	8	(36%)	14	(3%)
Moderate long-term relief	2	(9%)	14	(3%)
Temporary relief	2	(9%)	2	(9%)
No relief (ineffective)	9	(41%)	14	(63%)
Made participant feel worse	1	(5%)	0	(0%)

'The neurosurgeon operated on my neck,' wrote a retired public relations man from Ohio, 'because of bone spurs pinching a nerve and causing paralysis in my right arm. Now I can use the arm again, I can move my neck freely, which I couldn't do before, and I've had a major reduction in pain.'

An insurance agent from Louisiana consulted a neurosurgeon about the osteoarthritis in her spine, but, she said, 'He candidly tells me at this time there is no surgery that would help. He evaluates me every year or so in the event there has been a change in surgical options for me.' Meanwhile, she got her ongoing care from a rheumatologist who answered all her questions, prescribes drugs, and gave exercise advice.

If you have pain in your neck or back that hasn't responded to anyone else's care, consider discussing the problem with a neurosurgeon. If your doctor can't make such a referral, or you don't want to ask for one, check with your county medical society or with the hospitals in your area.

Allergy Specialist

Some people are allergic to certain foods which can aggravate arthritis. This varies greatly between individuals and only an allergy test can determine if particular foods are a problem for you. At the time of the original US survey insufficient numbers of participants had visited an allergy specialist for the results to be included, however in the 2005 UK survey a more significant proportion of people had visited an allergy specialist. As you can see the results don't suggest an allergy specialist can make an enormous difference to your arthritis, however it will at least establish if certain foods are or are not a problem for you. You can be referred to an allergy specialist by your GP.

Total number of allergy specialists seen	28	
Number rated by participants	27	(96%)
Outcome of treatment:		
Dramatic long-term relief	1	(4%)
Moderate long-term relief	0	(0%)
Temporary relief	3	(11%)
No relief (ineffective)	22	(81%)
Made participant feel worse	1	(4%)

For more information on arthritis and allergies contact the Arthritis Research Campaign or Allergy UK (see Useful Addresses, page 544)

Musculoskeletal Physicians

Musculoskeletal medicine is an emerging discipline. Currently eight hospitals in the UK have musculoskeletal departments. Musculoskeletal physicians are orthodox medical doctors who have done lengthy additional training in the specific diagnosis and treatment of conditions of the spine, muscles and joints. Their treatment may consist of manipulation and exercises but they are also able to perform injections, such as prolotherapy and epidurals and the more invasive techniques such as discography and intra-discal electro thermal therapy (IDETT) under X-ray guidance. The discipline is a fusion of skills and techniques from general practice, rheumatology, orthopaedics, pain management, physiotherapy, osteopathy and chiropractic, occupational health, sports medicine, rehabilitation, psychology, and psychiatry. Relatively few survey participants had visited a musculoskeletal physician reflecting the fact that this is a new branch of medicine, however 40 percent of participants at least received temporary relief or better, although 60 percent experienced no relief.

Total number of muscoskeletal physicians seen	28	
Number rated by participants	28	(100%)
Outcome of treatment:		
Dramatic long-term relief	3	(11%)
Moderate long-term relief	5	(18%)
Temporary relief	3	(11%)
No relief (ineffective)	17	(60%)
Made participant feel worse	0	(0%)

Pain Clinic Doctors

Pain Management Clinics are specialized clinics for the treatment of all forms of chronic pain including arthritis. Pain clinics take a multi-disciplinary approach to the treatment of pain and various options may be considered including nerve blocks, analgesics and psychological therapy. You will need to be referred by your GP. Your pain will be assessed and a treatment plan discussed with you; the plan will be sent to your general practitioner or to your referring consultant.

The aims of pain clinics are to reduce your level of pain, to restore your functioning and to improve your sense of well being. Pain clinics appear to be a reasonably effective form of treatment with over half the participants at least receiving temporary relief or better.

Total number of pain clinic doctors seen	33	
Number rated by participants	33	(100%)
Outcome of treatment:		
Dramatic long-term relief	6	(18%)
Moderate long-term relief	6	(18%)
Temporary relief	6	(18%)
No relief (ineffective)	13	(40%)
Made participant feel worse	2	(6%)

Other Practitioners

Survey participants saw many different kinds of physicians in addition to the ones already discussed, but they saw some of them too infrequently for them to be rated. We felt we needed participants' comments on at least twenty practitioners in any given specialty to be able to rate that field. The list of doctors who were seen too infrequently to be rated includes anaesthesiologists, cardiologists, dermatologists, emergency-room doctors, endocrinologists, gastroenterologists, general surgeons, haematologists, obstetrician/gynaecologists, oncologists, ophthalmologists, otolaryngologists, paediatricians, plastic surgeons, radiologists, and urologists. (Acupuncturists are covered in Chapter 4, and psychiatrists are considered together with other mental-health practitioners, also in Chapter 4.)

How to Get the Most out of Any Doctor Visit

'When my family doctor first diagnosed rheumatoid arthritis,' a forty-seven-year-old Florida housewife wrote, 'he told me to go home, take aspirin until my ears ring, and come back next year. When you feel frightened and awful, that's not very comforting.'

Surely *any* doctor has the responsibility to touch you gently, to treat you with respect, to explain your diagnosis, as well as the effects and side effects of various treatments, and to make suggestions of ways that you can further help yourself through exercise, for example, by taking warm baths or showers, and by protecting your joints. In the reality of a busy practice, however, there's a lot that never gets said. Often it is you, the patient, who – despite your pain, your fears, your personal problems, and your money worries – still must take responsibility for getting the information you need. Here are some tips from survey participants on how you can do this.

Communicate with your doctor

'I feel I have developed good communication skills over the years,' said a twenty-nine-year-old participant from Indiana who has had arthritis since she was fourteen. 'Communication is the key! It is the basis for choosing together what medication, exercises, and so on to try for your particular problems. Both the doctor and the patient have to work at this system. Communication is not always easy, but I'm sure it has been of benefit to me, *and* to the doctors and therapists who have worked with me.' You can do your half this way.

- Think about what you want to tell the doctor ahead of time, so you'll be prepared for the visit.
- If writing down your symptoms or questions helps you, then write them, but remember that many doctors react badly to the sight of a long list of items. It may be better to leave the list home altogether, but if you use it, try to refer to it, and *communicate*, instead of just reading aloud.
- Be as brief as possible, out of respect for the doctor's schedule, but don't be cowed into thinking he or she doesn't have time to listen to you.
- Make your descriptions of symptoms or reactions to medications as specific as you can.
- Ask questions about anything that isn't perfectly clear to you. Then tell the doctor, in your own words, what you think he or she said.

- If you get home and realize you still have questions, or new questions are forming in your mind, call up and ask them now. If the doctor can't come to the phone, tell your questions to the person who answers the phone so the doctor can consider them before calling you back.
- Follow your doctor's advice, or explain why you don't want to.

Keep your Perspective on the Doctor-Patient Relationship

'I have often found that doctors lose interest and rapport after a few treatments,' said a retired economist from California. 'I believe this happens because many practitioners become irritated with their ageing patients when they fail to deliver relief – and when the doctors realize that, in the course of time, they may find themselves in similar straits.' Doctors, no matter how knowledgeable, are only human. And they can get as frustrated and as frightened as the rest of us. Some of them have never gotten over their embarrassment at talking about sexual matters, for example, while others are dangerously impaired – either because of incompetence or addiction to drugs or alcohol. By striving to communicate with your doctor, you have the best chance of knowing whether he or she is just having a bad day, or whether it's time for you to find a new doctor.

Summary of Medical Practitioners

Highly Recommended for Diagnosis and Ongoing Care

Rheumatologists
Orthopaedic Surgeons

Recommended for Continuing Care of Arthritis

General or family practitioners
Pain clinics

Recommended for Special Types of Care

For most types of joint surgery: Orthopaedic surgeons
For neck or back surgery: Neurosurgeons
For rheumatoid arthritis: Rheumatologists

Chapter 4
Non-Medically Qualified Practitioners:

Which Ones Get the Best Results

• *What to learn from a physiotherapist* • *What to fear from a chiropractor*
• *What to look for in an acupuncturist* • *The virtues of exercise instructors
and mental health practitioners*

Some of the most successful programs for arthritis care use a team approach, with several kinds of professionals working together for a common goal – your well-being. Such a team might consist of (1) a **physician** who examines you, makes a diagnosis, prescribes drugs, and supervizes your care; (2) a **physiotherapist** who gives you wax or heat treatments, for example, and works out an exercise routine for you to follow at home; (3) an **occupational therapist** who shows you how to protect your joints and go about your daily activities with the help of special aids or smart tips on body mechanics; (4) a **psychologist** or counsellor who might teach you a self-hypnosis technique for pain control, and help you work through any emotional difficulties arthritis could be causing; and (5) a **nutritionist** who talks to you about your diet and weight, with specific suggestions about how you can improve your eating habits.

Few of our survey participants received this ideal level of attention, but many of them successfully assembled their own 'teams' over the years and enjoy the advantages of receiving several – totally different – kinds of care. Thanks to their efforts, we can give you the information you need to find your own 'players.' We've already examined the physician members of the team (in Chapter 3). Now let's look at the non-medical doctors who have the most to offer, starting with the ones most frequently seen.

Our participants rated each kind of practitioner on the basis of the amount of help they received from his or her care, whether it was dramatic long-term relief, moderate long-term relief, or temporary relief. They judged a practitioner ineffective if they got no relief, and found a few non-medical practitioners who left them feeling worse off than before. Of the two most popular non-medical practitioners seen in our survey, physiotherapists have the edge over chiropractors.

Physiotherapists

- Physiotherapists perform a wide variety of hands-on treatments that usually bring temporary relief.
- Their exercise advice can be the ticket to long-term improvement.

Most survey participants thoroughly enjoyed the whirlpool treatments they got from the physiotherapist; likewise the massage, the wax dips, the hot packs, the cold packs, the ultrasound, the diathermy, and the electrical stimulation. The variety was great, and sometimes the relief was, too.

'The hot packs were heaven,' wrote an investor from Idaho.

'The physiotherapist used heat and massage, plus traction for sciatica pain that was brought on by arthritis,' said a retired optometrist from Colorado. 'I feel the traction definitely helped, and I've not had sciatica since I took those treatments in 1979.'

'With a combination of cold pads, massage, and electrical stimulation,' reported an Ontario travel agent, 'I began to feel results in about three weeks. After five weeks, the pain in my knee was gone.'

Some people felt that exercise instruction from the physiotherapist had far greater value than any of the hands-on treatments – no matter how good they may have felt at the time. A thirty-seven-year-old mother of two from South Dakota wrote: 'The physiotherapist was fantastic for me – a lifesaver. After four years of severe rheumatoid arthritis and inactivity, I've experienced little, if any, loss of range of motion. I attribute that to the exercises I was taught. The exercises were painful at times, but very beneficial in the long run. The whirlpool, heat packs, and massages, on the other hand, were a great relief, but all very short-lived.'

Exercise advice, in fact, accounted for most of the long-term relief that physiotherapists were credited with providing.

	US Survey	US Percentage	UK Survey	UK Percentage
Total number of physiotherapists seen	440		137	
Number rated by participants	427	(97%)	137	(100%)
Outcome of care:				
Dramatic long-term relief	112	(26%)	33	(24%)
Moderate long-term relief	77	(18%)	35	(26%)
Temporary relief	183	(43%)	57	(42%)
No relief (ineffective)	30	(7%)	17	(12%)
Made participant feel worse	25	(6%)	5	(4%)

Physiotherapists typically used a combination of treatments, sometimes including splints or braces that participants wore on their hands or wrists, for example, to help prevent deformity. 'Physiotherapy was a godsend to me,' said a Texas teacher. 'It made me feel so much relief and helped me to regain some of the range of motion I had temporarily lost in my arms. The splints kept my wrists stable at night, so I could sleep.'

If your particular regimen calls for physiotherapy every week, or as often as seven days a week right after surgery, you'll probably spend more time with your therapist than with any other practitioner. This can be an emotional uplift, if you find someone who dispenses tender, loving care – or an educational bonanza, if you fill the time with talk as well as treatment. Moreover, a good physiotherapist is long on practical demonstrations. 'I had daily physiotherapy to strengthen my muscles after knee surgery,' wrote a retired teacher from South Carolina. 'The therapist also showed me how to use a paraffin bath for my hands, and gave me several gadgets for turning a doorknob, buttoning and unbuttoning my clothes, removing jar tops, and things like that.'

The extremely high scores for temporary relief (42–43 percent) result from the hands-on treatments that *do* ease pain – but only for a few hours, or less. 'The massage helped for a little while,' said a waitress from Nevada, 'but by the time I finished my work shift, the pain had returned.' A salesman from California described the brief relief situation this way: 'It's like driving your car. You're going like sixty when you're driving it, but when you stop, that's it.'

Physiotherapists *rarely* failed to help the people in their care. Some, however, caused harm by being incompetent, insensitive, or both. 'The therapists I saw,' noted an electronics technician from Oregon, 'all seemed to possess a sadistic streak. The treatment was only so much torture for me, and any relief was brought about when they *stopped*.' An administrative aide from Rhode Island wrote, 'Physiotherapy made my knee more painful to the point where I quit going after several appointments.'

While sound exercise instruction may serve you well for the rest of your life, the advice of an incompetent therapist can be disastrous. For example, a New York policewoman said that five weeks of performing prescribed exercises and going to the physiotherapist's office for treatments left her with debilitating low back pain – which she *did not have* in the first place.

How to Find a Good Physiotherapist

If you need a physiotherapist, your doctor or hospital consultant will refer you to one. Some GP practices have their own physiotherapist. Most orthopaedists and rheumatologists have their favourites and may give special instructions to the therapist about how to proceed in your particular case. If you are in a position to pay for your own treatment, there are a large number of physiotherapists across the UK offering treatment in dedicated physiotherapy and sports injury clinics as well as many who will treat people in their own homes. To find a local private practitioner within the UK consult the Chartered Society of Physiotherapy. The Organisation of Chartered Physiotherapists in Private Practice (OCPPP), an occupational group of the CSP for private practitioners, also has a listing service of private practitioners working in the UK. Some large employers run occupational health schemes for their employees that may include provision for physiotherapy treatment and private medical insurance schemes for individuals through the independent healthcare sector will often include physiotherapy treatment. Check with the scheme providers for eligibility.

Some physiotherapists may specialize in certain areas of rehabilitation, such as physiotherapy for cancer, heart conditions, or orthopaedic problems. Before you take any treatment from a physiotherapist you've found on your own, call and ask whether he or she has experience working with people who have arthritis. If not, ask to be referred to another one who does.

'The therapist I saw was not well versed in arthritis,' lamented a retired teacher from New York. 'He never supervized me in the exercises he suggested, so I overdid them and further injured my elbows.'

Many participants learnt from the professionals how to use *some* of the treatments safely at home, on their own. You can do this, too. (See the tips on wax dips, heat, ice, and other self-help strategies in Chapter 16.)

Osteopathy

Osteopaths diagnose and treat problems with muscles, ligaments, nerves and joints. Treatment involves gentle, manual techniques – easing pain, reducing swelling and improving mobility. Osteopaths spend a large amount of their time dealing with the pain and suffering caused by arthritis. In many cases they can help considerably in pain relief and lifestyle management. As well as advice on exercise you may also be given dietary advice. On your first visit the osteopath will discuss and record your medical history in detail. A series of observations on your mobility, posture and testing of points of weakness or excessive strain will then be made. Further investigations may include an x-ray or blood test. Osteopaths complete four or five years of training in anatomy, physiology, pathology, biomechanics and clinical methods.

The practice of osteopathy is quite different in the US (there, osteopaths are medical doctors who can prescribe drugs and perform surgery) so the US survey results for osteopathy are not included here. In the UK survey we found that osteopathy had a good track record for a majority of patients with 77 per cent experiencing at least temporary relief or better.

	UK Survey	UK Percentage
Total number of osteopaths seen	62	
Number rated by participants	62	(100%)
Outcome of care:		
Dramatic long-term relief	10	(15%)
Moderate long-term relief	11	(18%)
Temporary relief	27	(44%)
No relief (ineffective)	11	(18%)
Made participant feel worse	3	(5%)

Finding a Therapist

The majority of osteopaths work in private practice although an increasing number work alongside GPs so it may be possible for your doctor to refer you to an osteopath on the NHS. It may also be possible to claim for a course of osteopathy if you have private health insurance. To find an osteopath consult the General Osteopathic Council (see Useful Addresses, page 544). By law osteopaths must be registered to practice.

Chiropractors

- Chiropractors' non-medical approach is particularly appealing to some participants who can't take drugs.
- Chiropractors often provide good temporary relief, but their rate of making participants feel *worse* was higher than that of any other widely seen practitioner according to our survey.

In the UK some people may be confused about the difference between chiropractors and osteopaths, and the professions are similar in many ways. The main differences are:

- Chiropractors focus mostly on spinal integrity, using x-rays of the spine to form a diagnosis: osteopaths use palpation (touch) of soft tissues (muscles, ligaments and tendons) and spinal positioning in conjunction with overall postural balance to form a diagnosis
- Chiropractors work mainly on the spine; osteopaths work on the spine but also on the whole body, including peripheral joints

- Chiropractors use more manipulative techniques; osteopaths may use manipulation in conjunction with soft tissue and mobilization (stretching of joints) techniques.

There are basically two kinds of non-medical practitioners – those who work with or for physicians, as most nurses and physiotherapists do, and those who work independently of medical doctors on the basis of different healing philosophies, the way chiropractors tend to do. Medical practitioners, however, have in the past been sceptical of chiropractors' heavy emphasis on spinal manipulation.

'I had chiropractic manipulation when my arthritis began three years ago,' wrote a forty-five-year-old locksmith from New Jersey, 'but when I went to an orthopaedic surgeon, I was told I had taken a big risk by letting the chiropractor touch my back, and that in the future, only a medical specialist could treat me.' This anti-chiropractor bias may be changing, though, partly because of a lengthy legal battle that began in 1977, when chiropractors charged that the American Medical Association, the American College of Surgeons, and several other bastions of orthodox medicine had conspired to ruin the chiropractic profession. After ten years, a U.S. District Judge ruled in favour of the chiropractors, portraying them as the victims of 'systematic, long-term wrongdoing.' Recently, more than a dozen hospitals around the country have allowed chiropractors to join their staffs, or at least to treat some patients while they are in the hospital.

There are indeed good things to be said for chiropractic care. In addition to spinal manipulation, chiropractors may use heat, ultrasound, electrical stimulation, traction, massage, and give exercise and practical advice. They generally have five years of college study followed by post-graduate clinical training including studies in anatomy, nutrition, X ray, and physical therapeutics. They can be caring, and they can be good listeners, our participants avow. What's more, some people seek them out expressly *because* of their non-medical philosophy.

'Since I can't tolerate any of the arthritis drugs with my ulcer,' wrote a retired advertising director from Illinois, 'the chiropractor's gentle massage and heat gave marvellous, if temporary, relief.'

'The chiropractor was better than the medical doctor,' said a forty-one-year-old postal-service worker from Tennessee. 'The chiropractor tried to help the problem, not mask the symptoms with drugs.'

'I had a synovectomy on my right knee in 1981,' reported a thirty-nine-year-old Wisconsin housewife. 'My knee became even more stiff and painful after the operation. The chiropractor helped me get to walk again. I still go twice a week for relief.'

'In my particular experience,' said a fifty-four-year-old factory foreman from Pennsylvania, 'chiropractors are the only effective doctors to see. They know the muscular and skeletal systems of the body, plus they believe in proper nutrition, vitamin and mineral supplementation, and exercise. They will also admit it if they can do nothing, and send you to someone else for treatment – as opposed to the medical types, who will admit to no limitations of knowledge or experience.'

'Regular visits to the chiropractor has been the single most effective treatment for me,' wrote a sixty-two-year-old participant from Surrey.

A fifty-six year old woman from Ilfracombe reported, 'Exercise as indicated by my chiropractor helps me sleep at night if done just before I go to bed. Otherwise the pain keeps me awake.'

	US Survey	US Percentage	UK Survey	UK Percentage
Total number of chiropractors seen	349		77	
Number rated by participants	345	(99%)	77	(100%)
Outcome of care:				
Dramatic long-term relief	75	(22%)	15	(19%)
Moderate long-term relief	53	(15%)	12	(16%)
Temporary relief	118	(34%)	24	(31%)
No relief (ineffective)	50	(15%)	19	(25%)
Made participant feel worse	49	(14%)	7	(9%)

As the ratings show, chiropractors delivered most of their help in the form of temporary relief. Although some participants felt

improved for as long as three weeks after a chiropractic treatment, others found the effects disappear within a few days or a
few hours. 'I see a chiropractor because of arthritis in my neck
and back,' wrote a fifty-four-year-old former truck driver, now
disabled, from Illinois. 'I get relief for about three hours after
each treatment.' A seventy-one-year-old Nebraska homemaker
said, 'The chiropractor helped for some time, but it got to the
place where I would feel good after the treatment, and then the
next day I would be right back where I started from.' She eventually resolved her back pain with surgery and physiotherapy.

Chiropractors' record for making their patients feel worse –
14 percent in the US survey, 9 percent in the UK survey – was
the highest for any practitioner rated in either survey. And most
of the harm comes from manipulation. 'I went to a chiropractor
first,' said a retired glass worker from West Virginia, 'and that was
my big mistake, because I did not get better. I got worse. After a
few adjustments, I could not sit down to eat or watch TV, but
had to lie on the floor for relaxation, and it was painful to force
myself to sit in a car long enough to go for my treatment. When
I quit going, I got so I could sit again.'

'The manipulation made me feel like a cripple,' asserted a
sixty-nine-year-old Florida woman. 'The chiropractor told me
I would feel worse before getting better, but that never happened. I had to go back to my internist and get a shot of cortisone and medication to help me feel better.'

Comparing osteopaths with chiropractors, according to the
UK survey osteopaths provided better results in providing temporary and medium term relief and were less likely to be ineffective or to make the patient feel worse.

Nurses

- These professionals fill a variety of roles in several different
  settings, from hospitals to private homes.
- Nurses' positive attitude of caring and concern helps survey
  participants both physically and emotionally.

Nursing is called the caring profession, and the nurses who minister to our survey participants care for them in many different

ways – as attending nurses in hospitals where participants have had surgery, as assistants in doctors' offices where they go for regular exams, as visiting or practical nurses who come to their homes, as nurse practitioners who provide some form of treatment, and as instructors in courses aimed at helping them remain independent. No matter which role the nurses fill, they seemed to help most by sharing a personal warmth and an attitude of real concern. Here are the statistics.

	US Survey	US Percentage	UK Survey	UK Percentage
Total number of nurses seen	108		43	
Number rated by participants	100	(93%)	43	(100%)
Outcome of care:				
Dramatic long-term relief	22	(22%)	13	(30%)
Moderate long-term relief	24	(24%)	14	(33%)
Temporary relief	39	(39%)	6	(14%)
No relief (ineffective)	10	(10%)	9	(21%)
Made participant feel worse	5	(5%)	1	(2%)

Nurses are often the ones who take the time to give small bits of advice that make large differences in the quality of a participant's life. 'The nurse at my family doctor's office gives me moral support and a little praise,' said a forty-two-year-old homemaker from Montana. 'She gives me practical suggestions, too. Thanks to her I wear insulated mittens instead of gloves, insulated socks, and boys' shoes, usually, because they come with wider, rounder toes that keep my feet more comfortable.'

An escapee from city life, who now lives quietly in the woods of Wisconsin, got reflexology treatments, or foot massages aimed at resolving pain elsewhere in her body, from a nurse: 'The treatments bring relief for twelve to twenty-four hours. The nurse also taught me some stretching exercises and gave me a relaxation tape. When I exercise and use the tape, I get eight to twelve hours of relief. She has also recommended a diet/vitamin/mineral program that seems to be keeping my arthritis in check.'

Exercise Instructors

- Many kinds of exercise instructors help survey participants find long-term relief.
- A safe, sane approach to exercise is the deciding factor in their success – not the type of exercise they teach.

Exercise instructors come in all guises, from health-spa owners and track coaches to judo experts and Yoga teachers. In fact, in the US Survey more participants mentioned Yoga instructors than any other type of exercise teacher. Of the fifty-eight exercise instructors seen in the US Survey, twenty-seven were Yoga teachers, and thirteen of these (48 percent) helped their students find *lasting* relief.

Whether exercise instructors teach people individually or in groups, their record of success with our survey participants is impressive.

	US Survey	US Percentage	UK Survey	UK Percentage
Total number of exercise instructors seen	58		89	
Number rated by participants	55	(95%)	89	(100%)
Outcome of instruction:				
Dramatic long-term relief	18	(33%)	20	(23%)
Moderate long-term relief	12	(22%)	22	(25%)
Temporary relief	18	(33%)	29	(33%)
No relief (ineffective)	4	(7%)	13	(15%)
Made participant feel worse	3	(5%)	5	(6%)

One of the safest places to look for an exercise instructor is in a water-exercise class at a local pool. A gentle workout in water appears to be both pleasurable and possible, even for people who have a great deal of joint damage. It could be dangerous, however, to join an exercise class at a health club unless you tell the instructor that you have arthritis and may need some special modifications in the program. Many exercise instructors are experienced at working with people who have some kind of disability, and they are only too happy to oblige. 'I go to a workout studio where the owner takes time with each student to set up a special individual program,' said a writer from Missouri. 'He was crippled himself for ten years, and is truly an inspiration to all of us who learn from him.'

If your instructor is not sympathetic or knowledgeable about arthritis, proceed with caution, and let your body be your guide. A safe program starts out slowly and increases gradually. Many participants acknowledged that exercise may hurt a little before it brings relief. But movements that cause a lot of pain are not going to help you and may make matters worse. The slogan 'No pain, no gain' does *not* apply to people who are already in pain and are exercising to banish it!

Mental-Health Practitioners*

- These practitioners teach valuable techniques for controlling pain with mental energy.
- Their 'talk therapy' gets results, too, by helping participants accept themselves – and accept arthritis.

In the US Survey psychiatrists, psychologists, and counsellors were able to achieve more enduring pain relief for our participants than any other non-medical practitioners rated. The secret of their success seemed to lie in the techniques they taught for exercising the mind's power over the body, including self-hypnosis, imagery, biofeedback, and relaxation. All of these mental tools improve with use, and participants continued to control pain effectively with them years after their last visit to a mental-health practitioner. The UK results weren't so favourable for long-term relief, although visiting a mental health professional still proved very helpful for many. The results are similar to those recorded for people visiting pain clinics where many of the same techniques are taught.

The success of these practitioners does not imply that their patients' pain was 'all in their heads,' or milder than the norm.

---

* All types of mental-health practitioners seen by our participants, including psychiatrists (who are M.D.s), are considered together in this section.

	US Survey	US Percentage	UK Survey	UK Percentage
Total number of mental-health professionals seen	46		30	
Number rated by participants	45	(98%)	30	(100%)
Outcome of care:				
Dramatic long-term relief	180	(40%)	4	(13%)
Moderate long-term relief	12	(27%)	6	(20%)
Temporary relief	7	(15.5%)	7	(23%)
No relief (ineffective)	7	(15.5%)	11	(37%)
Made participant feel worse	1	(2%)	2	(7%)

Participants who praised mental-health practitioners included those with rheumatoid arthritis and those with osteoarthritis, old and young, with pain ranging from moderate to severe. Indeed, most participants who believed in the 'mind over matter' approach used it *along with* other kinds of treatment – medication, exercise, physical therapy – but reaped a special bonus for trying to will themselves well. 'I saw a psychiatrist who taught me how to use biofeedback,' said a forty-year-old housewife from Ohio. 'I can relax more and handle stress better because of it. I can also raise the temperature in various parts of my body, to decrease the pain there.'

Psychologists and psychiatrists are also frequently consulted for psychotherapy, or the attempt to solve emotional problems by talking about them to a qualified practitioner. Several participants found psychotherapy to be an effective part of their treatment, as arthritis pain is frequently aggravated by stress. Also, some of them have been plagued by problems of denial, depression, and loss of self-esteem that followed in the wake of their arthritis diagnosis. 'I had only one session with the psychologist,' said a retired receptionist from Arizona, 'but it helped change my self-image so that I was better able to deal with pain, and I became determined to help myself.'

A twenty-two-year-old California student wrote: 'I've had rheumatoid arthritis since I was fifteen. I don't want to have to live with it, but I have to learn to do it anyway. The psychiatrist has helped me cope with the fact of arthritis, and given me ways to relieve pain.'

There are so many kinds of mental-health professionals practising so many different forms of psychotherapy or behaviour modification that we could not even list all the types here. The best places to go for a referral are your doctor or a trusted friend. Knowing the type of help you want – self-hypnosis instruction, for example, or the chance to talk about your feelings – will speed the referral process along. If psychotherapy is your desire, a good recommendation is only the beginning, as *you* must determine, face-to-face, whether the therapist is the type of person who invites your trust and confidence. 'I saw a psychiatrist for a period of six months,' wrote an artist from Colorado, 'and she only made me feel worse. A psychiatrist who adds to the stress of an arthritis patient simply aggravates the problem.'

Acupuncturists

- Many kinds of practitioners offer acupuncture, but training separates the effective from the less so.
- Acupuncturists often achieve lasting results for those who seek their help.

As with mental health practitioners, the acupuncturists in the US survey were a mixed group of the medically qualified and non-medically qualifed. (Some chiropractors give acupuncture treatments, too, but ratings for all chiropractors are listed earlier in this chapter.) The treatment they offer, shrouded in history and mystery, has been used for thousands of years to assuage every imaginable symptom of illness, especially pain, and also to promote well-being in healthy individuals. Again the results differ for the US and UK surveys. In the US survey more than half of the acupuncturists who treated the survey participants helped them find enduring results. In the UK survey 41 per cent of people found the treatment to be ineffective; the biggest gains were made in temporary relief (31 per cent). This significant difference may be explained by the relatively small numbers of people who saw acupuncturists in the first survey (37) as opposed to the larger number in the UK survey (95). A larger sample minimizes the chances of results being skewed.

	US Survey	US Percentage	UK Survey	UK Percentage
Total number of acupuncturists seen	37		95	
Number rated by participants	37	(100%)	95	(100%)
Outcome of treatment:				
Dramatic long-term relief	12	(32%)	13	(14%)
Moderate long-term relief	7	(19%)	6	(6%)
Temporary relief	8	(22%)	34	(36%)
No relief (ineffective)	8	(22%)	39	(41%)
Made participant feel worse	2	(5%)	3	(3%)

'Although I have only been having acupuncture for about a month I feel that it has really helped with both the pain and stiffness,' reported a woman from Reading. 'The acupuncturist was the only one who knew what he was doing,' swore a retired claims examiner from New York City. 'In fact, the pain in my knee subsided after the first treatment. I am still visiting this gentle, knowledgeable Oriental medical doctor. I found the internist I consulted to be handicapped by his attitude on arthritis – "You'll have to live with it." No comments on the chiropractor I saw, except to say that his knowledge and know-how were limited.'

Teachers of acupuncture agree that the best practitioners are the ones educated in the *entire theory and use* of this ancient healing art. A GP or orthopaedic surgeon, who has taken a weekend seminar in the placement of acupuncture needles for pain relief, for example, is not likely to be as successful as another practitioner who has had several hundred hours of training in acupuncture's full scope and technique.

Ineffective acupuncturists were fairly common, both surveys showed. So if you decide to try acupuncture, make sure you get the most out of the venture by contacting the British Acupuncture Council for a list of recommended therapists in your area. There is no government legislation in the UK covering acupuncture at present. This means that unfortunately anyone can currently provide acupuncture treatment without any professional acupuncture training whatsoever. The British Acupuncture Council maintains standards of education, ethics, practice and discipline to ensure the health and safety of the public at all times. It is also committed to promoting research and enhancing the role that traditional acupuncture can play in the health and well-being of the nation.

You'll probably need to try several treatments before you can judge whether the acupuncturist is helping you. At the same time, no responsible acupuncturist would tell you to stop taking your arthritis drugs as a prerequisite for receiving treatment. Like any other approach, acupuncture for arthritis is one element in a comprehensive program.

Although the risks of acupuncture appear vanishingly small, practitioners did leave some people feeling worse than before. 'The acupuncturist did not help me,' wrote a thirty-five-year-old housing security officer from California, 'as I could not stand the needles and the treatment caused me a lot of stress.' Another participant reported negative results with one acupuncturist but then got a great deal of help when he went to a different practitioner.

Podiatrists

- These specialists can help solve arthritis-related foot problems.
- Orthotics (shoe inserts) prescribed by a podiatrist can make walking considerably more comfortable.

Although they are limited to treating the joints in the feet, podiatrists often get good results, and several of our participants thanked them for providing far-reaching help. A podiatrist's surgery, for example, helped a California housewife walk again.

'The podiatrist was the only one who would listen to me at first,' wrote a telephone operator from Arizona. 'He gave me physiotherapy on my feet and ankles, had orthotics made for my shoes, which helped a lot, and he insisted that my internist check me for osteoarthritis and osteoporosis. It turns out I have both.'

The sole participant to blame a podiatrist for making him feel worse was a licensed practical nurse from Ohio who underwent an unnecessary and damaging operation on his foot. 'Podiatrists can provide orthotics,' he said, 'which provide some relief. But

	US Survey	US Percentage	UK Survey	UK Percentage
Total number of podiatrists seen	21		41	
Number rated by participants	21	(100%)	41	(100%)
Outcome of care:				
Dramatic long-term relief	7	(33%)	7	(17%)
Moderate long-term relief	4	(19%)	11	(27%)
Temporary relief	7	(33%)	11	(27%)
No relief (ineffective)	2	(10%)	12	(29%)
Made participant feel worse	1	(5%)	0	0

in some communities, sporting-goods stores provide the same service – from people who are just as capable and certainly much less expensive!' Indeed, 'over-the-counter' arch supports are a familiar sight in pharmacies and variety stores, too.

Shoe insoles made a difference to a participant from Dorset. 'Shoe inserts correct the way I walk, ensuring the weight is evenly spread and that I maintain correct posture.'

Podiatrists sometimes prescribe drugs, such as Naprosyn or other anti-inflammatory agents. If you see a podiatrist who gives you a prescription, find out how it will mesh with the other medications you are taking.

Occupational Therapists

Although the number of people who saw occupational therapists in the US survey were too small to be included as a statistical sample, occupational therapists gave advice and practical tips that thirteen out of seventeen participants found extremely or moderately useful over the long run. The suggestions had to do with performing tasks more easily, both at home and at work, and with ways to protect the joints from further injury. Another two got temporary help from occupational therapists. At their worst, these practitioners were ineffective or failed to tell participants anything they didn't already know – they did however hurt two people in the US survey. In the UK survey we had more participants' experiences to draw on. The UK results were broadly similar although a larger percentage (31 percent) gained long term relief.

	UK Survey	UK Percentage
Total number of occupational therapists seen	68	
Number rated by participants	68	(100%)
Outcome of treatment:		
Dramatic long-term relief	21	(31%)
Moderate long-term relief	13	(19%)
Temporary relief	18	(26%)
No relief (ineffective)	14	(21%)
Made participant feel worse	2	(3%)

Dentists

Dentists may be able to provide relief from arthritic jaw pain. In the US survey two participants gained dramatic relief with the fitting of a plastic mouthpiece to wear during sleep. In the UK survey a larger sample had consulted a dentist; for 59 percent there was unfortunately no relief from the pain although a significant 15 percent gained long term relief.

	UK Survey	UK Percentage
Total number of dentists seen	27	
Number rated by participants	27	(100%)
Outcome of treatment:		
Dramatic long-term relief	4	(15%)
Moderate long-term relief	1	(4%)
Temporary relief	4	(15%)
No relief (ineffective)	16	(59%)
Made participant feel worse	2	(7%)

Nutritionists/Dietitians

Again, at the time of the US Survey insufficient people had visited a nutritionist to make the results statistically valid. However nutritionists and dietitians helped thirteen out of fourteen participants who sought their advice. 'The nutritionist changed my diet and told me to take vitamins E and C,' wrote a retired aluminium welder for Union Carbide. 'This eased the pain and made me feel much better. After three months, I found I could cut down on the aspirin.'

In the UK Survey 36 people had visited a nutritionist. For 47 percent the treatment made no difference to their arthritis, but 53 percent gained at least temporary relief or better.

	UK Survey	UK Percentage
Total number of nutritionists/dietitians seen	36	
Number rated by participants	37	(100%)
Outcome of treatment:		
Dramatic long-term relief	5	(14%)
Moderate long-term relief	6	(17%)
Temporary relief	8	(22%)
No relief (ineffective)	17	(47%)
Made participant feel worse	0	(0%)

Summary of Non-Medical Practitioners

Most highly recommended

Physiotherapist
Exercise instructor

Also highly recommended

Nurse
Occupational therapist

Worth a try

Acupuncturist
Podiatrist
Nutritionist or dietitian
Osteopath

Not recommended

Chiropractor

Section 3
The Value of Orthodox Treatments for Arthritis

All substances are poisons; there is none which is not a poison. The right dose differentiates a poison from a remedy.

— Philippus Aureolus Paracelsus (1493–1541)

An orthopaedic surgeon who fell asleep in 1947 and awoke in 1987 could not comprehend the vast advancements. … Management of joint diseases in the adult by total joint replacement is possibly the most significant development in orthopaedics in the past 40 years.

— Paul P. Griffin, M.D., from a retrospective in *Postgraduate Medicine*, July 1987

So far I have spent about $25,000 over 35 years with different doctors, medicines, etc. The rheumatologist finally told me that aspirin was the best medicine he could prescribe.

— Survey Participant #1050, a retired teacher from Virginia

Chapter 5
Rating and Comparing the Major Prescription Drugs:

The First Across-the-Board Evaluation of Arthritis Medications

• *Personal preferences in anti-inflammatory drugs* • *Breaking the steroid habit*
• *Going for the gold* • *The special uses of anti-rheumatic and cytotoxic drugs*

All the major prescription drugs for arthritis – some twenty products that we'll discuss in this chapter – fall into just two broad categories, called, simply, the first line and the second line.

The first-line drugs are used to control pain and inflammation in both osteoarthritis and rheumatoid arthritis. They include the non-steroidal anti-inflammatory drugs (NSAIDs), such as Feldene and Motrin, and the steroids, such as prednisone in pill form and cortisone injections into particularly troublesome joints. Aspirin, which is probably the most widely used and perhaps the most effective drug for arthritis, is also part of the first line. (However, since aspirin is an over-the-counter medication, not a prescription drug, it is covered in Chapter 6.)

The second-line treatments behave in mysterious ways that may slow the underlying disease process in rheumatoid arthritis: gold, in pills or shots; hydroxychloroquine, which is a malaria treatment that may slow down the destruction of the joints; penicillamine, a very different-acting relative of the famous antibiotic; and the cytotoxic drugs, originally developed for treating cancer.

Reports from the 1,051 participants in the US Arthritis Survey and the 460 participants in the UK survey allow us to rate and compare all these medications, both in terms of their positive effects on arthritis symptoms *and* their noisome side effects. At the end of this chapter, you'll find tips on buying and taking prescription drugs, including important questions for your doctor and inexpensive mail-order drug sources.

THE FIRST LINE

Non-Steroidal Anti-Inflammatory Drugs (NSAIDs)

As we've said before, the lowly aspirin is generally recognized as the most effective arthritis medication. In high doses of about ten or twelve 5-grain tablets a day, it can work to control both pain and inflammation, and it's cheap, too. The trouble with aspirin, though, is that it irritates the stomach more than many people can bear. The threat of gastrointestinal bleeding and full-blown ulcers is very real to those who take arthritis-strength doses of aspirin. Indeed, aspirin's often intolerable side effects created the market for today's NSAIDs, all of which aim to be easier on the gut but none of which substantially improves on the original.

Though these drugs all have to prove themselves against aspirin's benchmark, they take their class name from the other arthritis 'wonder drugs' – the steroids, including cortisone and prednisone. When cortisone was first isolated in the 1940s, it was hailed by some as the cure for rheumatoid arthritis because it banished inflammation so quickly and completely. It didn't really cure the disease, however, it only masked the symptoms. And as time passed, the ugly side effects of long-term use became all too obvious – cataracts, bone fractures, and thin fragile skin, to name a few. Today steroids are given more sparingly and cautiously. The NSAIDs do not approach their power for reducing inflammation, but their side effects are considered far less toxic.

The first widely used anti-inflammatory drug other than aspirin that was *not* a steroid was phenylbutazone (Butazolidin). It's considered part of the NSAID family today, but when it first came out in 1949, steroids were scarcely used, so it wasn't called 'non-steroidal.'

The first anti-inflammatory agent to appear in the wake of the wonders wrought (and havoc wreaked) by steroid drugs was indomethacin, known by its trade name, Indocin (Indocid). It is still widely used, although it now competes with other drugs including naproxen, ibuprofen, piroxicam, diclofenac and nabumetone.

If you read, as we've been reading, what doctors counsel other doctors about these drugs, you learn that there are no significant differences among them. And yet, one person with arthritis will thrive on Indocin, while the next person taking it will feel nothing but angry and nauseated until he tries Motrin (Naprosyn), which works perfectly for him, even though it did nothing for the first person. No one can account for the wide variation in the way people react to these medicines, and, unfortunately, no one can predict which one is most likely to work for you. This means that you are in for a trial-and-error period that may be tough in many respects. But it also means that if the first drug doesn't bring relief, you're likely to hit on one that will.

Cox-2 inhibitors are a type of NSAID, but have been developed to be safer for the stomach. According to the UK National Institute of Clinical Excellence they should only be prescribed instead of standard NSAIDs for people who may be at high risk of developing serious gastro-intestinal problems. There are different types of Cox-2s which are used for different kinds of arthritis. Celecoxib and etodolac can be used for rheumatoid and osteoarthritis, meloxicam is used for acute osteoarthritis and long-term treatment of rheumatoid arthritis while rofecoxib is licensed for osteoarthritis.

Our UK survey participants have experience with many of the NSAIDs, and their ratings allow us to compare them. We'll look first at the standard NSAIDs. The five most popular standard NSAIDs used by our UK survey participants are Ibuprofen, Diclofenac, Naproxen, Indometacin and Etoricoxib. Let's compare these on several features, beginning with popularity. Here's how they stack up.

NSAID NAME	BRAND NAME	NUMBER OF PARTICIPANTS
Ibuprofen	Advil;	229
	Anadin;	
	Ibuprofen;	
	Arthrofen;	
	Brufen;	
	Brufen Retard;	
	Care Ibuprofen;	
	Cuprofen;	
	Fenbid;	
	Fleximex;	
	Galprofen;	
	Hedex Ibuprofen;	
	Ibufem;	
	Librofem;	
	Mandafen;	
	Manorfen;	
	Migrafen;	
	Motrin;	
	Novaprin;	
	Nucare Ibuprofen;	
	Nurofen;	
	Obifen;	
	Pacifene;	
	Relcofen;	
	Taylors Ibuprofen	
Diclofenac		162
Naproxen	Naprosyn;	69
	Naprosyn SR;	
	Naprosyn EC;	
	Nycopren;	
	Synflex;	
	Napratec	
Indometacin	Indocin;	37
	Indomethacin	
Etoricoxib		20

The above listing actually reflects the drugs' popularity among *doctors*, since our participants can't take an NSAID unless their doctors prescribe it. To figure the drugs' relative popularity among our *participants*, we'll use the rating scale that appeared on the questionnaire (Appendix A). The following list puts the drugs in order of the greatest percentage of top ratings – 'plus 3,' or 'dramatic long-term relief.'

1. **Indometacin – 33% of those taking it.**
2. **Etoricoxib – 25% of those taking it.**
3. **Naproxen – 23% of those taking it.**
4. **Diclofenac – 22% of those taking it.**
5. **Ibuprofen – 13% of those taking it**

If we pool *all* the positive ratings for each of the drugs – 'plus 3' (dramatic long-term relief), 'plus 2' (moderate long-term relief), *and* 'plus 1' (temporary or minor relief) – the line-up takes this shape.

1. **Ibuprofen – 86%**
2. **Indometacin – 85%**
3. **Naproxen – 84%**
4. **Etoricoxib – 80%**
5. **Diclofenac – 79%**

These comparisons are interesting, but as mentioned said earlier, they don't predict the way the drugs will behave for you. It's more instructive to consider each one's record individually, in the light of what is known about the NSAIDs as a group. We'll also look at half a dozen other drugs in the non-steroidal anti-inflammatory family in addition to these 'top five.' The following products are listed according to their frequency of use, beginning with those taken by the greatest number of survey participants. We've included the US results for the same drug known there as Motrin.

Like all NSAIDs, **Ibuprofen** is both a pain reliever and an anti-inflammatory drug. It may work on your pain in a hurry, perhaps within a short time after you take your very first dose; but you may have to wait at least a week before you can tell how well it controls your inflammation. The same is true of the other

Motrin (Ibuprofen)

	US Survey	US Percentage	UK Survey	UK Percentage
Number of participants taking Ibuprofen	554		229	
Outcome:				
Dramatic relief	106	(19%)	30	(13%)
Moderate relief	96	(17%)	46	(20%)
Temporary or minor relief only	155	(28%)	121	(53%)
No relief (ineffective)	143	(26%)	32	(14%)
No rating*	54	10		
Most common drug reactions:				
No unpleasant side effects	210	(38%)	N/R	N/R
Stomach upset, pain, or indigestion	89	(16%)	N/R	N/R
Nausea and/or vomiting	72	(13%)	N/R	N/R
Dizziness or drowsiness	53	10	N/R	N/R

* Participants did not rate a drug they had just started taking, or one to which they reacted badly and stopped taking before they could judge its effectiveness.
† Side effects listed in these ratings were reported by at least 10% of the US participants on a given drug.

drugs in this class. This is why your doctor will encourage you to stay with **Ibuprofen**, for example, even if the first few weeks don't seem so promising. One strategy doctors use with NSAIDs is to prescribe them for two weeks, then, if there's no significant change, increase the dosage for another few weeks, and then, if there's still no improvement, try a different NSAID.

'While taking Indocin (Indomethacin) I suffered from nausea and abdominal pain,' said a North Carolina homemaker. 'Motrin (Ibuprofen) has helped more than the others, and with fewer side effects.'

The side effects from most NSAIDs centre on the gut, otherwise known as the gastrointestinal or GI tract. As you'll see from the ratings, nausea, vomiting, and stomach upset or pain are the most frequently mentioned side effects for the drugs in this class.

Indocin (Indomethacin)

	US Survey	US Percentage	UK Survey	UK Percentage
Number of participants taking Indocin	352		33	
Outcome:				
Dramatic relief	52	(15%)	12	(33%)
Moderate relief	61	(17%)	11	(30%)
Temporary or minor relief only	97	(28%)	8	(22%)
No relief (ineffective)	102	(29%)	6	(16%)
No rating	40	(11%)		
Most common drug reactions:	102	(17%)	N/R	
No unpleasant side effects	105	(30%)	N/R	
Nausea and/or vomiting	65	(18%)	N/R	
Stomach upset, pain, or indigestion	48	(14%)	N/R	
Dizziness or drowsiness	44	13	N/R	

And, as far as anyone can tell, the reason they cause so much grief is the *same* reason they bring so much relief. Aspirin and other NSAIDs apparently reduce inflammation and pain by blocking the body's production of substances called prostaglandins. There are *some* prostaglandins, however, that work to protect the stomach lining. The NSAIDs' shotgun destruction of them may leave the stomach open to injury.

What's more, since the NSAIDs are swallowed and spend some time inside the stomach, they get a chance to cause a little direct irritation while they're there. This is why your doctor has probably told you to take your medication with food or milk, so that you buffer the drug and hasten it along its way. Your chance of developing an ulcer if you have arthritis is at least one in five, due to these drugs. In fact, some of our survey participants listed a prescription ulcer drug – Tagamet (cimetidine), Zantac (ranitidine), or Carafate (sucralfate) – right under their arthritis medications.

'Of all the anti-inflammatories, Indocin (Indomethacin) is the most powerful,' wrote a thirty-six-year-old househusband and father with rheumatoid arthritis, who has taken Anaprox, Clinoril, Feldene, Meclomen, Motrin, Naprosyn, Oraflex, Orudis, and Tolectin. Indocin (Indomethacin) has helped him as much as Plaquenil and prednisone, he said. 'Sometimes I have to back off a little when I start getting dizzy and nauseous with it. Sometimes I get a little jumpy, too.'

Naprosyn (Naproxen)
(naproxen, Syntex)

	US Survey	US Percentage	UK Survey	UK Percentage
Number of participants taking Naprosyn	335		69	
Outcome:				
Dramatic relief	62	(19%)	16	(23%)
Moderate relief	61	(18%)	14	(20%)
Temporary or minor relief only	90	(27%)	28	(41%)
No relief (ineffective)	88	(26%)	9	(14%)
No rating	34	(10%)		
Most common drug reactions:				
No unpleasant side effects	128	(38%)	N/R	
Stomach upset, pain, or indigestion	55	(16%)	N/R	
Nausea and/or vomiting	45	(13%)	N/R	

Much is known about the different NSAIDs effectiveness and their side effects from the drug comparisons that have been done and from doctors' long experience in giving certain drugs to their patients and then hearing how they fared. This is how **Indocin** (Indomethacin) got its reputation for being more likely to bring on headaches and psychological effects, such as anger and confusion, and how **Meclomen** (Ponstan) became known for causing diarrhoea. These tendencies showed up the US survey data too. Fully 15 percent of those participants taking **Meclomen** said that it caused diarrhoea, while only 1 percent of those on **Motrin** (Ibuprofen) and 3 percent of those on **Indocin** were troubled with diarrhoea. As for causing headaches and psychological changes, **Indocin**, at 6 percent of those taking it, was more aggravating to participants than **Motrin** (2 percent), **Naprosyn** (Naproxen) (4 percent), and **Felden**e (2 percent). Other unfortunate associations reported by the drug manufacturers include **Tolectin** with allergic reactions and **Nalfon** with kidney damage. On the positive side, **Clinoril** is reputed to be kindest to the kidneys, although not completely benign, while **Meclomen** and **Feldene** are said to be easiest on the liver.

'I've been using Naprosyn (Naproxen) since the summer of 1985,' reported an electric-meter reader from California. 'The pain was reduced immediately, and the pills have never bothered me. Even if I take them on an empty stomach, I get only very slight nausea.'

Feldene (not rated in UK survey)
(piroxicam, Pfizer)

	US Survey	US Percentage
Number of participants taking Feldene	326	
Outcome:		
Dramatic relief	76	(23%)*
Moderate relief	46	(14%)
Temporary or minor relief only	73	(22%)
No relief (ineffective)	91	(28%)
No rating	40	(12%)
Most common drug reactions:		
No unpleasant side effects	110	(34%)
Stomach upset, pain, or indigestion	62	(19%)
Nausea and/or vomiting	44	(13%)

* Rather than carry out the percentages to decimal places, we round off, with the result that ratings for some drugs total 99 or 101%.

Feldene, although it is similar to other NSAIDs in most respects, has one advantage in that it's easy to swallow, or rather, you only have to swallow it once a day. Other NSAIDs have to be taken at least twice a day, or as often as four times a day, while aspirin users may need to down three or four tablets together at each dosage time. Some physicians – not to mention the manufacturer of **Feldene** – believe that making an arthritis drug easier to take makes it more likely that people will remember to take it, and therefore get the most benefit from it.

If you are over sixty-five, you may be more susceptible to any of the side effects from any of these drugs, and your doctor will have to prescribe them cautiously and watch you carefully.

'I've been taking Feldene for four and a half years,' said a sixty-six-year-old educator from Delaware who gave the drug high marks. 'Once I learned to take it in the morning with breakfast, I had no trouble with it. Last summer I had a complete upper and lower GI series, and the doctor said I was fine.'

Being fancier updates of aspirin, all the NSAIDs have appreciably higher price tags. Remember that the cost of the pill is not the only expense of taking the drug. Writing in *The Journal of Musculoskeletal Medicine*, rheumatologists Daniel O. Clegg, M.D., and John R. Ward, M.D., point out: 'If the cost of treatment for peptic ulcer disease and of hospitalization for GI hemorrhage is included, aspirin indeed may not be the least expensive anti-inflammatory medication.' In other words, the more expensive drugs *may* save you from other medical expenses later. After all, attempting to *minimize* side effects is the NSAIDs' whole reason for being. In general, they are thought to cause less bleeding and fewer ulcers than aspirin. Some of them, like aspirin, can make your ears ring. Others may change your appetite or your blood pressure. Most of them have the potential, like aspirin, to cause a rash, itching, or hives.

For all the help they provide, the NSAIDs do not cure arthritis. Since they do not cure, NSAIDs are long-term therapy. And yet, as you may have noticed, their effects can wear off with time. 'I used Motrin (Ibuprofen) successfully for fourteen years,' said a Weight Watchers lecturer from Delaware, 'and then it finally quit working.' A manager of a car dealership in Vermont wrote, 'I was on Clinoril (Sulindac) for nine years and got a great deal of relief, but I apparently built up a resistance and by the end of that time it did very little for me.'

NSAIDs may be prescribed for osteoarthritis or rheumatoid arthritis, to good effect, but the drugs play different roles in the

Clinoril (Sulindac) (Not rated in UK survey)

	US Survey	US Percentage
Number of participants taking Clinoril	120	
Outcome:		
Dramatic relief	31	(26%)
Moderate relief	25	(21%)
Temporary or minor relief only	22	(18%)
No relief (ineffective)	33	(28%)
No rating	9	(7%)
Most common drug reactions:		
No unpleasant side effects	40	(33%)
Dizziness or drowsiness	19	(16%)
Nausea and/or vomiting	15	(13%)
Stomach upset, pain, or indigestion	12	(10%)

two ailments. Rheumatoid arthritis is by definition an inflammatory disease, and NSAIDs are a mainstay of treatment. Even if you require one of the second-line drugs for rheumatoid arthritis, such as gold or penicillamine, your doctor will no doubt tell you to continue taking one of the NSAIDs.

The role of inflammation in osteoarthritis, on the other hand, is much foggier. Inflammation may be present *some* of the time, as opposed to most of the time, or it may be present in such a slight degree that only the most sensitive diagnostic measures can prove it's there. However, since the process of inflammation is thought to damage the joints, controlling it with NSAIDs when necessary makes sense – and, of course, the NSAIDs *also* act as painkillers. If you have osteoarthritis, your doctor will probably strive for the lowest dose possible, and he or she may suggest that you drop the NSAID from time to time, to see how you fare without it. This cautionary move is to avoid the risk of GI side effects. There is *no* danger of becoming addicted to any of the NSAIDs, as there is with narcotic painkillers.

'A few months ago, I stopped taking Dolobid (Diflunisal) for about a week at my doctor's suggestion,' wrote a retired nurse from New Jersey who has had osteoarthritis for ten years.

Dolobid (Diflunisal) (Not rated in UK survey)

	US Survey	US Percentage
Number of participants taking Dolobid (Diflunisal)	84	
Outcome:		
Dramatic relief	9	(11%)
Moderate relief	11	(13%)
Temporary or minor relief only	21	(25%)
No relief (ineffective)	27	(32%)
No rating	16	(19%)
Most common drug reactions:		
No unpleasant side effects	24	(28%)
Nausea and/or vomiting	12	(14%)
Stomach upset, pain, or indigestion	12	(14%)
Dizziness or drowsiness	9	(11%)

'But the pain in my hips and knees was much worse and more continuous then, so I went back on it.'

We've said that NSAIDs serve two functions: reducing inflammation and relieving pain. For most of them, a relatively small dose is all that's needed to unleash their full pain-relieving power. Higher doses bring on the anti-inflammatory effect. As a general rule, then, if the drug controls your inflammation, it is doing all it can do to relieve your pain. But what happens if you are getting good control of your inflammation with the drug you're taking and yet you still have pain from time to time? Should you take more of the drug?

Most experts say no. An extra measure of the same medicine will not only fail to help you but it will raise your chances of suffering some adverse side effect; nor can you call in another NSAID to boost the power of the one you're taking. Since the NSAIDs are so similar to each other, using two together multiplies the risks of all side effects. Remember, too, that over-the-counter drugs such as aspirin and ibuprofen are also anti-inflammatory agents. Check with your doctor before you mix any of these with your prescription pills. Acetaminophen (Tylenol or Datril, for example), since it's *not* an anti-inflammatory, is a safer bet for added pain relief. Or your doctor may recommend a prescription painkiller for you to use from time to time.

Nalfon (Fenoprofen) (not rated in UK Survey)

	US Survey	US Percentage
Number of participants taking Nalfon	38	
Outcome:		
Dramatic relief	15	(40%)
Moderate relief	9	(24%)
Temporary or minor relief only	2	(5%)
No relief (ineffective)	5	(13%)
No rating	7	(18%)
Most common drug reactions:		
No unpleasant side effects	16	(42%)
Dizziness or drowsiness	4	(11%)

One special category of drug fallout has not been mentioned yet, and that is the effect of the NSAIDs when used by pregnant or nursing women. According to the UK Arthritis Research Campaign NSAIDs are best avoided during pregnancy if at all possible, especially during the early months, and towards the end of the pregnancy, particularly during labour because of possible complications occurring during delivery, or to the infant after delivery. A low-dose NSAID is sometimes prescribed if pain is a problem and paracetamol is not sufficient. If you are planning to have a baby, you'll want to discuss your medication with your obstetrician and make any necessary adjustments. If you have rheumatoid arthritis, you may find that your joint pain and inflammation all but vanish during pregnancy, anyway, perhaps because of the natural changes in hormone levels and the immune system that keep your body from rejecting the half-foreign cells of your baby.

Although the NSAIDs make up a group, or family, of drugs, some of them are more closely related than others. For example, **Indomethacin** and **Sulindac** make up one chemical class, called indoles, while **Diflunisal** and aspirin are part of another, called

Orudis (Ketoprofen) (Not rated in UK survey)

	US Survey	US Percentage
Number of participants taking Orudis	38	
Outcome:		
Dramatic relief	2	(5%)
Moderate relief	9	(24%)
Temporary or minor relief only	12	(32%)
No relief (ineffective)	8	(21%)
No rating	7	(18%)
Most common drug reactions:		
No unpleasant side effects	9	(24%)
Stomach upset, pain, or indigestion	7	(18%)
Nausea and/or vomiting	4	(11%)

salicylates. Your doctor may use these class lists in trying to find the right NSAID for you. As the theory goes, if **Indomethacin** fails to help you, you probably wouldn't find much comfort in its classmates. That's the theory. In practice, however, the drugs continue to defy anybody's predictions. Often enough, the person who gets no comfort from **Indomethacin** goes on to have great success with **Sulindac**.

Of the six chemical classes of NSAIDs we mentioned above, one has fallen far behind the others in popularity. This is the class containing phenylbutazone (**Butazolidin**) and oxyphenbutazone (**Tandearil**). Ciba-Geigy took **Tandearil** off the market in 1985, and put new restrictions on the use of **Butazolidin** at that time. **Butazolidin** is no longer recommended as an early choice, but only as a last resort if other NSAIDs fail, and it is not to be used on a long-term basis. In addition to the usual risks, **Butazolidin** has the potential to block the bone marrow's life-sustaining production of new blood cells.

As we've seen, the cast of NSAID characters is a changing one, with new drugs entering frequently, and both old and new drugs making a command exit on occasion. Carol A. Warfield, M.D., director of the Pain Management Center at Boston's Beth Israel Hospital and assistant professor at

Phenylbutazone (Butazolidin) (Not rated in UK Survey)

	US Survey	US Percentage
Number of participants taking Butazolidin	33	
Outcome:		
Dramatic relief	10	(30%)*
Moderate relief	3	(9%)
Temporary or minor relief only	11	(33%)
No relief (ineffective)	7	(21%)
No rating	2	(6%)
Most common drug reactions:		
No unpleasant side effects	10	(30%)
Stomach upset, pain, or indigestion	4	(12%)

* Percentages have been rounded to the nearest whole number over the next few pages, with the result that ratings for some drugs do not total 100%.

Harvard Medical School, advised in *Hospital Practice* that doctors 'refrain from using newer NSAIDs until a track record of safety is established.'

Voltaren (Diclofenac) (Not rated in US Survey)

	UK Survey	UK Percentage
Number of participants taking diclofenac	162	
Outcome:		
Dramatic relief	36	(22%)*
Moderate relief	48	(30%)
Temporary or minor relief only	44	(27%)
No relief (ineffective)	34	(21%)

A sixty-four-year-old school custodian from Ontario said that Voltaren (Diclofenac) makes him feel 'very good,' and causes no side effects of any kind. A forty-three-year-old New Hampshire real estate agent said: 'It's easier on the stomach than the other drugs I've tried and its effects seem to last longer.'

Cox-2 Inhibitors

As stated above Cox-2 inhibitors are a type of NSAID, but have been developed to be safer for the stomach. Some frequently prescribed drugs in this group include etodolac, meloxicam, rofecoxib and celecoxib. In our UK survey meloxicam proved very effective.

Meloxicam

	UK Survey	UK Percentage
Number of participants taking meloxicam	86	
Outcome:		
Dramatic relief	37	(43%)*
Moderate relief	29	(34%)
Temporary or minor relief only	13	(15%)
No relief (ineffective)	7	(8%)

Celecoxib

	UK Survey	UK Percentage
Number of participants taking celecoxib	112	
Outcome:		
Dramatic relief	34	(30%)*
Moderate relief	23	(20%)
Temporary or minor relief only	42	(38%)
No relief (ineffective)	13	(12%)

Steroids

The drugs in this group, though also part of the first line, are no longer offered first. Their impressive power is held in reserve until other first-line measures have been tried. And while it was once common practice to prescribe large doses of steroids for long periods of time, most doctors today use low doses for safety's sake, and frequently set up an every-other-day dosage regimen to further minimize drug side effects. You may be offered a short course of steroids to get you through an arthritis flare-up, or to tide you over a period of switching from one slow-acting drug to another, but your doctor will probably move to reduce the dose fairly quickly or get you off the drug altogether. From time to time, you may also have steroids injected directly into a severely affected joint. This technique gets the drug right to the site where it's needed most.

The steroid family drugs are synthetic copies of hormones that our bodies normally produce. Other names for them are corticosteroids, glucocorticoids, and adrenocortical steroids. The drugs themselves include dexamethasone (Decadron is one example), hydrocortisone or cortisol (Cortef, for one), methyl-prednisolone (Medrol), prednisolone (such as Delta-Cortef), and prednisone (Deltasone and others).

All of the steroids date from the 1940s and 1950s, and they all have a history of use in the treatment of many conditions other than arthritis, from asthma to cancer. Indeed, a few of the participants got their first taste of prednisone for a totally unrelated problem, and found arthritis pain relief to be the chief side effect of the drug. 'Two years ago I had bypass surgery, after which I developed pericarditis [inflammation of the membrane around the heart],' wrote a sixty-two-year-old homemaker from North Carolina. 'I was treated with prednisone for five months, from August through December, and I had no pain from arthritis during that time.'

Prednisone and Other Pills
Compared to the NSAIDs, the steroids are far more effective at relieving pain and reducing inflammation. As the ratings show, 52 percent of the US survey participants taking steroid pills got dramatic relief, and another 33 percent reported moderate or temporary relief. No NSAID comes close to that score. Steroids work so well, in fact, that many participants willingly put up with any number of troublesome side effects in exchange for the relief they got. 'I have taken prednisone continuously for about eight years,' wrote a forty-four-year-old Texas police officer, 'and I guess the side effects have come from it. My kidneys hurt, I have blurred vision because of cataracts, growth of excessive hair, and lots of water retention, causing me to swell up at the face.' Puffed-out cheeks or 'moon-face' is a common side effect of these drugs. Less obvious but

more insidious is the high blood pressure that can also come with fluid retention.

	US Survey	US Percentage
Number of participants taking oral steroids	133*	
Outcome:		
Dramatic relief	69	(52%)
Moderate relief	25	(19%)
Temporary or minor relief only	19	(14%)
No relief (ineffective)	5	(4%)
No rating	15	(11%)
Most common drug reactions:		
No unpleasant side effects	33	(25%)
Fluid retention, with hypertension or moon-face	22	(17%)
Thin fragile skin, bones, muscles, or tendons	15	(11%)

* 'Steroids' include prednisone (110 participants), cortisone acetate (9 participants), methylprednisolone (7 participants), dexamethasone (3 participants), prednisolone (3 participants), and triamcinolone (1 participant).

The UK survey concentrated on one steroid, prednisolone. The ratings for that drug were impressive.

Prednisolone

	UK Survey	UK Percentage
Number of participants taking prednisolone	43	
Outcome:		
Dramatic relief	23	(53%)*
Moderate relief	5	(12%)
Temporary or minor relief only	9	(21%)
No relief (ineffective)	6	(14%)

Conspicuous by its absence in the list of side effects mentioned in the US survey was any mention of gastrointestinal distress, which is so common with the NSAIDs. Only five participants taking steroids complained of nausea (4 percent), three of stomach upset or cramps (2 percent), and one of diarrhoea (less than 1 percent). The more serious side effects of steroid use, in addition to the ones listed in the ratings, include the risk of eye damage, diabetes, and increased susceptibility to infection. Some people have reportedly developed ulcers, too, from steroid use, although no one in our survey complained of ulcers from this source. Depression, anxiety, and other psychological fallout from steroids is well documented in clinical studies, and was reported by nine of our participants (7 percent).

'I hate prednisone,' wrote a homemaker from Connecticut. 'Yes, it did help me through the bad flare-ups, but it made me jumpy and edgy, snapping at people for no real reason. I had trouble sleeping, too.'

Steroids are also known to create a kind of drug habit called functional dependence. Because they are so similar to the natural hormones produced by the adrenal glands, steroid drugs may shut down the body's own production of those hormones. This means that if you've been taking prednisone for a while, you can't suddenly stop, lest you leave yourself virtually defenseless against infection, and find your arthritis symptoms much, much worse. Instead, you must be 'weaned' off slowly, under close medical supervision.

'I took prednisolone for almost four years,' wrote a fifty-five-year-old farm wife from Ohio. 'It made me feel wonderful at first. I could do things I couldn't do before. But the doctor didn't tell me it could cause diabetes, which I now have, or that it was dangerous to go off the medicine suddenly. At one time, I decided to quit taking it because of some of the changes that were occurring with me. I became miserable with pain and high fever, and I was practically crippled. It took me a while to realize the connection between stopping the medicine and the horrible way I felt.'

Today, prednisolone is used along with other treatments, including NSAIDs. Getting down to the lowest dose possible, experts agree, should be the goal for anyone taking prednisolone or other steroids.

Cortisone and Related Injections

Steroids can also be given as a shot in the arm – or the knee, the hip, the wrist, whichever part hurts most. For a joint that has been immobilized by pain or stiffness, steroid injections can bring dramatic relief that typically lasts anywhere from a few days to a few months. A fifty-six-year-old man from Woking reported, 'Cortisone injections bring immediate relief.' 'Cortisone shots gave me instant relief,' said a retired telephone operator from Louisiana, 'and the relief lasted from a week to six months. Once I remember I couldn't even lift my arm, and as soon as I received the injection in my shoulder, my arm was free from pain and I could raise it.' The best practitioners capitalize on this startling degree of relief by coupling the injections with physical therapy and safe exercises that are likely to bring about long-term improvement. They will also warn you that overuse of a suddenly pain-free joint may cause more damage in the long run.

Steroid shots promise only temporary help, but a few of our participants found themselves enjoying extremely lasting benefits from shots they took years ago. A Florida homemaker reported: 'The doctor said the cortisone injection in my knee would last for four or five months, but I have been very fortunate in that the knee has not given me any great pain that can't be helped with Ascriptin [aspirin] tablets.' A retired social agency director from Seattle wrote: 'I find the shots are a blessing to me, and last several years. They say it's dangerous to take them, but as far as I'm concerned, it's better than crying all the time with pain or being in a wheelchair. I don't see how it's hurt me.'

By the same token, 'temporary help' from steroid shots can be relatively long-lived, compared to other treatments. A nurse from Illinois, for example, said she gets 'temporary relief' lasting from three to six months after an injection of cortisone. Keep this in mind as you look at the ratings for 'temporary' help. However an English woman from Runcorn said that she only gets a week's relief after cortisone injections.

'I've had many, many injections in all the affected joints during bad flare-ups over the years,' wrote a thirty-four-year-old homemaker from Maryland. 'The injections help after several hours, although the spot where the needle goes in always hurts

	US Survey	US Percentage
Number of reports on steroid shots	485*	
Outcome:		
Dramatic relief	183	(38%)
Moderate relief	103	(21%)
Temporary or minor relief only	95	(20%)
No relief (ineffective)	57	(12%)
Participant felt worse after injection	27	(5%)
No rating	20	(4%)

* For at least twenty-three of our participants, results from steroid shots differed so greatly from one injection to the next that they listed two or more separate ratings for this treatment. Because of the way steroid shots are given – in different joints at different times, and spread out over intervals of months or years – the experience and the amount of relief may vary greatly for some people. 'I got some pain relief from cortisone in my knee,' recalls a retired postal clerk from Wisconsin, 'and the first time I had a shot in my hip it gave me relief for months. But the second injection in my hip six months later brought no relief at all. The pain even seemed to get worse.'

In the UK survey the type of steroid being injected was specified. Overall prednisolone emerged as the most effective if we combine all three measures of pain relief from dramatic, to moderate and temporary (88 percent). Cortisone was the next most effective at 87 percent and Hydrocortisone not far behind at 84 percent.

Prednisolone injection

	UK Survey	UK Percentage
Number of participants injected with prednisolone	24	
Outcome:		
Dramatic relief	6	(25%)*
Moderate relief	3	(12.5%)
Temporary or minor relief only	12	(50%)
No relief (ineffective)	3	(12.5%)
Made participant feel worse	0	(0%)

Cortisone injection

	UK Survey	UK Percentage
Number of participants injected with cortisone	122	
Outcome:		
Dramatic relief	22	(18%)*
Moderate relief	26	(21%)
Temporary or minor relief only	59	(48%)
No relief (ineffective)	12	(10%)
Made participant feel worse	3	(3%)

Hydrocortisone injection

	UK Survey	UK Percentage
Number of participants injected with hydrocortisone	32	
Outcome:		
Dramatic relief	8	(25%)*
Moderate relief	7	(22%)
Temporary or minor relief only	12	(37%)
No relief (ineffective)	5	(16%)
Made participant feel worse	0	(0%)

for a day or two. Cortisone will usually settle my hips, knees, ankles, and elbows, but it has no effect on my back, shoulders, and neck.' Cortisone definitely helps some joints more than others for several participants who have tried shots in various painful places. And while the places vary from one person to the next, the US survey had more reports of ineffectiveness for cortisone shots to the joints of the back and neck than to any other part of the body. This is apparently true because the joint spaces of the spine are not accessible by injection, and getting the drug into the surrounding tissue does little good, if any, according to the manufacturers.

Another, perhaps obvious point is that the effectiveness of any steroid injection depends to a large extent on the skill of the person giving the shot. Since the needle must be properly positioned inside the joint space, the practitioner must be ultra familiar with the anatomy of the joint.

Cortisone shots, as mentioned before, are not a cure. Even if they work for you, they will likely have to be repeated someday. 'Cortisone shots help me a lot for about two months,' said a Texas carpenter, 'then I need another one.' There is a limit to the number of times any one joint can be injected, however, before the procedure poses a threat of damage to the cartilage or bone there, or both. And, although steroids that are specially prepared for injection into the joints are considered safer than pills or intramuscular shots that spread steroids through the bloodstream, the drug still builds up in the body, and its effects are cumulative. In other words, the more you take, the greater your risk of long-term difficulties, which include osteoporosis and cataracts. 'I was taking shots of Depo-Medrol every two months in each thumb,' wrote a retired salesman from Florida. 'It was the most effective medication I've ever had, but after a couple of years, I was advised by another doctor that it might be destroying my bones.'

Aside from the dangers of long-term use, a few of our participants noted that steroid shots eventually lose their effectiveness anyway. 'The cortisone injections gave instant relief,' wrote a nun from Missouri, 'but in time the effects lasted only a day or two, instead of weeks.' A joint that is crying out for repeated injections is probably a candidate for surgery. 'I had three cortisone shots in my left knee before my total joint replacement,' said a thirty-six-year-old New York freelance writer with rheumatoid arthritis. 'The first was a miracle, the second great, and the third so-so, as the disease progressed.'

Steroid injections rarely fail to bring relief, but some people do find them useless, and others actually feel worse after having one. 'The cortisone injection I had did not help the pain,' recalled a restaurant owner from Staten Island, 'and I couldn't move my arm at all for almost two weeks.' Here's another negative report from an Idaho homemaker: 'Cortisone in my knee made it get black and blue and more painful. The only relief I had came when the bruised area healed.' And an Ohio teacher reports that she has lost the use of the joint where cortisone was injected.

THE SECOND LINE

The drugs that make up the second line are reserved almost exclusively for the treatment of rheumatoid arthritis. They are also called remittive, or disease-modifying anti-rheumatic drugs (DMARDs), because they may bring about a remission by countering the disease process itself, although no one can say just how they do so. Another name for them is slow-acting, and they do take a long time – weeks or months – to take effect. The oldest and most popular among them is the injection of gold salts. This treatment has become the standard against which all other second-line drugs are judged.

Gold: The Gold Standard

Gold was first used to treat rheumatoid arthritis for the wrong reasons. That was in the 1920s, when the disease was thought to be a chronic infection in the joints. Renowned German bacteriologist Robert Koch had shown that gold and other heavy metals, such as arsenic and mercury, could fight the tuberculosis germ in the test tube, and it was only natural to try the novel therapy on other infectious diseases. Gold looked promising against rheumatoid arthritis, and doctors quickly built up evidence to support its use. But by the mid-1940s, when gold had proven itself effective, most scientists had abandoned the belief that arthritis was an infectious disease. So gold was then *rejected* by doctors because it didn't fit the prevailing theory of the day. A few diehards continued to use it anyway, however, and a couple of decades later, gold resurfaced in the 1960s as a standard treatment. No theory yet explains its effectiveness, but that doesn't stop anyone from using it, since gold works, after all, and since the cause of rheumatoid arthritis remains a mystery.

Gold Injections

'After three or four months on gold injections,' wrote a retired teacher from New York, 'the miracle started and I was a new person. I now take one injection a month, and in general I feel well with very occasional bouts of pain.'

Although gold is the standard, it does not stand alone. If used, it is but one element in a regimen including, for example, exercise, physiotherapy, and other medications. 'I have been on gold almost from the onset of the arthritis twenty-two years ago,' said a salesman from Pennsylvania, who stretches and walks regularly – on his doctor's advice – to keep limber. 'I credit the gold, plus a combination of Indocin or Feldene and some other medications, for keeping me as well as can be.'

Gold injections carry weighty risks, and your doctor will no doubt talk to you about these before you start the therapy. You'll be seeing a lot of your doctor if you take gold injections, most likely going to the office for a shot every week during the first few months. You'll also be tested at each visit for any of the toxic side effects the gold may cause. These include kidney problems and bone-marrow suppression. Much more common side effects, which you will see for yourself if they develop, are itchy skin rashes and sores in the mouth. 'I had gold shots for six months,' wrote a housewife from Iowa, 'and they did wonders for me. But after six months I broke out all over my body and the rash itched something terrible. That was a year and a half ago, and I still have some of the spots.' A credit analyst from New York said, 'Gold injections seemed to put the rheumatoid arthritis into remission. Then, after thirteen injections, I broke out in a rash, and the doctor stopped the treatment.' Even if you can tolerate the itching, the rash signifies that the drug is causing a toxic reaction, and it will do worse damage unless you stop taking it.

Several researchers have shown that gold controls pain and inflammation, and prevents further deformity, for as many as two-thirds of those who try it. It is such a well-liked therapy that you may be encouraged to take a series of gold *again* if an earlier trial failed to help you. Several of our participants reported two or even three experiences with gold injections. 'I tried gold three times in different cities, with different doctors, but it was no help,' wrote a librarian from Missouri. A retired tax representative from California recalled, 'Gold gave me so much help that I discontinued treatment. I had to resume the injections at a later date, and they had absolutely no effect then. I often wonder if further damage could have been prevented had I not stopped gold in the first place.' Although still used as a treatment in the UK insufficient numbers of participants in the UK survey had had gold injections for us to be able to tabulate the results.

	US Survey	US Percentage
Number of participant trials of gold shots*	146	
Outcome:		
Dramatic relief	50	(34%)
Moderate relief	25	(17%)
Minor or temporary relief only	15	(10%)
No relief (ineffective)	35	(24%)
No rating	21	(14%)
Most common drug reactions:		
No unpleasant side effects reported	62	(42%)
Allergic reaction, including rash, itching, or sores in the mouth	34	(23%)

* The product used is either gold sodium thiomalate (**Myochrysine**, Merek Sharp & Dohme) or aurothioglucose (**Solganal**, Schering Corporation).

A small minority of practitioners today believe in the value of gold treatments for osteoarthritis, but only eleven of our participants with osteoarthritis got the chance to try gold injections, and just one of them got any lasting help. Gold may also fail to help people with rheumatoid arthritis, and it makes some of them feel worse. The following account comes from a retired specialized clerk for the armed forces: 'I had three gold injections, and each time I could not move my body the next day because all of my joints hurt too much. In those three weeks, I missed three days of work because of the shots.'

Several of our participants used gold successfully for long periods of time – ten, twenty, or even thirty years – before it finally lost its effectiveness for them. They never developed any side effects, they just woke up one day to find that the treatment didn't work any more, and it was time to try something else. Others got good results for several years before a toxic reaction ended the therapy. 'Gold did the best,' claimed a housewife from Michigan, 'but I developed a rash and ulcers in my mouth. Now I'm on oral gold.'

Gold in Pill Form

Auranofin tablets mean the end of the bothersome rear-end injections for many people with rheumatoid arthritis. It's thought to be a little safer than the shots but also a little less effective, and some doctors don't trust it because they like the chance to see and evaluate their patients before each dose of gold. If you take the capsules, you simply swallow them yourself although you still need to see your doctor every month for blood and urine tests. Auranofin carries the same dangers as injectable gold, and already it has a reputation for being a more frequent cause of diarrhoea.

	US Survey	US Percentage
Number of participants taking auranofin	41	
Outcome:		
Dramatic relief	8	(20%)
Moderate relief	7	(17%)
Minor or temporary relief only	6	(15%)
No relief (ineffective)	14	(34%)
No rating	6	(15%)
Most common drug reactions:		
No unpleasant side effects	11	(27%)
Diarrhoea	8	(20%)
Rash, itching, or mouth sores	6	(15%)
Nausea	4	(10%)

Hydroxychloroquine: The Antimalarial Drug

The primary use for hydroxychloroquine (**Plaquenil Sulfate**) is in the treatment of malaria, but it can also tackle rheumatoid arthritis, for reasons no one really understands. Like gold, hydroxychloroquine and chloroquine are slow-acting and may take as long as four to six months to make any appreciable difference in the way you feel. Doctors consider it to be less effective than gold or penicillamine, but then, it's quite a bit safer. The major threat from hydroxychloroquine and chloroquine is to the retina of the eye because the drug winds up in that tissue, where it can disturb your vision. Three US survey participants who took **Plaquenil** (8 percent) mentioned this problem.

'Before I started on Plaquenil,' wrote a retired Canadian research chemist, 'all the prescription drugs I took made my white blood cell count too low. I get good relief from Plaquenil, with no noticeable side effects. But, since the drug may damage the retina, I see an ophthalmologist twice a year who tests my eyes for colour vision and visual field.' A social worker from Indiana, after four years on Plaquenil and regular eye exams every four to six months, said she was doing well on both counts.

	US Survey	US Percentage	UK Survey	UK Percentage
Number of participants taking hydroxychloroquine	39		36	
Outcome:				
Dramatic relief	11	(288%)	6	(17%)
Moderate relief	6	(15%)	11	(31%)
Minor or temporary relief	2	(5%)	9	(25%)
No relief (ineffective)	8	(21%)	10	(28%)
No rating	12	(31%)		
Most common drug reactions:				
No unpleasant side effects	16	(41%)	N/R	
Nausea	4	(10%)	N/R	

Sulfasalazine

Another comparatively safe disease-modifying drug favoured by some rheumatologists is sulfasalazine, which is an anti-inflammatory agent approved by the FDA for the treatment of ulcerative colitis, and used sporadically for forty years to treat rheumatoid arthritis. Insufficient numbers of people had used the drug in the US survey for the results to be included, however the UK survey produced some impressive results for this drug. Thirty-six percent gained dramatic relief, while 23 percent gained at least moderate relief.

	UK Survey	UK Percentage
Number of participants taking sulfasalazine	66	
Outcome:		
Dramatic relief	24	(36%)
Moderate relief	15	(23%)
Minor or temporary relief	10	(15%)
No relief (ineffective)	17	(26%)
No rating	0	(0%)

Penicillamine and the Copper Connection

If you've ever thought about wearing a copper bracelet, you know that the copper leaching into your skin from the jewellery is rumoured to have healing powers. This is just a rumour, though, and survey participants' experience shows the copper bracelet for what it is: a piece of jewellery. (See Chapter 9.) Penicillamine, on the other hand, *removes* copper from the body. This makes it the ideal treatment for people with the extremely rare illness called Wilson's disease, who build up too much copper in their body organs and then suffer brain damage, cirrhosis of the liver, kidney dysfunction, and other potentially fatal problems. What penicillamine does that makes it so effective in reducing the pain and inflammation of *arthritis*, however, is unknown. It appears to quiet the disease by influencing the immune system. Copper removal may have everything or nothing to do with the fact that penicillamine works.

'Before trying penicillamine,' wrote a sixty-one-year-old accountant from New York, 'I used a cane and was hardly able to walk. Now I am almost free of pain and swelling.' Insufficient numbers of UK participants had used penicillamine for us to report the results.

	US Survey	US Percentage
Number of participants taking penicillamine*	36	
Outcome:		
Dramatic relief	13	(36%)
Moderate relief	8	(22%)
Minor or temporary relief	3	(8%)
No relief (ineffective)	8	(22%)
No rating	4	(11%)
Most common drug reactions:		
No unpleasant side effects	8	(22%)
Nausea and/or vomiting	5	(14%)

* Penicillamine is also known by the trade names Distamine or Pendramine.

Unlike the vast majority of arthritis drugs, penicillamine must be taken on an *empty* stomach – at least an hour before meals or after any other drug, food, or milk – for it to have maximum effect. Penicillamine is used *with* other drugs and treatments. 'I have been taking the combination of **Feldene** and penicillamine for nearly three years now,' said a thirty-five-year-old librarian from West Virginia, 'and am *very* pleased with the results. I have had no side effects other than some light-headedness and occasional nausea.' For others, penicillamine's noxious side effects included kidney problems (8 percent of our participants), rashes (6 percent), muscle weakness (6 percent), as well as bone-marrow suppression and syndromes that resemble other diseases, including systemic lupus erythematosus, which is characterized by arthritis and other disorders.

It takes two or three months of treatment to tell whether penicillamine will work for you. This is the case with all the slow-acting agents, as we've seen. Aside from their long start-up time, these drugs pose a problem for doctors in deciding which one to try first. As a general rule, X ray evidence of serious joint damage is the signal to go for gold, but many doctors like to start with Plaquenil because, if it works, it offers the safest treatment. Penicillamine is probably the least popular of all, and is usually reserved for those who get no help from gold.

Cytotoxic Drugs: Chemotherapy for Arthritis

The drugs in this group have been used to halt the uncontrolled cell growth that characterizes cancer, to help keep transplanted organs from being rejected by their new hosts, and, more recently, to slow the runaway inflammation of rheumatoid arthritis. They are praised for their demonstrated ability to bring relief when all else fails. And they are feared for their awesome side effects. Some of them can *cause* cancer, strangely enough, as well as bone-marrow suppression, sterility, or cirrhosis of the liver.

The cytotoxic drugs include azathioprine (Imuran, Azamune), cyclophosphamide (Endoxana), and methotrexate (Emtexate and Maxtrex).

Methotrexate

Methotrexate was developed for leukaemia therapy in the 1940s, and a report of the first attempt to pit it against rheumatoid arthritis appeared in 1951 – more than fifty years ago. It has taken all this time for other studies to prove the claims of that first report. Methotrexate was once considered an experimental treatment for rheumatoid arthritis. Practitioners worried about its severe and potentially lethal side effects (more about these later), which become a tremendous concern for people with arthritis, who, unlike cancer patients, may take the medication for a long, long time.

In fact, as more and more rheumatologists have tried methotrexate on patients with the most destructive cases of rheumatoid arthritis, the drug has proved to be safer than they expected. The dread toxic reactions have not shown up as frequently or as severely as had been feared. This is probably because the dosage level used for arthritis is so much lower than the dosages required for cancer chemotherapy – about 1/100 of the amount.

Together with the drug you will also usually be prescribed a weekly tablet of folic acid (5 mg). This is to be taken three days after taking the methotrexate. It counteracts some of the possible side effects of methotrexate. If you forget to take tablets on your regular day, take them the next day. Alcohol can increase the risk of side-effects and is best kept to a minimum.

Methotrexate is by all means a *long-term* treatment. It seems to perform a miracle within the first month or two of use for many people with arthritis, relieving even the most intractable pain and all but eliminating stiffness. A good number of these individuals keep on improving steadily as they continue the treatment over successive months, and they may stay on it for years. Withdraw the drug, however, as doctors have done in studies, and all signs of improvement vanish in a blazing flare-up within a few weeks. At Albany (NY) Medical College, five patients stopped receiving methotrexate in 1987 after three years of steady use. As a group, they suddenly had more than twice as many painful joints as they'd had while taking methotrexate, and their period of morning stiffness *quintupled* in length. Every way the five individuals and attending doctors looked at the situation, their arthritis was definitely as bad as it had been before they began the treatment. The experiment completed, they went back on methotrexate and were feeling much better one month later.

Here's how our US and UK survey participants rated methotrexate.

	US Survey	US Percentage	UK Survey	UK Percentage
Number who tried methotrexate	48		26	
Outcome:				
Dramatic improvement	24	(50%)*	11	(42%)
Moderate improvement over time	3	(6%)	7	(27%)
Temporary or minor improvement	1	(2%)†	3	(12%)
No improvement (ineffective)	5	(10%)	3	(12%)
No rating (too soon to tell, or toxic reaction	15	(31%)	Not rated	Not rated
forced individual off drug before any benefit could be achieved)			Not rated	Not rated
Made participant feel worse			2	(7%)

* These percentages have been rounded to the nearest whole number, with the result that ratings for some treatments do not total 100%.
† This participant, a fifty-eight-year-old homemaker from Michigan, actually received methotrexate for her psoriasis, but she also has both rheumatoid and osteoarthritis. 'Methotrexate helps my psoriasis a lot,' she says, 'but gives little help for my pain.'

These numbers, drawn from the survey, approximate the results from formal clinical trials. In 1984, for example, in a large study organized at the University of Utah, slightly more than 50 percent of the 189 patients enjoyed a significant reduction of pain and swelling on methotrexate.

Methotrexate works. That's the good news. And it works where all else has failed, because methotrexate is not given to anyone who hasn't already tried a whole series of strategies, typically including aspirin, other non-steroidal anti-inflammatory drugs, steroids, gold shots, and antimalarial drugs or penicillamine.

A thirty-six year old man from Huddersfield commented that, 'Methotrexate worked wonders over the four years that I took it.'

'Methotrexate gives a great deal of relief for several days after taking the weekly medication,' a participant from Canada reported. And a fifty-nine-year-old woman from Oxford wrote, 'In combination with methotrexate of 6×2.5 mg tablets I take Adalimumab injections and at the moment I am very well indeed, the best I have been for 17 years since the onset of the arthritis.'

'Methotrexate is helping me a great deal. It has given me back the strength in my wrists and hands,' wrote a sixty-two-year-old retired government official from Tennessee who took gold injections for seventeen years until they lost their effectiveness for him. A sixty-seven-year-old medical technician from New York who has had arthritis for twelve years said, 'This is the first time that something has worked. I'm on my third year.'

Methotrexate may be prescribed along with other drugs in treating your condition. Some drugs interact with methotrexate and particular care is needed with NSAIDs. You may only take these if they are prescribed to you by your doctor. Methotrexate is not a painkiller so if you are on painkillers you may continue to take them unless your doctor advises otherwise. Do not take 'over-the-counter' preparations without first discussing this with your doctor.

Just what, exactly, methotrexate does in rheumatoid arthritis remains a mystery; but then, no one can say for sure how most of the common arthritis drugs achieve their benefits. If they *work*, they are used. And while it would be very nice to know *how* they work, scientific understanding has not kept pace with practical experience.

The names applied to methotrexate and the other drugs in its class – they are called, by turns, cytotoxic drugs, immuno-suppressives, antimetabolites, and immunomodulatory drugs – all hint at their possible actions in the body. For example, 'cyto-toxic' means 'poisonous to the cells.' By interfering with cell reproduction, these drugs can halt the uncontrolled growth that characterizes cancer, or, as in rheumatoid arthritis, the runaway inflammation and destruction of the joints. 'Immunosuppressive' means they can damp the immune response. Since rheumatoid arthritis is believed to be an immune-system attack on one's own body, it stands to reason that suppressing the immune system might quiet the disease. Again, the mechanism by which methotrexate brings arthritis relief is simply not known.

What are the Side Effects of Methotrexate?

The most common side effect of methotrexate – in clinical studies and among our participants – is nausea. Eleven US survey participants mentioned it, three of whom said the nausea was only occasional or slight. Nausea, unfortunately, is nothing new to people who have run the gamut of non-steroidal anti-inflammatory drugs, as most methotrexate recipients have done. But that doesn't make it any easier to bear. The nausea from methotrexate, however, often disappears on its own, and if not, it may be controlled by lowering the dose or by spreading it out – that is, by taking the three or four tablets of methotrexate every few hours over the course of the appointed day, instead of swallowing them all at once. Another option is to take the drug as an injection instead of a pill, but that necessitates a weekly trip to the doctor.

A weekly trip to the doctor may be avoidable, but a monthly one is *mandatory* if you are on methotrexate. Every few weeks, you must undergo the tests that show whether the drug is causing any of the more hidden noxious kinds of damage of which it is capable. You need a complete blood count because methotrexate can suppress the production of new blood cells and lead to severe forms of anaemia. You also get a blood test to point up possible ill effects in the liver, called a liver-chemistry profile. Liver damage is one of the worst threats of methotrexate, because the damage, once begun, cannot be undone. The blood-chemistry profile, moreover, is not a complete check for liver problems, since the most serious damage does not show up in a blood test. Only an actual biopsy can tell for sure, and if you take methotrexate, you are supposed to undergo a liver biopsy after about two years of treatment. The other worrisome fallout from methotrexate is lung disease. If you take the drug, you are warned to be on the lookout for a dry cough accompanied by fever and shortness of breath. If you notice these symptoms, you need to see your doctor and have a chest X ray *immediately*.

'Methotrexate dramatically relieved my arthritis,' wrote a fifty-six-year-old communications consultant from North Carolina, 'but it also brought extreme tiredness, inability to eat, weight loss, lowered resistance to infection, and depressed spirits. I had to discontinue it because the side effects were unacceptable to me.' She now manages her arthritis with prednisone and penicillamine.

Some people on methotrexate develop sores on their skin or inside their mouths. These are signs of a toxic reaction to the drug, and mean, 'Get off it at once.' Others begin to lose their hair. Here's a rundown of the side effects reported by our US participants.

Problem	US Survey Number Affected	US Percentage
Nausea or vomiting	11	(23%)*
Lowered disease resistance	4	(8%)
Lost or thinning hair	3	(6%)
Sores in mouth	3	(6%)
Liver dysfunction	3	(6%)
Hives or skin lesions	3	(6%)
Depression	2	(4%)
Shingles (herpes zoster)	2	(4%)
Stomach pain or burning	2	(4%)
Eye problems	2	(4%)
Low blood count	1	(2%)
Anorexia and weight loss	1	(2%)
Intestinal cramps	1	(2%)
Bladder ulcers	1	(2%)
Dry skin	1	(2%)
Extreme fatigue	1	(2%)
Dizziness	1	(2%)
Swelling of legs and feet	1	(2%)
Difficulty breathing	1	(2%)
No side effects	8	(17%)

* Some participants reported two or more side effects.

Who Can Take Methotrexate?

Methotrexate is not for everybody. The decision to prescribe it is not made lightly, and the drug is reserved for those with the most severe cases of rheumatoid arthritis. In other words, you have to have a great deal of pain, stiffness, and swelling in several joints, plus fatigue. You also have to have proved yourself a reliable patient, since it takes a fair degree of responsibility on your part to follow the treatment plan, both in taking the drug on schedule and showing up at the doctor's office for frequent checkups to test for danger signs.

You cannot take methotrexate if you are pregnant or planning to have a baby. This warning also applies to men who are planning to become fathers, since the drug may cause birth defects and even sterility. A few other physical conditions would rule out using methotrexate. If you drink a lot of alcohol, for example, the danger of cirrhosis of the liver rises dramatically.

Tips on Drug Safety and Purchase

The following suggestions are based on survey participants' comments and material from the US National Council on Patient Information and Education.

At the doctor's office

- Learn the *name* of any drug your doctor prescribes for you, and ask what it is supposed to do for you.
- Make sure you understand how and when to take it (before meals, after meals, with milk, etc.).
- Determine how long you are supposed to stay on the drug – and what would happen if you stopped taking it for any reason on your own.
- Ask whether there are any foods or drinks that might interfere with the drug's action (milk, for example) or multiply its side effects (alcohol, perhaps). Also find out whether the drug makes it dangerous for you to drive.
- Get an idea of the possible side effects to look for, and what you should do if you experience any of them.
- Get your own copy of any written information that the doctor has available about the drug.

- Mention to the doctor the names of the medications you already take, whether they are prescription drugs or over-the-counter staples in your medicine chest. It's also very important to mention any allergic reactions you've ever had to any drug.

At the Pharmacy

- Read the prescription before you hand it over, and check the drug you get to make sure it's what the doctor ordered. Some pharmacists substitute generic drugs for brand names, and while these are usually less expensive, they may not be the equal of the original. If your prescription says 'DAW,' or 'Dispense as Written,' it means your doctor does not want you to take the generic version.
- If your pharmacist is accessible, repeat your questions about the drug and any precautions about taking it. The pharmacist may tell you something the doctor overlooked.

At Home

- Take the drugs as directed.
- If you forget some of your doctor's directions, call and ask for a reminder.
- If you develop problems while taking the drug, report them to your doctor immediately.

Summary of Prescription Drug Treatments for Arthritis

The First Line

NSAIDs – Good control of pain and inflammation, although finding the best one for you may take some time.

Steroids: Oral – Great relief, but dangerous as high-dose or long-term therapy.

Intra-articular injections – Excellent spot relief for painful joints.

Intramuscular injections – Effective for control of severe arthritis flares or during start-up period of second-line drugs.

The Second Line

Gold: Injections – Time-honoured treatment for advanced rheumatoid arthritis.

Pills – Easier to take but not quite as effective.

Sulfasalazine – Effective for many.

Penicillamine – Useful for rheumatoid arthritis when gold fails to help.

Methotrexate – Excellent results and fewer side effects

WARNING: All drug treatments carry the risk of side effects, and not one of them constitutes a cure in itself. Whatever you take, take it along with exercise, proper diet, rest, physiotherapy, and all necessary precautions.

Chapter 6
Over-the-Counter Drugs:

From the Miraculous to the Preposterous

• *Aspirin* • *Acetaminophen* • *Ibuprofen* • *Rub-on balms*

One of the most widely used and well regarded treatments for arthritis is an over-the-counter drug. Its name, of course, is aspirin, and more than half of the 1,051 US survey participants relied on it every single day. Many of them gave aspirin a 'plus-3' rating – the highest on the scale used. This was not the case according to the results of our UK survey where many more participants used ibuprofen or paracetamol and rated both drugs more highly than aspirin.

Most participants are thrilled that they can buy aspirin or ibuprofen without a prescription because it means their favourite drug stays cheap and readily available. But they hate the myth, spawned by some aspirin or paracetamol advertisements, that arthritis is nothing more than 'minor aches and pains' – easily managed by the same pills everyone else uses to chase a headache or a fever.

Separating the facts from the myths, the misleading claims of manufacturers, and the well-meaning advice of friends who swear by some non-prescription treatment, whether it's Tylenol or Tiger Balm, is what this chapter is all about. In it, you'll find the benefit of participants' experience with over-the-counter drugs, from tablets and tonics to creams, lotions, and sprays. Their testimony is backed with reports from the medical literature, and there are tips on how to buy and use these products with savvy and safety.

Aspirin
Perhaps the most important thing to say about aspirin, simply, is that it works, and works well for many arthritis sufferers.

Here's how the original wonder drug fared statistically in the US and UK surveys.

	US Survey	US Percentage	UK Survey	UK Percentage
Number of participants using aspirin	598		80	
Outcome:				
A great deal of help that lasted a year or more	121	(20%)	8	(10%)
A little help that lasted a year or more	239	(40%)	7	(9%)
Minor or temporary relief only	210	(35%)	44	(55%)
Didn't help at all	19	(3%)	21	(26%)
No rating	9	(2%)	0	0

As you can see there is a marked difference between the US and UK surveys. Totalling the positive ratings for the US survey reveals that aspirin gave at least some relief to 95 percent of those who use it; the figure drops to 74 percent in the UK survey. However that is still a very positive result. 'I have tried several arthritis drugs prescribed by my doctor,' wrote a retired businessman from California, 'but aspirin seems as good as anything.'

Aspirin is not only good medicine. It's cheap. The brand you choose and the place you shop may drive the expense up or down, but not by much when you compare aspirin prices to the cost of other anti-inflammatory drugs.

Although it is used for every imaginable pain, from toothache to cancer, aspirin remains uniquely suited to the treatment of arthritis. All three of aspirin's major actions are called into play in arthritis. It acts as: (1) an analgesic to ease pain, the hallmark of the disease; (2) an anti-inflammatory to control inflammation, the culprit responsible for much joint damage; and (3) an antipyretic to reduce fever, which frequently plagues people with rheumatoid arthritis.

The amount of aspirin you take probably depends on the type of arthritis you have. For osteoarthritis, for example, aspirin is mostly a pain reliever, and you use it as often as your pain demands. But to treat rheumatoid arthritis, aspirin levels have to build up in your body, and you may be urged to take as many as a dozen or even two dozen a day to get the full anti-inflammatory effect.

You'd almost think aspirin had been tailor-made for arthritis, but it came about as a failed attempt to create a man-made substitute for quinine. In the 1800s, when malaria was rampant and supplies of natural quinine couldn't fill the need, German chemists set out to synthesize quinine in the laboratory. They did not succeed. None of their concoctions cured malaria. But one of them, acetylsalicylic acid, the drug we now call aspirin (or A.S.A. in Canada), did prove to quell fever and pain.

Although acetylsalicylic acid was synthesized in 1853, it did not become commercially available until decades later, in 1899, when the Bayer Pharmaceutical Co. introduced it and coined the trade name 'aspirin.' Another half a century passed before scientists learned through animal experiments in the mid-1950s that aspirin could also control inflammation. And it has been only relatively recently that medical researchers began to fathom *how* aspirin works its various wonders apparently by blocking the body's production of substances called prostaglandins, some of which cause pain and inflammation.

Aspirin's Most Common Side Effect . . . and What to Do About It

The dark side of aspirin therapy lurks in the stomach, where even one tablet can cause a little bleeding, and where prolonged heavy use has lead to ulcers. If you depend on large quantities of aspirin for controlling your arthritis, then the chance of your developing an ulcer is probably somewhere between one in four and one in five. In hospitals where doctors have studied the effects of long-term aspirin use, as many as 25 percent of their patients with rheumatoid arthritis have ulcers from the treatment.

The 598 participants who rated aspirin in the US survey have osteoarthritis or rheumatoid arthritis or both, and they take anywhere from one to thirty-six tablets a day. Of these, 151 (25 percent) complained of some kind of gastric distress, whether it was upset stomach, heartburn, or ulcers.

Aspirin manufacturers have tried to protect their customers' stomachs with several strategies, but each one has its shortcomings. *Buffering* the aspirin with an antacid, for instance, may keep you from feeling that you have an upset stomach but doesn't seem to ward off ulcers in the long run. Some examples of buffered aspirin are Bufferin (including Arthritis Strength Bufferin), Ascriptin, and Arthritis Pain Formula. The very highly buffered aspirin products that must be dissolved in water, such as Alka-Seltzer, *do* succeed in sparing and even protecting the stomach. There's a catch, though. They contain so much sodium that no one on a low-salt diet can use them, and no one should use them on a regular long-term basis. They also cost more than plain aspirin.

Coated aspirin keeps itself under wraps as long as it stays in the stomach. The protective coating around Ecotrin, for example, does not dissolve until *after* the pill leaves your stomach. This makes it a poor bet for fast pain relief but fine for many people taking large daily doses of aspirin. A thirty-four-year-old Florida homemaker rated Ecotrin higher than any of the twenty prescription drugs she's taken for rheumatoid arthritis, saying it eased the pain and didn't bother her stomach. For some people, though, the coating and delayed dissolving can cut down the amount of aspirin that actually gets into the bloodstream.

Aspirin *suppositories* only switch the irritation from the stomach to the rectum, and what's more, they don't deliver the drug reliably.

So what else *can* you do to protect yourself? Here are a few suggestions, based on a combination of survey participants', doctors', and pharmacists' advice:

- *Drink a full glass of liquid* with your aspirin, to dilute its irritating effect. Water and milk are the best choices. Anything alcoholic is the worst because it doubles the damage that can be dealt to your stomach. Never mix aspirin with alcohol.
- *Eat something* to act as a buffer. Be aware, though, that a big meal can slow down the aspirin's entry into your bloodstream. This shouldn't matter at all if you are taking large doses regularly to build up a high level of aspirin in your body. However, if you're swallowing two tablets in the hope of quick pain relief, don't eat more than a small snack.

- *Take an additional drug to protect your stomach*, such as **Maalox** or **Mylanta** or **Tagamet** or **Carafate**, which are anti-ulcer medications your doctor may prescribe. Another approach is to take aspirin with misoprostol (**Cytotec**), a drug that apparently undoes the stomach damage aspirin causes but without blocking its good effects.

Less Common Side Effects

Another unpleasant aspirin side effect is the ringing, clicking, or humming sound that you may hear as an accompaniment to aspirin therapy. The noise is a signal that you've had too much, and you must try to use less. It often turns out, however, that the people who are the most susceptible to tinnitus, or ringing in the ears, are also the ones who get the greatest benefit from aspirin. Among the 598 US survey participants who used aspirin, 57 (nearly 10 percent) complained that their ears rang.

A few participants noticed that they bruised easily, apparently because of aspirin's blood-thinning effect, and that the bruises tended to last a long time. (See Chapter 14 for information on how vitamin C may counteract this effect.) Others found themselves growing drowsy after they took aspirin, but they didn't necessarily object to the feeling. Indeed, for every participant who complained of daytime drowsiness, there's another who counted on aspirin for help with relaxing and getting to sleep at night.

According to the US Aspirin Foundation, about one person in five hundred is truly allergic to the drug and suffers an attack of asthma or hives upon taking it. In our group of 1,051 US survey participants, however, 8 individuals (about 4 in 500) said they did not use aspirin because they are allergic to it.

Aspirin by Other Names, in Other Forms ... and Even by Prescription

Aspirin is aspirin, whether it's **Norwich** or **Bayer** or any other brand. Name brands cost more than generic, or so-called 'house' brands, but the price difference reflects each product's packaging and marketing, not its content. Most drug companies, in fact, get their raw material – acetylsalicylic acid – from the same supplier, mix it with starch and other inactive ingredients, and then shape the mixture into aspirin tablets etched with their own company name. As long as the product you buy is labelled 'USP aspirin,'* you can be sure it measures up to the government's quality standards. Aspirin is *not* just aspirin, however, when it's **Anacin, Excedrin**, or **Vanquish**, all of which count caffeine among their ingredients.

Typical aspirin tablets give you 325 milligrams (mg), or 5 grains of the drug. Most 'extra strength' formulas contain 500 milligrams, or about half again as much aspirin per pill.

After all we've said about aspirin's being an over-the-counter drug, we have to mention the exceptions to this rule. Several US survey participants took one of the high-dose formulations sold only by prescription: Easprin, a coated aspirin that is the equivalent of three ordinary tablets (975 milligrams, or 15 grains), and Zorprin, which contains 800 milligrams of aspirin in another kind of stomach-sparing coat. Convenience is a major advantage of prescription-strength aspirin, especially for those participants who would otherwise have to swallow three or more pills every few hours. Another advantage is the fact that they can have their drug costs reimbursed by medical insurance.

Aspirin and Other Drugs

Aspirin doesn't mix well with several other drugs in general, and with a number of arthritis drugs in particular. If you take medication for diabetes or a heart condition, don't take aspirin unless you clear it with your doctor. The same goes for anticoagulants (blood thinners), diuretics, and drugs that lower blood pressure.

I can't take aspirin because I take Clinoril, some participants said, or *because I take Naprosyn,* or some other prescription product in the NSAID (non-steroidal anti-inflammatory drug) family. And they're right. These drugs are so closely related to aspirin that taking them both together does little good, if any – and dangerously increases the likelihood of suffering the bad side effects of each. All of the NSAIDs, as aspirin itself, are designed to relieve pain *and* control inflammation, so take one *or* the other, and discuss the decision with your doctor.

* USP stands for United States Pharmacopeia, the agency that sets the drug standards enforced by the Food and Drug Administration.

Over-the-counter products made of ibuprofen, such as Nuprin or Advil, behave just like their prescription-strength parents, the NSAIDs Rufen and Motrin. Mixed with aspirin, they may produce double-whammy side effects.

Methotrexate (Methotrexate, Rheumatrex), used by a number of the participants to control severe rheumatoid arthritis, can have toxic side effects all by itself. Aspirin may aggravate them.

The steroid drugs, including prednisone, may undermine the effect of aspirin, so there's no point in taking both. And if you combine aspirin with gout medications such as Benemid or Anturane, then the aspirin can wipe out the good effects of those drugs – and make your gout feel worse.

Also, if you plan to have surgery, whether for arthritis or any other condition, talk to your surgeon about cutting back on aspirin as a pre-op precaution. This could save you from a serious loss of blood during your operation.

Paracetamol (Acetaminophen): The 'Aspirin Substitute'

Paracetamol is definitely effective against arthritis pain, our participants report, although for most of our UK participants it was for temporary relief. The fact that it has little or no power to combat inflammation simply didn't bother many of them.

	US Survey	US Percentage	UK Survey	UK Percentage
Number of participants taking paracetamol (acetaminophen)	201		132	
Outcome:				
Find it moderately to dramatically helpful	177	(88%)	38	(28%)
Find it provides temporary relief			67	(51%)
Find it of no use (ineffective)	14	(7%)	27	(21%)
No rating	10	(5%)		

Paracetamol has very few side effects. It rarely upsets anyone's stomach and it doesn't cause ulcers. This made it the treatment of choice for many participants who have been burned by aspirin or other anti-inflammatory drugs. 'I tried **Naprosyn** and **Indocin**,' wrote a housewife from North Carolina, 'but I was nauseated all the time. **Paracetamol** is helpful for me.' A gardener from New York said, '**Paracetamol** has the same effect on my pain as aspirin, and it doesn't seem to retard blood clotting the way aspirin does.' Overuse of paracetamol over long periods of time, however, can do serious, perhaps even fatal damage to your liver. And a one-shot overdose may be just as dangerous.

Tablet for tablet, paracetamol works at the same dosage level as aspirin – 325 milligrams in a regular-strength tablet and 500 milligrams in most extra-strength products.

Some of our participants took paracetamol because it is so *un*likely to interfere with the drugs they had to take for their other health problems. Indeed, paracetamol is hardly ever to blame for intensifying the side effects of another drug. Exceptions are Dolobid, a non-steroidal anti-inflammatory, and members of the anticoagulant family, including medications such as Coumadin. If you take one of these blood-thinning drugs, check with your doctor before using paracetamol.

'I take Tylenol Extra Strength,' wrote a retired teacher from Louisiana, 'and I get just as much relief as I did from Indocin, Motrin, and Naprosyn – without the internal bleeding. My only complaint is that six to eight pills per day can get expensive.' Other participants lower the expense by using generic brands of paracetamol, which may sell for half the price of nationally advertised names. Regular-strength tablets of any brand cost less than 'extra strength' formulas, so it also makes sense to try taking two of the regular strength before deciding to buy the larger-dose pills.

Ibuprofen: The Aspirin Rival

Anything aspirin can do, ibuprofen can, too, including fight inflammation, relieve pain, reduce fever, and upset the stomach.

Ibuprofen was first marketed as a prescription drug in Europe by Boots, under the name Rufen, before Upjohn introduced it to the United States in 1974 as Motrin. Within a decade, however, ibuprofen found its way around the prescription pad and over the counter, where some of the US participants bought it in packages labelled Advil, Medipren, and Nuprin. Some participants considered it the best arthritis drug of all: 'Ibruprofen seems to work well for temporary pain relief,' said one man from Orpington. Similarly, one woman from Cardiff reported, 'I find that Co-codomol & Brufen ease the pain and discomfort.' 'Ibuprofen has given me a period of freedom from all pain,' wrote a sixty-one-year-old secretary from Washington, who had switched from aspirin to ibuprofen five months before joining our survey. 'There were a couple of days when it didn't seem to help, and then suddenly I realized my hands weren't hurting for the first time in ten years.'

	US Survey	US Percentage	UK Survey	UK Percentage
Number of participants taking ibuprofen*	120		229	
Outcome:				
Find it moderately to dramatically helpful	93	(77%)	76	(33%)
It gave only temporary relief	NR	NR	121	(53%)
It didn't help at all	13	(11%)	32	(14%)
No rating	14	(12%)	0	0

* This is the number of US participants who take over-the-counter ibuprofen in the form of **Advil, Medipren, Nuprin**, or other brands.

The over-the-counter brands of ibuprofen rated here *coexist* in the marketplace with the original prescription products which remain among the all-time most popular drugs for arthritis. Indeed, more than half of our US survey participants filled at least one prescription for ibuprofen. (See Chapter 5 for more information about ibuprofen, plus ratings.) What separates the prescription drug from the non-prescription is the amount of ibuprofen in each tablet. Over-the-counter brands contain 200 milligrams of ibuprofen per pill, while a prescription has 400, 600, or 800 milligrams, depending on which strength your doctor prescribes. But obviously, you can take enough 200-milligram tablets to give yourself a prescription-strength dose of ibuprofen.

As a rule, it is best to take just enough of an anti-inflammatory drug to get the most help with the least trouble. Taking a lot does not necessarily produce added relief, but it *does* leave you more vulnerable to side effects. The advice to 'Take two aspirin and call me in the morning' has been repeated so often that most people think one aspirin is only half a dose. But 325 milligrams of aspirin or paracetamol, or 200 milligrams of ibuprofen – the amount in one regular-strength tablet of these drugs – may be all you need at any one time.

Just as ibuprofen mimics aspirin's pain-relieving and anti-inflammatory effects, it often produces the same unwanted side effects: upset stomach (with the potential to cause ulcers) and ringing in the ears. 'Midiron is great for me,' said a twenty-two-year-old housewife and mother from Kansas. 'It doesn't cost as much as my other medicine. But it bothers my stomach.' If your stomach is sensitive to ibuprofen, you can try to ward off an upset with the same steps that apply to aspirin, such as taking the pill with food or milk. A 75-year-old woman from London said, 'Voltarol and ibuprofen helped but I was unable to continue taking them due to severe bouts of stomach upsets and diarrhoea.'

Rub-on Balms

Only about 10 percent of the UK survey participants have sought pain relief by rubbing some kind of lotion, liniment, cream, oil, or gel on a painful part. However more than 70 percent of the US survey group said that they have used a rub on balm. According to most of them, the rest of the group is missing out on something good.

There is no scientific proof that any of these home remedies provides any substantive help. But there is a measure of relief to be had here, our participants say, even if it's only temporary, and there's no serious harm in trying.

Many of these products are counter-irritants. That is, they try to make you forget about pain by irritating your skin to make it feel hot. The heat, in turn, may soothe some soreness and stiffness. Survey participants who understood this relationship still enjoyed the sensation: 'I don't think my liniment does any real good,' said a retired teacher from Indiana, 'but the warmth it produces makes you feel better.' Several participants shared a different theory about how and why such liniments help: 'You rub on the Aspercreme,' a Colorado homemaker explained, 'and the *massage* is the truly effective part.'

Balms and liniments are the particular favourites of participants who didn't get any help from drug treatments. 'No drug has ever helped me,' said a housewife from Florida. 'I find the best remedy for temporary relief that works for me is Absorbine Jr. I carry it at all times.' Other participants found rubs to be of special help at certain times, such as immediately before or after exercising, or at bedtime: 'BenGay and Sloan's Liniment are wonderful for me,' wrote a shipping clerk from California. 'If I take a scalding hot bath, cover my knees and ankles with liniment and wrap them in Ace bandages, I can sleep for a few hours with no discomfort.'

Several of these products contain salicylates. The implication is that aspirin, or other members of its drug family, could relieve pain in a certain area by being applied directly to the surface of the skin there. As we've seen, however, aspirin *irritates* the stomach if it's swallowed, or sometimes the rectum if it's used in suppository form. On the skin, too, it is irritating, not anaesthetizing. Aspirin can relieve pain only by getting into the bloodstream. True, some aspirin may be absorbed through the skin and into the blood when applied this way, but mostly it just rubs the skin the wrong way. 'At first I tried a lot of different liniments,' wrote a dry cleaner from Arizona, 'but some of them felt like they would burn my skin off, so I stopped using them.'

WARNING: If you are allergic to aspirin or other salicylates, then you must avoid using rubs that contain them, too.

In all, participants tried about thirty brands of balms and got at least some temporary relief or sense of well-being from all of them.

The differences in effectiveness among these products are not striking enough to serve as strong recommendations for one brand over another – especially when you consider the other differences among them, including cost and *smell*. A veterinary assistant from Florida insisted, 'If it doesn't smell strong, it doesn't help!' The aroma of wintergreen or menthol, however, really offended some participants who denounced the 'smelly relief' offered in a rub. Take a whiff if you can, before you buy.

Summary of Over-the-Counter Treatments for Arthritis

Aspirin – Aspirin is an effective and inexpensive way to control pain and inflammation. Even though it is sold without a prescription, its potency calls for caution if you use a lot, or if you take it with other types of over-the-counter or prescription medicine.

Paracetamol – One of the safest pain-relieving drugs available, paracetamol is not effective for the inflammation that often accompanies arthritis. Its kindness to the stomach, however, may make it the best available drug for people who have arthritis and ulcers.

Ibuprofen – Ibuprofen works much the way aspirin does to relieve pain and inflammation. Some people find that it even surpasses aspirin, but, like aspirin, it can upset your stomach and sound bells in your ears.

Rub-on balms – Even though there is no scientific justification for finding relief in any of the lotions, liquids, creams, or gels sold for arthritis relief, these products do have a soothing effect on joint pain for most of the people who try them. Choose one in your price range that doesn't hurt your skin or offend your nose.

Chapter 7
Surgery for Arthritis:

A Surprisingly Successful Solution

• *Dramatic results from joint replacement* • *Fusion* • *Arthroscopic surgery*
• *Facts about procedures and risks* • *How to prepare yourself for surgery*

To walk without a cane, or even a limp.

To move without pain for the first time in years.

These are the outcomes of surgery that the Arthritis Survey participants called 'miraculous.' And they are commonplace miracles. Indeed, success and satisfaction are by far the most common results reported by those participants who had one or more joints replaced or repaired. As most of them tell the story, the end result is well worth all the pre-op anxiety they suffered and all the post-op inconvenience.

'The outcome of my two operations – total left hip replacement in 1984 and total left knee replacement in 1986 – has been a vast improvement in the quality of my life,' said a freelance writer from New York. 'A five-mile walk is no big deal to me now. Going from nearly being in a wheelchair to limpless walking is nothing short of miraculous.' 'The hip replacement operation was wonderful – it gave me back ten years of my life. Everything else was just palliative,' reported one woman from London.

If you are currently facing a decision about joint surgery, this chapter will tell you the encouraging truth about the level of improvement you can expect from various types of operations, and why some procedures get better results than others. You'll learn the risks involved, too, and the things *you* can do in preparation for surgery to assure yourself of the best possible outcome.

In all, 194 participants, or slightly more than 18 percent of the 1051 members of the US survey group, and 102 participants, or 23 percent of the UK survey group had joint surgery. Many of them had two or more operations because, for example, both their hips, both their knees, or all their knuckles had been badly damaged by arthritis. Others had their wrists fused, bone spurs removed, or tendons repaired. Most of the operations fall into one of these major categories, all of which are covered in this chapter:

arthroplasty – the replacement (partial or total) or resurfacing of damaged joints

arthrodesis – the fusing together of bones to make a joint more stable

arthroscopy – the technique for accomplishing surgical procedures through small incisions, using fibre optics and miniature tools

synovectomy – the removal of the joint lining

Arthroplasty

Total joint replacement is the flashiest, most dramatic achievement in arthritis treatment of the past several decades. Many people swear that the surgery gives unparalleled pain relief and a return to near-normal function. Yet, most surgeons still consider it the *last resort* for people with arthritis – an option to hold in reserve until all else fails. This is because an artificial joint, no matter how well it works, has a limited life span. If it is cemented in place, it can come unstuck. If it is pushed too hard through strenuous activity, it may break. In either case, it will have to be replaced, and the bones that support the replacement's replacement will have to be further cut – and further compromised.

The challenge of total joint replacement is to copy nature with materials that are not really the equal of bone and cartilage. Metal implants have been used to repair the living skeleton, historians say, for as long as humans have practised surgery. But not until this century were the materials and techniques available to make replacement parts work well in the body's hostile environment. Most metals crack under the pressure, or corrode, or cause infection. Even stainless steel can *break* when it has to do the work of a person's shoulder.

Most total joint replacements are hips and knees made of metal alloys (cobalt chromium is one) and tough plastics, or finger joints fashioned from silicone rubber. Scores of specially engineered joints already compete in the marketplace, and new modifications are constantly being introduced, so that the replacements ever more closely approximate the form and function of the original (nature's) design. One of the early artificial knees, for example, created in the 1950s, was a hinge that replaced the worn-out surfaces of the joint and anchored itself with long metal shafts driven into the bones of the leg. A human knee, however, doesn't open and shut like a door on a hinge, but rolls, glides, and rotates in an extremely complex fashion. Current designs allow for this freer, more natural kind of movement.

Total Knee Replacement

At the knee, the bottom of the thigh bone (femur) meets the top of the shin bone (tibia), and the two move effortlessly in tandem, thanks to their caps of glistening cartilage. When arthritis destroys the cartilage, however, the bones are left to grind painfully against each other. A surgeon performing a total knee arthroplasty cuts away the damaged bone ends and replaces them with a matched set of implants that let the bones glide smoothly once again.

The overall results survey participants reported were excellent, and some of those who were the most satisfied with their surgery were walking around with no trouble on artificial knees that have been in place for ten or twelve years. 'Surgery will not restore 100 percent natural movement,' said a forty-two-year-old writer from Kentucky who had both her knees replaced, 'but it will relieve pain drastically and restore a major portion of lost mobility. The psychological effect of all this for me has been a greater feeling of self-esteem and self-worth.'

We present here the findings of the UK survey only as asked participants were to rate both pain relief and mobility after surgery, a question not asked in the original US survey.

As you can see an impressive 54 percent achieved pain relief as a result and 40 percent achieved greater mobility.

The period immediately after surgery is quite painful for some people, and most participants said that full recovery takes three to six months. 'I was very fortunate,' wrote a sixty-seven-year-old Iowa housewife who had one knee replaced in March and the

	US Survey	US Percentage
Number of total knee replacements	33	
Outcome:		
Pain relief	18	(54%)
Same amount of pain	1	(3%)
Greater pain	0	(0%)
Greater mobility	13	(40%)
Reduced mobility	1	(3%)
No improvement in mobility	1	(3%)

other in April of 1986, 'as my recovery was painless after the first eighteen hours each time. I had full use of both knees in about two and a half months.'

What kind of replacement will I get? Surgeons choose styles of knees from a wide array of models. The choice of joint implant depends a lot on the type and degree of destruction in the original joint, not to mention the surgeon's personal preference. At some hospitals, in fact, surgeons work with bioengineers to help put their own ideas for new joint designs into production.

What happens after surgery? The implanting of the new joint is only the beginning of a successful replacement. Physiotherapy is the next phase, and it covers everything from teaching you how to use crutches or a walker to demonstrating and supervizing exercises that will strengthen the muscles that make your new knee go. (These muscles, including the quadriceps at the front of the thigh and hamstrings at the back, may be quite weak if pain has kept you inactive before surgery.) The exercises participants describe include both *active* movements, such as extending the knee while wearing small weights around the ankle, and *passive* motion. 'After my total knee replacement,' wrote a retired electrician from West Virginia, 'my left leg was put in a motion machine that moved my leg as if I was riding a bicycle. I used this for several days and it kept my knee flexible. I was also given exercises and instructions as to what I should and shouldn't do with my new joint.' Even after some participants left the hospital, they returned two or three times a week for physiotherapy and then continued exercising regularly on their own, mostly by walking, swimming, or riding a bike.

What risks do I face? Total joint replacement is major surgery and patients face all the known risks of being put under general anaesthesia or numbed with a spinal. Over the long run, the special risk of replacement is the possibility that the new joint will come loose and the pain return. 'I was one of the first men to have two total knees and two total hips,' said a thirty-five-year-old artist from Ohio. 'Actually, I've had three total knees over the years, the first two in 1972 and 1973, and one redone in 1983.'

Loosening is the most common risk with joint replacements, but infection is the most serious. It is quite rare today, thanks to the extreme precautions taken at most hospitals. Despite all the safeguards, infection can sometimes undermine the new joint by spreading to it from some other part of the body days or weeks after the operation. A fifty-six-year-old teacher from Massachusetts told how her artificial knee was undone by a tooth:

'In June of 1982, I had a total knee replacement and an uneventful hospital stay that lasted eleven days. But five days later, at home, severe pain set in. I took a series of tests that revealed a strep infection in my knee. The doctors determined the source to be some dental work I'd had done, for which my dentist should have given me penicillin. I had to be treated with intravenous antibiotics for forty-nine days – yes, seven full weeks. Then I had another operation in October. The surgeon found then that the bone around the new joint had become soft, brittle, and jagged with multiple fractures. The cement had cracked and so the prosthesis was loosened. Ligaments, too, had been destroyed. The second joint replacement took seven and one-half hours, and I spent more than eight months on crutches. Physiotherapy is *still* going on, because of the damage to the ligaments. But this experience is just a fluke. Most of the time a knee replacement gives a great deal of pain relief and greater mobility. It's like a new lease on life. I know because I had surgery on my other knee the year before all this happened, and that knee is fine.'

Total Hip Replacement

The hip was the first joint to be successfully replaced on a wide-scale basis, thanks mostly to the brilliant efforts of British surgeon Sir John Charnley, who figured out the best combination of materials for creating an artificial joint and implanted a series of them in his patients in the early 1960s.

Previously, hip parts had been made of everything from wood and hand-carved ivory to Pyrex, Bakelite, and Teflon, as well as metals such as gold, silver, aluminium, lead, copper, iron, and zinc. But no combination was ideal. Even the best of the metal-on-metal designs, though precision-ground for a perfect fit of ball in socket, wore each other down and dumped metal debris into the joint space. They also squeaked. Dr. Charnley became 'the father of modern total hip arthroplasty' by designing a hip that was part metal and part polyethylene, with virtually no friction between the moving parts.

Although Dr. Charnley's concept was readily applied to the knee and other joints, hip replacement remains the most successful of the arthroplasties. The reason lies in the anatomy of the hip. The bones there are large enough to accommodate prosthetic parts that hardly ever break. And the ball-and-socket action of the joint has proved easier to imitate than the complex workings of the wrist, for example, or the ankle. In total hip arthroplasty, the surgeon cuts away the top of the thighbone, with its ball-shaped knob, and replaces it with a metal one that has a long shank to fit inside the bone. The damaged socket (acetabulum) also gets cut out and a new cup is screwed or cemented into the pelvis. Again we present the findings of the UK survey which asked participants to rate mobility as well as pain relief. As you can see from the results surgery achieved excellent results in pain relief for the vast majority of participants.

	US Survey	US Percentage
Number of total hip replacements	21	
Outcome:		
Pain relief	20	(95%)
Same amount of pain	1	(5%)
Greater pain	1	(5%)
Greater mobility	6	(27%)
Reduced mobility	1	(1%)
No improvement in mobility	0	(0%)

Dr. Charnley cemented his implants in place with an acrylic bone cement called polymethyl methacrylate, or PMMA, which added an element of solidity to the surgery. Instead of sinking the shaft of the hip ball into the thighbone, for example, and counting on a perfect fit to hold it there, surgeons could shoot some cement into the bone along with the implant. When it hardened, it would create a solid bond. Surgeons have found ever better ways over the years to improve PMMA's performance – mixing it in a vacuum chamber or whirling it in a centrifuge to get the air bubbles out, then applying it with a high-pressure caulking gun that drives it into all the nooks and crannies of the surrounding bone. Even so, some experts now claim that the *cement* eventually makes the replacement come *unstuck* by engendering a barrier between itself and the bone.

When surgeons set about performing re-replacement of implants that have loosened, they often discover that a membrane has grown all around the cement, resembling the synovial membrane that normally surrounds the joint. Inside the membrane they find tiny particles of PMMA cement – and evidence that the membrane is doing chemical battle with these particles, releasing substances that cause the bone around the cement to retreat, or resorb, and the implant to grow progressively looser.

Uncemented Stems

In the course of the 1980s and with younger orthopaedic patients emerging, surgeons developed a new surgical procedure to prolong the life of a total hip replacement. They designed a stem of the prosthetic joint that would fit so tightly into the patient's femur that cementing would be unnecessary. With a younger patient the living bone tissue would grow in and around the prosthesis and forge a permanent fusion. Although the recovery period may be lengthier, waiting for the new joint to take hold, the cementless implant generally lasts longer – perhaps indefinitely. Bony-ingrowth joints should also stand up to the stresses and strains of a more active lifestyle, making them a more likely choice for younger people. Most surgeons accept that the critical age for preferring an uncemented stem is sixty-five, however heavy smokers as young as sixty may have to be given a cemented stem due to weakness in the bone.

Finger-Joint Replacement

What Dr. Charnley did for the hip, Dr. Alfred B. Swanson did for the joints of the fingers in the mid-1960s, and at least fifteen of the US participants were able to fill out their survey questionnaires in longhand thanks to the implants that bear his name.

Dr. Swanson discovered early on that metal replacements wouldn't do for the fine bones of the hands or feet. His success, like Dr. Charnley's, depended partly on his own creativity, and partly on finding the right material for the job. This was a flexible and durable synthetic rubber called silicone (and later dubbed 'Silastic'), created by the Dow-Corning Corporation, and made available to Dr. Swanson for his research. The revolutionary finger joints he devised turned out so well that Dr. Swanson went on to fashion some two dozen other kinds of replacements out of silicone, including toe joints, wrist bones, and parts of the elbow.

The Swanson finger joint is a one-piece design that roughly resembles a flower with two stems – one at the bottom and one growing out the top. If the implant replaces the knuckle of your index finger, for example, one of its stems will extend into the bone of that finger and the other into the adjoining bone of your hand, leaving the wider middle portion to cushion and hold the proper space between these bones. The middle part is also a flexible hinge, easily operated by your muscles and ligaments. Once implanted, it should not only restore pain-free motion but also stabilize the joint, keeping the bones properly aligned. Survey participants whose hands were deformed by rheumatoid arthritis, with their fingers skewed at an exaggerated tilt, were pleased with the change in their appearance after surgery.

The finger joints take no cement. In fact, the stems actually glide, just a fraction of an inch, inside the bones as they move, like pistons in cylinders. To fix the implants rigidly in place, Dr. Swanson explained, would put intolerable strain on them. Only two of the participants of the UK survey had had knuckles replaced, so it was not possible to rate them; however here are the US survey results.

An eighty-one-year-old retired accountant from upstate New York described the exercises he did after receiving artificial joints in the thumb and fingers of both hands: 'The physiotherapist brought me a glove that had small lead weights attached to it.

	US Survey	US Percentage
Number of knuckle replacements	75	
Outcome:		
Dramatic pain relief	62	(83%)
Moderate relief	1	(1%)
Minor or temporary relief	10	(13%)
No relief	1	(1%)
Made participant feel worse than before	1	(1%)

I would put on this glove and then raise and lower each finger ten or fifteen times. I did this twice a day for several weeks, then once a day for a fairly long time.' This participant also spoke frankly about the difficulties of recuperating from his hand operations, which were done in the fall of 1984 and the spring of 1985: 'I was sent home four days after the operation with my whole arm immobile and held straight up in a foam cushion. I had to have complete care, including washing, feeding, and bathroom, for weeks. It was very hard on me and on my wife.'

Several people judged the recovery period, with all its disability and dependence, to be as much of a trial for their families as for themselves. 'I was fortunate to have an understanding family,' wrote a fifty-five-year-old Michigan homemaker whose surgery entailed four operations within ten months: both wrists and all the fingers on both hands, including two tendon transplants to make her fingers functional. 'After surgery there was very little I was able to do for myself, and I had to rely on family members. For a while, all I could manage was to squeeze a Nerf ball or therapeutic putty for exercise, and soak my hands in warm water. It's been a year now, and though I guess I'm still recovering, my hands get stronger with use. I can once again cook, do laundry, some limited gardening, shop, run errands, clean the house, and even crochet and do other handcrafts. I have about 60 percent function in my hands at this point. However, the *pain is gone!*'

For the accountant mentioned, unfortunately, the trying recovery period did not end so happily. 'There was pain relief for about a year,' he said. 'After that, although my fingers *looked* better, the mobility was not helped. My wife is typing the answers on the questionnaire because I am unable to write or even hold a pen.'

Other Partial and Total Replacements

The hips, knees, and knuckles are far and away the most frequent sites for total joint replacement, and the results are usually excellent. Several other participants in the US survey had some of the less commonly performed joint replacements, including the shoulder, elbow, wrist, and ankle. There were too few of these operations for us to rate them individually, but it's worth noting what happened with each type of joint.

Total Ankle Replacement

All four US survey participants who'd had a total ankle replacement were very pleased with the outcome. The design of the prosthetic ankle implants began to improve in the late 1980s and ankle replacement is now evolving as a viable option for the management of end-stage ankle arthritis. More recent prostheses have had encouraging intermediate results because of improved surgical techniques and improved designs. Acceptable results have been reported in older, non-obese patients who have osteoarthritis or rheumatoid arthritis. However a significant percentage of patients with end-stage ankle arthritis are younger patients with arthritis due to trauma. The use of ankle replacement in younger, more physically active patients and in those with significant deformity in the ankle or hind foot remains controversial because the risks and complications are still significant. However as the prostheses and surgical techniques continue to improve it now seems inevitable that ankle joint replacements will be offered to an increasing number of patients with rheumatoid arthritis, osteoarthritis and post-traumatic arthritis.

Total Shoulder Replacement

Five out of the six total shoulder replacements were successful, and the one that failed was redone to become one of the five successes. 'Although my first right shoulder replacement did not work out,' reported this wholesale paper dealer from Virginia, 'the second time was perfect. I have almost complete relief, but limited use of the joint. I've also had total replacement of my right hip and knee, with complete relief of pain in both. My advice is: *Do not delay*. Have surgery performed *mit schnell, muy pronto*, after obtaining the best surgeons.'

Elbow Replacement
A retired teacher from Kansas underwent elbow replacement twice, once in 1986 and then over again in 1987. 'My orthopedic surgeon has helped me more than anyone,' she said, after two total knee replacements, surgery on both hands, and left shoulder, in addition to the two elbow operations.

Wrist Replacement
'It does relieve the pain,' reported a thirty-three-year-old nurse from Pennsylvania who had a total wrist replacement, 'but I have very little mobility and the joint feels fake. I'd think twice before having the other wrist done, whereas my artificial hip brought me total pain relief, much greater mobility and generally made me feel like new.'

Partial Joint Replacement
Nine US survey participants had a partial joint replacement of the hip or knee, seven of whom reported dramatic relief. Partial replacements work well for people whose joint damage is not so extensive as to require total replacement. In the hip, for example, the ball part alone may be replaced. Or the joint can be resurfaced by scraping the ball part smooth and capping it with metal, and also cleaning the socket and putting in a new plastic lining. It is also possible to replace one side of the joint and resurface the other. Partial replacement leaves the door open, so to speak, for total replacement later, if the joint continues to deteriorate.

'I had a partial hip replacement that made me feel fine for a year,' wrote a sixty-nine-year-old housewife from Wisconsin, 'but then it came loose and had to be redone, so my partial hip replacement was followed eighteen months later by a total one. After the second surgery I gained weight, probably from inactivity, and my prosthesis has come loose again – this time after six years. I have much pain now and remain inactive. I doubt that I will have another operation because I have emphysema, and the prognosis is not good.'

Overall, the US survey showed that nine out of ten joint replacements provide at least some relief, and about a quarter of these can be of dramatic help.

Resection

Resection arthroplasty is the removal of damaged bone and cartilage at the joint without replacing them. Before Dr. Swanson invented his Silastic hinges, many people's severely affected hand and finger joints were treated this way. Today, some of the joints in the feet are still relieved by resection arthroplasty, as this forty-seven-year-old Florida housewife explained: 'In March of 1986 I had a Hoffman resection of both feet. My metatarsal bones were cut off where they were unjointed and protruding on the bottom, and my toes realigned. I have about 80 percent pain relief now, and walk at least a mile a day, plus I can wear more normal shoes. It took almost a year to recover, during which time I was quite dependent and immobile, having had surgery on both feet, but I would do it again in a minute.'

An equally enthusiastic photographer from Massachusetts, age sixty-nine, called the outcome of her two 1975 metatarsal resections 'a total miracle.' 'I had screaming pain upon walking,' she recalled. 'The surgery gave me back my life.'

Another successful use of resection is the cutting away of painful, disfiguring bunions from the base of the big toe. The following ratings combine the experiences of fifteen US participants, ten of whom had metatarsal resection on one or both feet, and five who had one or two bunions removed.

	US Survey	US Percentage
Number of resections	27	
Outcome:		
Dramatic relief	23	(85%)
Moderate relief	2	(7%)
Minor or temporary relief	1	(4%)
No relief	0	–
Made participant feel worse than before	1	(4%)
No rating	0	–

Arthrodesis

Before joint replacement became popular, surgery often relieved arthritis pain by fusing the bones at their meeting place. A fused joint lost natural motion, it's true, but it gained strength, and besides, the promised freedom from pain was worth the sacrifice for many people. Today, fusion, or arthrodesis, is still regarded as the best surgical treatment for certain joints, especially the ankle and wrist, where several small bones come together, and where replacement is far from routine. In the spine, where replacements are not even attempted, fusion of two or three vertebrae may bring relief of severe neck pain or lower back pain. 'Cervical fusion brought me total pain relief,' reported a Rhode Island secretary, 'although I now have much less range of motion in my neck.'

Arthrodesis is also preferred in certain *situations*. A person with recurrent infections, for example, who faces a greater-than-average risk of losing an artificial joint because of loosening after infection, might be better off with a fused shoulder than a new shoulder.

The participants in the US survey who had one or more joints fused are extremely pleased with the results. Insufficient numbers of UK participants had experienced this treatment to allow us to rate the results.

	US Survey	US Percentage
Number of fusion procedures*	35	
Outcome:		
Dramatic relief	30	(86%)
Moderate relief	3	(8%)
Minor or temporary relief		
No relief	1	(3%)
Made participant feel worse than before	0	(0%)
No rating	1	(3%)

* This number combines the wrist, ankle, finger, toe, and spinal (including cervical spine) fusions reported by 18 survey participants, most of whom also had joint replacement surgery on their hips or knees.

No glue or cement is used to make the bones of a fused joint stick together. Instead, the surgeon cuts away all the damaged cartilage and bone, shaping the joint so that the bones interlock in the ideal position. The joints closest to the fingertips, for example, may be fused, if need be, in a slight crook – a position that lets you use them to write, or button your coat, or pick up coins from a countertop. 'Ten years ago I had the knuckles in my right hand replaced, and the joints of my fingers fused to make them bendable,' wrote a housewife from Tennessee. 'Before the operation, they wouldn't bend and I couldn't hold anything in that hand at all. Now it works great.'

Once the bones to be fused are positioned just so, they get fixed in place with a bit of wire. The wire stays in for several weeks until new bone has a chance to grow around the joint and form a natural seal. Often, small bone chips are also inserted at the fused joint, because they encourage new bone to grow. The bone graft may come from elsewhere in your own body – from the top of your pelvis, for example – or from a 'bone bank,' just as blood for transfusions comes from a blood bank.

New versions of arthrodesis in the wrist combine the best advantages of fusion and joint replacement. The joint between the arm bone and wrist can be fused, while other small bones of the wrist are resurfaced or replaced with silicone implants. This combination can relieve pain and shore up a weak wrist while leaving the natural motion of the hand intact. 'I had a total fusion in my right wrist,' said a Michigan homemaker, 'and a partial fusion on the left with an artificial joint. This is a new surgical procedure that gives me some movement.'

A fifty-three-year-old travel agent from Washington reported that the first twenty-four hours after her ankle fusion were extremely painful, and full recovery took about a year. Now, however, her exercise regimen includes low-impact aerobics three times a week, tennis once or twice a week, depending on the weather, and a daily walk.

Arthroscopy

The arthroscope is the device that has opened up the knee and selected other joints to lights, cameras, and surgical implements – and all without opening them very wide. Through an incision as small as a quarter of an inch, a surgeon can now get the best possible diagnostic picture of the inside of a joint, and, if necessary, perform surgery through another small hole with specially designed microtools.

The small scale of the procedure – the tiny incision, the short hospital stay – lead many people to believe that arthroscopy is a minor matter. But surgery via arthroscopy is still surgery and usually calls for general anaesthesia. What's more, the recovery period may last just as long as recovery from other types of surgery, depending on what gets done with the arthroscope. If you hear of someone who is up and about the morning after, you can bet that person had little more than a diagnostic look-see with a local anaesthetic.

Despite all the fanfare surrounding arthroscopy, however, especially the exciting stories of world-class athletes whose careers were saved by arthroscopic surgery, participants had less success with it than with the other forms of surgery they rated. Some of the operations carried out with arthroscopy simply don't improve life as dramatically as a joint replacement, say, or a fusion procedure. Here are the things that surgeons can do with arthroscopy to help people with arthritis: remove debris from inside the joint, scrape off bone spurs, and take out the joint lining (synovium). A salesman from Illinois described his arthroscopy the way it felt to him, as 'microsurgery of right knee to remove sand and gravel.' Here are the results of the US and UK surveys.

	US Survey	US Percentage	UK Survey	UK Percentage
Number of arthroscopic procedures	22		30	
Outcome:				
Pain relief	14	(64%)	13	(43%)
Same amount of pain	5	(23%)	9	(30%)
Greater pain/made patient feel worse than before	1	(5%)	1	(3%)
Greater mobility	Not rated		7	(23%)
Reduced mobility	Not rated		4	(13%)
No improvement in mobility	Not rated		5	(17%)

Synovectomy

In rheumatoid arthritis, the main culprit responsible for pain and swelling is thought to be the paper-thin membrane that surrounds and lubricates the joint, called the synovium. Inflammation can spur this membrane on to wild overgrowth, until it becomes so thick and unwieldy that it fills the joint space, puffs out the surrounding skin, moves bones, and ruptures tendons. As inflammation rages, the synovium also secretes enzymes that eat up the cartilage. Little wonder, then, that surgeons thought to stem the destruction by *synovectomy* – removing the synovium. 'I had a synovectomy on my right knee in 1962,' wrote a former coal miner from West Virginia. 'All of the inflammation, swelling, and practically all of the severe pain left, and full mobility in the knee returned.' An executive recruiter from Texas, who had a wrist synovectomy in 1978, said it relieved about 90 percent of his pain. Unfortunately only three participants in the UK survey had had a synovectomy so the results are not included here; however here are the results of the US survey.

	US Survey	US Percentage
Number of synovectomies*	25	
Outcome:		
Dramatic relief	11	(44%)
Moderate relief	5	(20%)
Minor or temporary relief	1	(4%)
No relief	6	(24%)
Made participant feel worse than before	1	(4%)
No rating	1	(4%)

* Sixteen participants had one or more synovectomies. The joints operated on were 11 knees, 4 hands, 3 wrists, 2 feet, 1 finger and 1 that was not specified.

Synovectomy is not performed as frequently as it used to be, partly because doctors have found that the membrane often grows back. 'I had greater mobility for a year after the synovectomy on my left knee in 1970,' said a fifty-eight-year-old homemaker from Minnesota, 'but then the diseased synovial membrane grew back, and there is very little mobility now.'

Even if the membrane does not overgrow the joint space again, the joint destruction may continue to get worse after synovectomy. 'I had synovectomy on one knee in 1967, and then the other knee the next year,' reported a retired engineer from Tennessee. 'After these operations I had less pain and I got around better for years, until my knees completely deteriorated and I had to have them both replaced, one in 1985 and the other in 1986. The replacements have given me total pain relief and good mobility.'

Other Surgical Procedures

The participants underwent several other kinds of surgery for arthritis, but not in large enough numbers to evaluate their relative effectiveness. **Osteotomy**, for one, was a popular way to relieve hip and knee pain in the late 1950s and early 1960s, but it got upstaged by joint replacement. Now, according to articles in the medical literature, it may be making a comeback, especially for people who are considered too young to receive an artificial joint.

Osteotomy entails cutting a bone to correct the alignment of the joint. At the knee, for example, if the thighbone and shin don't abut squarely, there may be too much stress on one part of the joint, and the cartilage and bone at the overloaded meeting place will wear unevenly. By cutting a wedge-shaped piece out of either bone, a surgeon may tip the balance, so to speak, and get the person's weight distributed evenly across the joint, the way it should be.

Two participants were relieved to have their rheumatoid nodules removed. These are lumps that form under the skin of some people with rheumatoid arthritis. They may appear on the fingers, or near the knees or elbows, and they may hurt anytime they are touched.

Other surgical procedures include attempts, most of them successful, to repair or release tendons and ligaments, and a couple of highly unusual procedures for rare complications of rheumatoid arthritis. A forty-three-year-old Washington real estate agent began losing his voice very soon after he developed rheumatoid arthritis. Surgery freed his vocal cords, he wrote, restoring 75 percent of his voice. A thirty-five-year-old Pennsylvania lab technician needed surgery to remove inflamed tissue around her heart.

Survey Participants' Advice About Surgery

No matter what their operations entailed, most of the surgery veterans among our survey participants agreed on certain points about joint surgery – including preparations and follow-up procedures that can increase the likelihood of a successful outcome. If you are considering surgery for arthritis, consider their suggestions.

1. *Have it done!* This was the most frequently offered advice about surgery from the group of participants who'd been through it, and the most common comment was, *I'm glad I did it. It was definitely worthwhile.*
2. *Give the whole process your most serious consideration.* Surgery for arthritis is *elective* surgery, which means that you must choose whether and when to go through with it. The pain and disability that bring you to this decision have likely been worsening over a period of years, so there's no need to make snap judgments now.
3. *Get a second, and even a third opinion.* By all means get the opinion of at least one other doctor. A second surgeon's analysis is valuable, but so is the opinion of a physician who's used to dealing with joint problems *non*-surgically, like a rheumatologist or a doctor of physical medicine and rehabilitation. The expert opinions should cover whether or not you need surgery, and if so, which type of procedure is likely to help most.
4. *Choose your surgeon carefully if you have the opportunity.* It's a simple case of practice making perfect. The more elbows that surgeons replace, the more proficient they become with the technique. Many orthopaedic surgeons specialize in treating certain areas of the body, for this very reason, and you owe it to yourself to try to find one who is especially adept at doing whatever you need done.
5. *Pick the best available hospital if possible.* The fact is that hospitals, like specialists, differ in their track records for safely accomplishing certain procedures. Some of the US participants chose the hospital first, for its fine reputation in joint surgery, secure in the assumption that any surgeon affiliated with that institution would be well qualified.

6. *Learn all you can about your surgery beforehand* by questioning your doctor(s), reading any available information, and talking to one or two people who have undergone the same type of operation. This will help you form a realistic picture of what's to be done, what the immediate aftermath may be like for you, how much time you may need to fully recover from surgery, and what long-term results you can expect.

7. *Get in shape for surgery.* If you are overweight and need surgery on your hips, knees, or feet, this is the time to try to shed extra pounds. A low-calorie but nutritious diet makes the most sense, because you need to reduce the strain on your weight-bearing joints *and* keep up your general health to withstand the physical stress of surgery. A crash diet could leave you dangerously weakened. Also talk to your doctor about all the *medications* you take regularly, such as aspirin, as some may need to be cut back or stopped altogether in preparation for surgery. Ask about food supplements, too, such as adding vitamins A and C, as well as iron, to help speed your recovery, or cutting out fish oil because it might prolong bleeding.

8. *Prepare your family for the role they will play.* Although the goal of your operation may be to restore your physical independence, the immediate recovery period could call for more help from your family than you've ever needed before. Involve them in the planning stages, and help them find out what will be expected of them.

9. *Follow post-op directions.* Exercise the joint according to the instructions you receive from your doctor or physiotherapist. Make sure you understand what you can and can't do during the recovery period and beyond, and, again, if it's a weight-bearing joint that's had surgery, don't give it any added weight to bear.

10. *Think positively.* There is every reason to believe that the surgery will turn out well, so try to keep that thought uppermost in your mind – before the operation and during the recovery period. A fifty-four-year-old housewife from Tennessee observes, 'I would highly recommend these operations [she's had eight] for people who have a good attitude toward this sort of thing. The attitude is very important.

It takes nerve to go through surgery. Confidence in your doctor helps, and the moral support of family and friends.'

Summary of Arthritis Surgery

Arthroplasty – Total hip replacements are the most successful surgery in this category, followed closely by knee and knuckle replacement. Replacement of other joints, such as the shoulder, is performed less frequently but can also be quite successful. Where the joint damage is not too extensive, partial replacements or resurfacing may be all that's needed to relieve pain.

Arthrodesis – Wrist, ankle, or neck fusion may give pain relief and joint stability in exchange for full range of motion. Arthrodesis may also be favoured over joint replacement for people with recurrent infections who would face a high risk of losing a replacement joint.

Arthroscopy – Microsurgery techniques enable surgeons to perform diagnostic exploratory surgery inside certain joints, and also to remove joint debris and scrape off bone spurs.

Synovectomy – Removing the grossly inflamed synovial lining of the joint may bring great relief, but the membrane sometimes grows back.

Osteotomy – Cutting the bones near the joint to correct misalignment may be better than joint replacement for younger people.

Other – Operations to remove rheumatoid nodules, to repair tendons and ligaments, free the vocal cords, and remove inflamed tissue around the heart were also successful for some US participants.

Chapter 8
Eleven Effective Extra Treatments for Reducing Arthritis Pain

• Exercise • Hydrotherapy • Heat / Cold • Ultrasound • Psychological Counselling • Wax • Massage • Traction • TENS • Splints • Biofeedback

The best of the current treatments for arthritis are combination plans – mixtures of methods that work *together* to bring pain relief, keep joints flexible, and slow the progress of the disease. The medicine prescribed or the surgery performed by your doctor, no matter how dramatically effective, does not stand alone. The truth is that the exercises you've learned to do at home for fifteen or twenty minutes a day are every bit as important. And exercise instruction is just one of a variety of other professional treatments, neither medicinal nor surgical, that helped Arthritis Survey participants to feel and function well. The list of these additional treatments includes many forms of physiotherapy, such as diathermy, hydrotherapy, massage, and ultrasound, as well as psychological counselling and biofeedback. (See Chapter 10 for information about the unconventional extras – acupuncture, manipulation, and Yoga.)

Some of these extra treatments work better than others, of course. A few bring at least some measure of relief to nearly everyone, while others work about half or three-quarters of the time. There were some differences between the US survey results and the UK survey. Psychological counselling and ultrasound were more effective for the US group, while wax dips, massage, TENS and splints were more effective for the UK group.

Treatment	US Survey Number of Participants Who Tried it	US number and percentage helped by it with improved mobility	UK Survey	UK number and percentage helped by it
Exercise	836	794 (95%)	450	See separate rating for individual exercises (p.302)
Hydrotherapy	83*	75 (90%)	67	61 (91%)
Heat/Cold	123*	104 (85%)	115	97 (84%)
Ultrasound	47*	38 (81%)	82	60 (73%)
Psychological Counselling	46	37 (80%)	28	13 (46%)
Wax	30	22 (73%)	Not rated	Not rated
Massage	298	211 (71%)	147	130 (88%)
Traction	46	29 (63%)	Not rated	Not rated
TENS	30	18 (60%)	85	60 (71%)
Splints	125	74 (59%)	62	48 (78%)
Biofeedback	42	20 (48%)	Not rated	Not rated

* These numbers may be underestimates, as 371 of the US survey participants who received physiotherapy did not say what the treatments entailed. Hydrotherapy and heat were likely included in the sessions, and perhaps ultrasound as well.

Exercise

The overwhelming majority of both groups of survey participants said they exercised regularly because of arthritis, and the
effort pays off. The chief benefits they got from exercise were
increased flexibility of their affected joints and some measure of
pain relief. Exercise also improved their general health, participants said, lifted their spirits, and kept their weight down. A few
even credited exercise with helping them fight stress, giving them
more energy during the day, and helping them sleep better at
night.

'Even though exercise is the last thing I feel like doing when my arthritis is unbearable,' wrote a teacher from Illinois, 'I always feel better later on after I force myself to get up and move around. Exercise doesn't aggravate the joint; it loosens up the stiffness.' A retired physician from Mississippi said, 'I believe that without the exercising I have done over the years I would now be in a wheelchair!' (See Chapter 17 for a rundown of the fitness exercises favoured by our participants.)

In general, activity is better than inactivity, but the wrong exercise can sometimes be as dangerous as the wrong medication. Out of 1,051 participants in the US survey, 174 (17 percent) reported being harmed at least once by inappropriate or overzealous workouts. Getting and following expert exercise advice is a good way to help you avoid injury. But where do you go for suggestions?

You can expect the most helpful individual attention to come from a practitioner who knows about your medical history, about exercise in general, and about the particulars of exercise designed to preserve range of motion in joints threatened by arthritis. Here are a few of the best choices.

- **Your doctor**, especially if you're seeing a rheumatologist (see Chapter 3). Doctors who are not exercise experts can at least advise you on safe limits and refer you to someone who knows how to teach the specifics, such as a physiotherapist.*
- **A physiotherapist** who has both interest and skill in helping people with arthritis. Sound exercise advice from these practitioners often led to long-term improvement for the survey participants. (See Chapter 4.)
- **The exercise instructor** at your local fitness centre. If you enrol in a general exercise class, make sure to tell the instructor that you have arthritis and that you may need to do some exercises differently or not at all. Many exercise instructors, including Yoga teachers, have the ability to provide such individualized help. (See Chapter 4.)

* Some chiropractors are quite knowledgeable about exercise for arthritis, on the whole, US participants did not fare well under chiropractic care. (See Chapter 4.)

- **Group classes** specially designed for people with limited movement, such as aquatic exercise at a community pool.

In recent years, DVDs and videos that can be played at home have become popular substitutes for exercise classes. Survey participants mentioned several exercise tapes produced especially for people with arthritis and sold in the US through the Arthritis Foundation (1314 Spring Street N.W., Atlanta, GA 30309).

The amount of time participants devoted to exercise varies from a few minutes to a few hours a day, depending on their family obligations, business demands, age, and physical fitness – including the degree of joint damage they had. 'I spend fifteen minutes a day on range-of-motion exercises,' wrote a forty-year-old Iowa homemaker, 'because I tend to get stiff and sore if I don't do them daily.' A retired car dealer from Florida, age sixty, followed a much more ambitious routine: 'I bicycle five miles per day, walk two miles per day, do stretching exercises in bed for half an hour every day, and type – to keep my fingers active – for about two hours a day.' There is no simple formula for determining an optimum amount of exercise time, but there are rules for safe exercise that seem to apply to just about everyone, whether your routine involves moving your fingers in warm water or walking miles at a time. Indeed, so many participants offered the same advice that we were able to create this list of exercise guidelines.

- *Don't overdo it.* 'Know your limits,' wrote a store manager from Texas. A Georgia housewife added: 'Learn to pace yourself. You may have to change your daily routine on bad days.'
- *Exercise regularly – every day if possible.* 'A little bit daily, faithfully and regularly, is much more effective than more exercise done sporadically,' explained an editor from New York.
- *Listen to your body.* 'Don't push through pain,' advised a retired purchasing agent from Maryland. 'If you start to hurt, *stop!*'
- *Start any new exercise program slowly, and increase gradually.* 'Set your own goals and don't be influenced by jocks or normal know-it-alls,' said a freelance writer from New Mexico.

- *Choose exercises that are easy on the joints.* 'And never try to exercise or force a joint when it is swollen,' wrote a factory worker from Virginia.
- *Learn to exercise properly, and follow the instructions you receive.* 'Find a good person who is knowledgeable and can relate to your individual body problems,' a New York psychotherapist suggested.
- *Get your doctor's OK before you embark on a new exercise regimen.*
- *Warm up before and cool down afterward.* 'Always warm up thoroughly,' said an insurance secretary from Texas. 'Cool-down is also important, and should contain some easy stretching, just like the warm-up.'
- *Don't give up.* 'Exercise can get very discouraging when you are alone and have to do it,' sympathized a retired postal worker from New Jersey. 'You seldom see immediate results, but sometimes you have to keep at it just to stay even. When you don't exercise, you tend to limit yourself more each day.'

Among the 215 US participants who did *not* exercise regularly, many found their jobs or daily activities to be so physically taxing that they had neither the time nor the energy for a structured exercise period. 'I just do all I can,' wrote a forty-nine year-old teacher from Nebraska. 'I recommend: Keep moving; keep living, don't stop!' Others said they were hoping or planning to start an exercise program soon. And a small minority said they find exercise too painful to pursue.

Hydrotherapy (Water)

Baths, spas, springs, tanks, and tubs that deliver the soothing powers of water all worked well for our participants. Hydrotherapy ranks among the oldest forms of medical treatment and remains one of the best-loved. Even though its good effects are temporary, the sensation is so pleasant that immersion became a daily ritual for many of our participants. When they were not receiving whirlpool or Hubbard tank* treatments from

---

* What separates the Hubbard tank from an ordinary whirlpool bath is the special apparatus that can lower you into the water and lift you out again.

their physiotherapists, they sought the hydrotherapy of their own bathtubs at home or the hot tub at a nearby health club. 'Hydrotherapy and activity keeps my pain at bay,' reported one woman from Cambridge.

Hydrotherapy can be considered a form of whole-body heat treatment – an extremely efficient way to warm up many painful joints at one time. Survey participants said the warmth relieved both pain and stiffness. (Inflammation, however, is better served by cold, as explained on page 135.) Participants also found that the buoyancy of the water takes the strain off their weight-bearing joints, while the whirlpool's churning action gave them a gentle, thorough massage. 'I've had chiropractic, acupressure, massage, and physical therapy with diathermy and hydrotherapy,' wrote a retired proofreader from New York. 'The whirlpool hydrotherapy is the only treatment that helps me significantly. In fact, it helps a great deal.'

Some of our participants reported that they did their exercises in the whirlpool because the water makes movement easier. 'This feels great while I'm doing it,' reported an Indiana social worker, 'and also gives me carryover mobility later in the day.'

Most hydrotherapy makes do with ordinary tap water, but a few of our participants got the chance to bathe in renowned mineral springs. 'Three years ago I spent four days at Hot Springs, Arkansas,' wrote a retired salesman from Illinois, 'and had hot-bath treatments at the spa there. On the third day I had a full body massage that, along with the hot baths, did make me feel great. But as soon as I would cool off or get chilled, my muscles would tighten and my joints would again become sore and tender.'

Thermotherapy (Heat) – and Cryotherapy (Cold)

Many survey participants found relief from pain and stiffness with thermotherapy, because heat increases the circulation where it is applied and helps the muscles relax. Professional methods for getting heat to affected joints include hot compresses, heat packs (sometimes called hydrocollators), heat lamps fitted with infrared bulbs, and devices that beam a comforting dose of warmth in the form of shortwave or microwave diathermy.

'An Army physiotherapist taught me how to survive in an environment where I have to use aching joints,' wrote a forty-five-year-old commissioned infantry officer from Hawaii. 'I find that direct heat on my shoulders and elbows, applied with a hot cloth, improves the mobility and gives temporary relief.'

'Heat always helps, particularly with exercise,' wrote one UK survey participant.

A forty-seven-year-old woman from Berkshire reported, 'I find warmth on a painful joint very comforting and helps to ease the pain. If I could afford it I would buy a hot tub as I use this at the gym on occasions as it brings great relief.'

Most participants who enjoyed professional heat treatments found that they could be helped just as much with the hot pads, hot-water bottles, or heat lamps they used at home. Heat is heat, after all, and it usually helps. An advantage of the professional thermotherapy is that it often comes complete with another form of treatment, such as massage or muscle stimulation. And a good practitioner, mindful of the real danger of burning you, may be more careful than you would be about where the heat source is placed and the length of time you are exposed to it. For example, most professionals say you should never lie on a heating pad, but put it on top of the painful part, and never use heat on a joint that is already hot and swollen. They also advise stopping any heat treatment session at the twenty- or thirty-minute mark.

The opposite of thermotherapy is cryotherapy, which aims to put the freeze on pain. Many doctors and therapists believe that cold is actually more effective for pain relief than heat. Some survey participants strongly agreed, although more of them used heat than use ice.

Cold treatments penetrate farther and last longer than most forms of heat, and cold has the added advantage of working to *reduce inflammation*. Professionals apply it much the way you would, with gel-filled, refreezable cold packs, or plastic bags filled with ice or a mixture of water and ice. They make sure to protect your skin from frostbite with a thin cloth and keep an eye on the clock – limiting cold treatments to twenty minutes every few hours. And they sometimes alternate heat and cold to maximize the benefits of both.

Ultrasound (Deep Heat)

The penetrating waves of ultrasound can heat small areas of the body so quickly that a treatment may go from start to finish in just *two* minutes, or ten at the most. Indeed, ultrasound is the only form of thermotherapy that has been shown to raise the temperature of tissues underneath the surface muscles. Heat pads, packs, and lamps, on the other hand, warm just the skin and surface muscles, letting the increased blood flow do the rest of the work.

Physiotherapists and chiropractors were the most likely sources of ultrasound treatments for our participants, some of whom enjoyed relatively long-lasting benefits. 'I found ultrasound the most beneficial of all therapeutic aids,' wrote a twenty-year-old college student with rheumatoid arthritis. 'Ultrasound gave me relief from the pain in my hips for about twenty-four to thirty-six hours.'

As any form of heat, however, ultrasound can *aggravate inflammation*. 'The ultrasound was very painful for me because of my inflamed nerves,' reported a former legal secretary from California who fares much better with ice and TENS (see pages 139–140).

Psychological Counselling

The medical literature is full of conflicting reports about the role of psychological counselling in the treatment of arthritis. In studies conducted at medical schools and hospitals, various types of psychological dishes have been added to the treatment menu – supportive group therapy, for example, or relaxation training – while doctors tried to see whether the treatments affected people with arthritis in ways that could be measured, such as their grip strength, pain level, and degree of inflammation. Some experts show objective proof that treating the mind helps the body, while others argue that the evidence is weak or wanting.

The nature of the US survey research was fundamentally different from these studies, since it relied totally on the participants' accounts of what happened to them and not on laboratory results or the observations of clinic personnel. By their own reckoning, US survey participants *did* find psychological intervention to be of value. It actually relieved pain for some of them and it helped others overcome emotional problems that have burgeoned around the fact of their arthritis, such as anxiety or depression. It is important to note that the UK survey did not find such a high rate of success for psychological counselling; however, pain clinics were highly recommended, and psychological therapy does form part of the pain clinic approach. UK survey participants also rated mental health practitioners specializing in pain management highly.

Forms of psychological counselling that are directly aimed at pain control include relaxation training, guided imagery, and self-hypnosis. (Biofeedback is also a pain-control strategy taught by some psychologists, and is described separately on page 141.) All of these approaches require that you marshal your powers of concentration to alter your perception of pain or even to change the course of your illness. For example, you might be asked to picture yourself in some much-loved place as a way to take your mind off the pain you feel, or you might be encouraged to conjure up a healing image – the fire in your joints, perhaps, being doused by guardian cells travelling through your body. Some of our participants regularly practised such techniques of thought control and they knew that their success did not mean their pain was minor or imaginary. 'I use self-hypnosis taught to me by a psychologist,' wrote an insurance underwriter from Louisiana. 'It works better than some medications I've tried for helping me deal with the pain.'

Treatments that address arthritis-related psychological problems include behaviour modification and the many forms of individual or group psychotherapy. These gave some of the participants the help they needed to regain a lost measure of self-assurance or self-esteem. 'During one of my very worst struggles with rheumatoid arthritis,' said a secretary and mother of four from Texas, 'I was given the number of a psychologist who has rheumatoid arthritis and who had led groups for the Arthritis Foundation. I was too ill for an office session, so she agreed to counsel me on the telephone. From talking with this kind lady, I realized that I was not alone in my disease or in the emotional havoc it causes.'

Wax (Heat)

Heat pads may be fine for the neck and back, and ultrasound ideal on an elbow, but some participants said there's nothing like a coating of wax to warm their hands and feet – over, under, and around every single joint of every finger or toe. Here's how it works: You dip your hands several times into the molten wax of the paraffin bath, then lift them out. The warm wax hardens immediately and you must hold the coated parts still, lest you crack the wax and let out the heat. The therapist then wraps your hands in plastic bags and heated towels, leaving you to enjoy the effect for about fifteen to twenty minutes. At the end of the treatment time, the wax peels off easily, since it is premixed with mineral oil.

Several participants found wax dips such a high point of physiotherapy that they bought or learned how to make their own paraffin baths at home. (See Chapter 16 for full instructions.)

Wax treatments tend to be kinder to your skin than repeated soaking in hot water.

Massage

Massage may work some of its good effects by the heat and increased circulation it generates. Some experts in pain control further believe that rubbing a painful area sends a different sort of message along nerves that travel to the brain. In other words, the 'massage message' blots out, or at least interferes with, the 'pain message.'

'I had massage treatments for six months from a physiotherapist,' wrote a homemaker from Oregon. 'These began very gradually, massaging only my feet at first, and then the rest of my body after a few weeks. The treatment helped me a great deal.' A former USDA inspector from Colorado added, 'I don't much like to get bent in the directions the physiotherapist bends me in. It doesn't feel all that great, but the massage part feels great anytime, and is really relaxing.'

Survey participants who praised massage said they liked it because it felt good – soothing and relaxing – even when it did not relieve pain. From the wrong hands, however, massage can make pain more pronounced. US survey participants preferred massages from physiotherapists, chiropractors, and osteopaths to those given by massage therapists who didn't understand the sensitivity of arthritis-stressed joints. 'Massage by a holistic massage therapist did me in,' said a retail buyer from New York. 'I've had trouble with my hernia ever since.'

Traction

Whether it's performed with weights and pulleys or a motorized machine, traction is supposed to relieve pressure and pain by pulling apart joint spaces that have narrowed and by freeing nerves that may be pinched. The vertebrae in the back and neck are the most frequent sites targeted for traction, although one of our participants was greatly helped by traction treatments on her legs during a hospital stay. 'In 1980 I became completely bedridden,' the forty-six-year-old Wisconsin housewife recalled. 'My rheumatologist put me in the hospital for a six-week stay with drug treatments and physiotherapy, including traction on my legs. I believe the traction is what helped me most to walk again.'

A few participants who received and benefited from traction said that the treatments sometimes caused nausea, headache, or jaw pain. Others found their original problem made worse by traction: 'I feel traction harmed me,' wrote a receptionist from Florida. 'It's as though my neck has been stretched so far that there is no elasticity left.' People with rheumatoid arthritis need to be cautious about traction, especially neck traction.

Two of the participants who were helped by traction received a form known as 'inversion traction' or 'gravity inversion,' which involves lying for short periods of time in a head-down tilted position. With their feet up and heads down, they found that the ever-present tug of gravity became a therapeutic device.

UK survey participants did not rate traction.

TENS (Transcutaneous Electrical Nerve Stimulation)

The fact that electricity can ease or erase pain has been known for many centuries – ever since the times when electric fish or eels were used as physicians' assistants. The compact ultramodern way to pit electricity against pain is with a device called a TENS unit, which has been around for only a few decades but has proven effective for some participants' arthritis pain. 'TENS diminishes my pain considerably,' said a college professor from Massachusetts.

The doctor or physical therapist who introduces you to TENS hooks you up to the device by taping its electrode-tipped wires to your skin at carefully selected points, depending on where you hurt. Turning on the battery-operated device delivers the electric current through your skin to the nerves. The relief you may feel within a few minutes is real, and it may last hours or days, although technology cannot explain why. The current may somehow short-circuit your perception of pain, or it may precipitate a flood of endorphins – your brain's own internally manufactured morphine.

'The TENS unit is the only thing that I've found effective,' wrote a housewife from Utah, 'and it has no side effects.' Actually, the gels and tapes used to secure the electrodes may cause skin irritations, if you're susceptible to them, and using the unit at the wrong setting can throw your muscles into spasm. But if you receive good instruction, and you respond to the treatment, you may want to purchase your own TENS unit for home use. 'I'm on my second one,' said a Michigan housewife. 'I had the first for eight years until I just wore it out.' TENS units can be bought in many pharmacists or on-line.

Splints

A strap-on mechanical aid that rests a joint, or keeps it stable while you work, or prevents deformity – or all three – is called a splint. Some of our participants say that splints also give them pain relief and protection from further injury. 'I've had at least four splints on my right hand,' said a nutritionist from South Carolina. 'The orthopaedist kept changing them as my hand changed, and those splints saved me from surgery.'

The function of a splint determines its form, and each one can be fashioned from a variety of materials, such as a combination of plastic, cloth, and metal, with Velcro fasteners.

Splints are often used 'as needed,' while driving or dressing, for example, or at night to keep the joint in the safest, most comfortable position. 'I have received a splint for my ankle,' wrote one sixty-seven year old UK participant. 'This helps in stabilizing the joint (the orthopaedist wanted to fuse the joint!). Thus far the splint has helped.'

'The wrist splints help, but I hate them,' wrote a Pennsylvania piano teacher. 'They aren't very romantic to wear at night, and once I accidentally hit my husband on the head with the metal plate in my sleep.'

This may sound like a truism, but splints can't help you unless you wear them. A California dental assistant reported 'immense' help from her splints, 'particularly after I decided to wear them religiously.' In contrast, a Connecticut housewife gave them up, even though they helped, because they just got in her way, especially when she was caring for her children.

A few participants levelled serious charges against splints for undermining the joint they were supposed to support. A retired tax assessor from Rhode Island said, 'After four months of wearing a splint on my left wrist, I felt that my wrist was getting weaker, so I discontinued wearing it.'

Biofeedback

A biofeedback device gives voice to the unseen, unheard vital processes that your body carries out without your conscious control. An ordinary thermometer is a biofeedback device – a meter that can show how your body temperature fluctuates over the course of a day. With practice, several of our participants have learned to use biofeedback devices to gain control over one or more of the body's automatic functions, and gain pain control as well.

One kind of hand-held biofeedback device gives a shrill whistle, for example, in response to a microscopic amount of perspiration on your palm. If, upon hearing the tone, you bend the powers of your mind to relaxation, you can stem the flow of sweat and make the machine hum quietly. More important, however, is the beneficial effect of relaxation on body tension and pain perception. 'I have tried biofeedback for the arthritis pain in my jaw,' wrote a Colorado homemaker, 'and I find it helps me a lot. I listen to the general relaxation tape the psychologist gave me, and work on relaxing my facial muscles, and this seems to relieve the tension and pain in my jaw.'

It should be clear by now that the biofeedback device is a means to an end. It is simply a monitor, no matter how elaborate it may be. The real painkiller in biofeedback is the relaxation technique you master. This may take a lot of work. 'Biofeedback does help,' said a high school chaplain and counsellor from Ohio, 'but it takes an extreme investment of time and concentration.' 'It's useless at the workplace,' added a California electrician, 'and also very expensive!'

Biofeedback was not rated in the UK survey.

Summary of Additional Orthodox Treatments

1. *Exercise* is the best, provided it's tailored to your needs. You may want to seek professional advice for instruction, while letting your own body be your guide to what exercise (and how much) you can do.
2. *Hydrotherapy* feels great while you're wet, and whirlpool treatments are especially helpful for reducing pain and increasing mobility, but the effects are temporary.
3. *Heat* is an effective treatment for pain and stiffness. *Cold* works even better than heat for some people's pain, and it also helps relieve inflammation.
4. *Ultrasound*, the most penetrating form of heat therapy, may achieve even better results in less time, with more lasting effects.
5. *Psychological Counselling* is a worthwhile adjunct to arthritis care, whether the therapist focuses on strategies for pain control or on the emotional problems arthritis can create.
6. *Wax* treatments in paraffin baths literally seal the hands (or feet) in warmth, and thereby provide a respite from pain.
7. *Massage* is at least soothing and relaxing, and may also relieve pain when it is performed by a knowledgeable practitioner.
8. *Traction* can relieve some kinds of pain by taking pressure off pinched nerves. In the wrong hands, this treatment can hurt as much as help.
9. *TENS*, the electrical painkiller, works by interfering with the brain's perception of pain.
10. *Splints* can relieve pain through physical support, while protecting a joint from injury and deformity.
11. *Biofeedback* requires your own finely honed powers of concentration to help you achieve relaxation and pain relief.

Section 4
What You Need to Know About Unconventional Treatments and Alternative Remedies for Arthritis

Be not the first by whom the new are tried, Nor yet the last to lay the old aside.

– Alexander Pope, from *An Essay on Criticism* (1711)

'I didn't say there was nothing better,*' the king replied. 'I said there was nothing* like *it.'*

– Lewis Carroll, from *Through the Looking Glass* (1872)

My experiences would indicate that what helps is often an individual thing, and each new treatment must be approached with cautious *enthusiasm.*

– Survey Participant #388, a school cafeteria server from Colorado

Chapter 9
Unorthodox Treatments

*• What is quackery, anyway? • The green wrist effect • The solvent solution
• Folk medicine • The sting*

There has probably been more haranguing, more breast-beating, and more outrage expressed on the subject of quack remedies for arthritis than on any other aspect of the disease. Estimates of the number of people with arthritis who have tried foolish or dangerous remedies run higher than 90 percent. And estimates of the money wasted on these quests are routinely figured in the billions of dollars per year.* Physicians often depict quackery as a boogeyman that preys on people in pain, making them discard proven treatments in favour of overblown promises. Some physicians blame themselves for the quack crisis. Dr. James F. Fries, director of the Stanford Arthritis Clinic, has said: 'The fact that patients try unorthodox treatments and go to quacks is an indictment of medical care. It smacks of poor communication on the part of physicians, lack of results, and a failure to deliver hope to patients.' Whatever the reason, the medical consensus is that quackery is pervasive and pernicious.

The nationwide US Arthritis Survey offered no support for these claims or fears. The 1,051 survey participants avoided quackery, for the most part, despite self-assessed pain ratings of 10 (the highest on our scale) and disease duration of more than twenty years in some cases. Of the one-third that did report using an unproven treatment, the majority had limited themselves to wearing a copper bracelet – on a lark, on the urging of a friend, or on the grounds that a five-dollar piece of junk jewellery couldn't hurt, so why not? The conclusion is that either the threat of

---

* This amount of money would buy several hundred copper bracelets for every man, woman, and child in this country with any of the one hundred forms of arthritis.

quackery is a fabrication – a straw man set up to divert attention from other issues in arthritis – or the haranguing has had its desired effect. In any case, people from every level of income and education are appropriately suspicious of mail-order miracles.

Quackery versus Alternative Treatments

The most useful definition of quackery hinges on the spirit in which a treatment is offered and the attitude with which it is tried. Anything that *promises* a cure is suspect, and anyone who ignores medical treatment while embracing such promises is asking for trouble; however, that leaves a lot of room for personal experimentation with a variety of products and plans that not only do no harm but may do a lot of good. A change in diet that actually improves the way you eat is a prime example. (See Chapters 12 and 13.)

Why I Decided (Not) to Try It

US Survey participants' attitudes on unproven remedies varied widely, from the few who were ever willing to try something new to the majority who rejected unproven remedies out of hand.

'I've tried every concoction friends would tell me about,' wrote an Oregon woman disabled by rheumatoid arthritis, 'from honey, vinegar, and iodine to gin-soaked raisins, with no results. The copper bracelet didn't help. The DMSO didn't help either, and it makes you stink. But when you have RA – and the pain and the emotional and physical problems it causes – you're willing to try anything to be the old you again.'

'Arthritis is enough of a problem without becoming a guinea pig for quack medicine,' said an adult-education instructor from New Mexico. 'Take nothing unless it's approved by the *New England Journal of Medicine*. If a cure is found, I'll know it by the six-inch headlines in my daily newspaper.'

The Most Popular Unproven Remedies

Copper Bracelets

Many people in the survey tried wearing a copper bracelet. A few participants wore copper rings, too, copper earrings, or even a copper insole in their shoes. But it was mostly for naught.

'The copper bracelet did nothing,' reported an audiologist from Indiana. 'I also wore a copper insole in one shoe for one day, and it was the worst day I'd had in months. On top of that, it gave me a metallic taste in my mouth and caused a run in my nylons.' Rating copper bracelets on the basis of our participants' reports showed the jewellery to have *less* than a placebo effect.

The term *placebo effect* comes from clinical research in medicine. To test the value of a new drug, for example, doctors gather a group of volunteers who have the illness the drug is supposed to treat. Then they give the new treatment to half the volunteers, while the other half get a placebo, or sugar pill – something that's really nothing but that looks and tastes just like the actual treatment. If the real drug is effective, then the people getting it should improve, and the people getting the placebo should feel no different from before. But a strange thing happens in these studies, as years of research have revealed. That is, some number of volunteers taking the placebo begin to feel better for reasons no one can explain. This is the placebo effect. It is probably a mixture of hope, faith, and good fortune. Thus, the bottom line in drug studies is that the new drug, to prove itself, must get whopping-good results compared to the placebo.

Even in studies where a new drug is *not* compared to a placebo, there can still be a placebo effect. That is, some number of people taking the drug may feel better by virtue of the placebo effect and not because the drug is really helping them. Scientists expect this to happen to as many as one-third of the volunteers involved.

In the US survey, copper bracelets proved more useless than a sugar pill. It might have been expected that there would have been a placebo effect alone for about 70 of the 211 participants who wore them. As it turned out, however, only 31 got any kind of help at all, whether it was pain relief or a boost for their morale. The UK results found a higher rating for copper bracelets, although the overwhelming majority of people who used them found them ineffective – 71 percent.

Although the bracelets appear to do no good, they do no real harm either. 'I once got a copper bracelet for kicks,' said a free-lance writer from New York, 'and kicks are all I got! It was an interesting piece of jewellery in which I invested a few bucks.'

	US Survey	US Percentage	UK Survey	UK Percentage
Number of participants trying copper jewellery	211		91	
Outcome:				
It helped	13	(6%)	26	(29%)
It may help	14	(7%)	Not rated	Not rated
It helped my morale	4	(2%)	Not rated	Not rated
No relief (ineffective)	180	(85%)	65	(71%)
Made participant feel worse	0	0	0	0

'I've used a copper bracelet for sentimental reasons,' reported a childcare giver from South Dakota. 'My pretty grandma always wore one. She was hopelessly handicapped with arthritis, however, and her hands were useless claws by her sixties, so I can't say I have much faith in the copper.'

'Copper bracelets are really neat,' quipped a novelist from Florida. 'They turn your arms green! They jingle and get caught on things, too. I wore them on each wrist for approximately two months, with no relief.'

'Sure I've tried copper bracelets,' wrote an Arthritis Foundation Self-Help Course instructor from Indiana. 'But other than 'psychological relief,' you only get green wrists. There's no harm in them, so if they make you "feel better," then it might be worth having green wrists!'

DMSO

DMSO (dimethyl sulfoxide) had its heyday in the 1960s and 1970s, when it was called an unproven remedy in the best sense of the term – that is, an experimental treatment under clinical investigation for a variety of problems ranging from athletic injuries to rheumatoid arthritis. After an exhaustive review of this research, however, a special committee of the National Academy of Sciences declared DMSO too iffy and too risky to become a prescription drug. The FDA has since *approved* it for treating the symptoms of one particular illness – a rare bladder disease called interstitial cystitis. But as far as arthritis is concerned, DMSO is considered more unproven than ever.

Prescription DMSO for cystitis is sold under the name Rimso-50 in the US. It is a 50-percent solution, prepared to be instilled directly into the bladder. Most DMSO available in the United States is less pure and more strong, though, meant to be used either as a solvent (99-percent solution) or for veterinary treatment (90-percent gel) of bruises, sprains, and other ills that befall horses and dogs. That doesn't stop people from trying to see if it works to relieve arthritis pain though. About half of the US survey participants who used it found that it did help, albeit temporarily. It was not rated in the UK survey.

	US Survey	US Percentage
Number of participants who tried DMSO	47	
Outcome:		
'It helped.'	23	(49%)
'It did nothing.'	24	(51%)
Most frequently mentioned side effects:		
Garlic/onion breath	7	(15%)

DMSO is colourless and odourless by itself, but once applied, it may make your breath reek within a few minutes, and the smell may persist for hours. A magazine editor from New Jersey said it made her smell like 'ripe pizza,' while several other participants complained of a strong garlic taste after use, or 'onion breath.' The odour foils the best efforts of researchers, since no placebo gives quite the characteristic flavour of real DMSO. Some studies have been done by giving DMSO to all of the volunteers and then tallying up the number who improve. But the results have not been convincing.

Our results were not convincing, either. At 49-percent effectiveness, DMSO certainly does *not* outperform standard arthritis treatments. For comparison, most of the prescription anti-inflammatory drugs help 60 to 80 percent of those taking them. (See Chapter 5.) We cannot recommend the use of DMSO, but if you are determined to test it on yourself anyway, please consider these warnings and tips from survey participants.

- Try to find DMSO that has been formulated for human or veterinary use, and not as a commercial solvent, so as to avoid impurities.
- DMSO can cause skin rash. Researchers say that a 70-percent solution of DMSO (with 30 percent water) is the best compromise between effectiveness and irritation. People with fair complexions, however, may not be able to tolerate more than a 50-percent solution.
- Because DMSO carries anything *on* your skin *into* your bloodstream, make sure your hands and the area to be treated are very clean.
- The threat of DMSO is to the lens of the eye, although real damage has been shown only in animal tests. Even if you never touch the solution to your eyes, it may wind up there, and the long-term effects are unknown.
- Beware of foreign clinics offering DMSO injections, as some of these have been found to mix steroids and other drugs with the DMSO, and to give shots without medical supervision.*

Remember that even DMSO's most ardent promoters, including Dr. Stanley Jacob, who did the pioneering research at the University of Oregon Medical School in Portland, do not claim that DMSO is a cure for arthritis. At best, it can reduce pain and increase mobility for some people, but it does not affect the course of the disease. Nor can anyone explain how it works to achieve its good effects. In the authorized account of his work, *DMSO: The True Story of a Remarkable Pain-Killing Drug* by Barry Tarshis, Dr. Jacob said, 'We've found that DMSO works better for arthritis above the waist than below the waist, and found that the most resistant part of the body to DMSO treatment is the hip.' (More than one-third of participants had arthritis in at least one hip, and well over half said their knees were affected.)

One of the participants, a fifty-six-year-old Oregon homemaker with osteoarthritis, received periodic DMSO injections

* 'Three days of an IV in a clinic in Mexico gave miraculous results,' writes a retired aerospace engineer from California, 'but within six months I had a massive haemorrhage in the abdominal cavity that put me very close to death.'

from Dr. Jacob several years ago as part of an experiment. 'The shots really helped me,' she recalled. 'I would limp in, and then be able to drive home myself. One shot lasted a couple of months, while the rub-on helped me only temporarily.'

Honey (and Apple-Cider Vinegar, too)

Is honey just a more natural sweetener than table sugar, or does it have healing powers? The results of the US survey show that the 'effectiveness' of honey as a remedy is about the same as any other sugar pill. It was not rated in the UK survey.

	US Survey	US Percentage
Number of participants who used honey*	20	
Outcome:		
'It helped.'	7	(35%)
'It did nothing.'	6	(30%)
No comment	7	(35%)

* Most of these used honey alone, but six participants combined it with vinegar, and one with willow tea.

'I had an herbalist girlfriend who used to give me willow tea with honey,' wrote an electronics technician from California. 'This does work for a short time, but beware of overdoing it, as too much upsets the tummy.' It's quite possible that both the relief and the stomach upset this man experienced had more to do with the willow tea than the honey. Thousands of years before aspirin was created, physicians advised people in pain to chew willow bark for the aspirin-like painkiller it contains.

'We raise our own honey,' said a cook/bartender from upstate New York, 'and I eat the yellow edge from the comb. It doesn't help.'

The popularity of honey with cider vinegar, such as it is, can probably be traced to Dr. D. C. Jarvis's 1960 book titled *Arthritis and Folk Medicine*, in which he aimed to distil some two hundred years of homey Vermont health wisdom into a program of arthritis self-care. That program consisted largely of two teaspoons of apple-cider vinegar and two teaspoons of honey dissolved in a glass of water – or sometimes just the honey, dissolved in a glass of apple juice and sipped like coffee with meals. The advice seems easy to follow, its philosophy is appealingly natural, and Dr. Jarvis himself comes across as an earnest character of great goodwill. Unfortunately, the plan didn't work out for most of the survey participants who tried it. 'I have taken apple-cider vinegar with honey for eight years,' wrote a retired postal clerk from Georgia, 'with no knowledge of any benefit or any harm.'

In all, sixteen participants said they had used cider vinegar, either alone or with honey. Most found it unremarkable, such as this retired carpenter from Ohio: 'I started drinking Dr. Jarvis's apple-cider vinegar three months ago, and the pains have not gotten worse.' An Illinois businessman had a little more luck: 'Honey and cider vinegar with water did nothing for the arthritis, but my ulcer got better.' The best report came from a sixty-six-year-old Ohio homemaker who has had arthritis for three years: 'I dissolve one-third of a cup of vinegar and one-third of a cup of honey in two quarts of water, and take one glass daily. It seems to work for me. Since I've been drinking this, I've been able to stop taking Feldene, which I used successfully for two and one-half years.'

Bee Venom

Once we dismiss honey, there is still the other end of the bee to consider – the stinging part. It turned out to be sweeter than the honey for several of the US participants who found relief in this unusual therapy. 'Bee venom cured the crippling arthritis in my toe joint immediately and completely,' said a computer consultant from New Jersey. 'My husband and I caught a few bees in a mayonnaise jar and shook them gently till they were dizzy and vulnerable. Then we used long tweezers to hold them around the middle and place them within the circle I had drawn in Magic Marker to show the area of pain on my foot. Bingo!'

At least three of the individuals who found relief with bee venom were not seeking therapy at all, but were stung accidentally. 'I raise bees,' explained a millwright and welder from Maine, 'and find that their sting on a hand or arm does seem to help, but I have not tried this on purpose.' Another beekeeper, however, who is a Missouri dairy farmer, wrote, 'I have received bee stings, of course, but couldn't see that it made any difference in my arthritis.'

According to Charles Mraz of Middlebury, Vermont, who has provided free treatments with live bee stings for more than fifty years to the many people with arthritis who visit his home, getting stung accidentally is *not* therapy. Mr. Mraz said that he must sometimes administer as many as two to three *thousand* stings over the course of a year or longer to achieve the desired result.

A few participants got their bee venom from the sting of a hypodermic needle in a doctor's office. One, a retired public school principal from Philadelphia, took shots first in London in the 1930s, and in 1941 from one of the leading American proponents of bee venom for arthritis, the late Dr. Joseph Broadman. 'I had to go to New York two to three times a week for several months while Dr. Broadman gave me the injection series,' she recalled, 'but I never had to return after that. While in his office, I saw people unable to walk across the room, who were walking on their own two weeks later.' Insufficient numbers of people had tried bee venom in our UK survey to enable us to rate it.

	US Survey	US Percentage
Number of participants who tried bee venom	23	
Outcome:		
Effective, sometimes dramatically so	11	(48%)
Ineffective	11	(48%)
Made participant feel worse	1	(4%)

Even those participants who seek out bee stings, however, warn of the dangers of allergic reaction and anaphylactic shock. This complication is rare, but it can be fatal, making the treatment entirely too risky for some people. 'I had no idea of my allergy to insect venom,' wrote an air force officer from North Carolina, 'until four years ago when I was stung by a yellow jacket and had to be rushed to the hospital emergency room for treatment.'

Motor oil and more

The brevity of this chapter and the small number of treatments that found even twenty tryers is, again, a testimonial to the caution and good sense exercised by participants. Based on the research done before conducting the survey, we had expected to write a much lengthier chapter on quackery, including such exotica as fetal lamb-cell injections and extract of the New Zealand green-lipped mussel – two of the treatments tried by world-famous heart surgeon Dr. Christiaan Barnard and described in his *Program for Living with Arthritis.*

There is nothing laughable or shameful in a person's trying an unproven approach, although there may be danger, or frustration, or both. Sometimes the cost of an unorthodox treatment is so high as to effectively limit the number of people who can try it. For example, Dr. Barnard had to travel to a private clinic in Switzerland for his lamb shots. On the other hand, the cost of conventional medical care in the US drove some people to seek a cheaper alternative. 'My husband died three years ago,' wrote a housewife from Michigan, 'and my insurance was dropped. I had been seeing a rheumatologist and was doing well on Plaquenil, but in these past three years I've not been to the doctor or had a prescription filled. I take honey and use Ben·Gay and aspirin. I've not had a bad flare-up, but the pain is still there.'

For whatever reason, eight of the US participants tried to loosen up their joints with a squirt of a lubricant called WD-40. 'In my line of work,' said an auto mechanic from Tennessee, 'I deal with lots of silicones, and I've used WD-40 for several years. This stuff really works when sprayed on an inflamed joint. Please don't think I'm too silly.' The problem is that for each participant who liked the effect of WD-40, another found it useless or worse: 'The cold of the spray caused extreme pain,' reported the owner of a gift shop in North Dakota, 'to say nothing of the smell.'

The rest of the survey reports on unproven techniques – including magnets, electricity, turpentine, and uranium rocks – are anecdotes, not supported by enough people's experience to be anything more than interesting stories.

Summary of Popular Unproven Treatments

Copper jewellery – less than a 'placebo effect' in the US survey, although 29% gained some benefit in the UK survey

DMSO – of some use to about half those who tried it

Honey – no better than a sugar pill

Bee venom – tempting but dangerous

Chapter 10
Three Widely Used Complementary Treatments for Arthritis:

What Is Their Value?

• *Manipulation* • *Acupuncture* • *Yoga*

Somewhere between the mainstream treatments and the fringe therapies lies a large grey area of popular, complementary approaches to arthritis care. These techniques include manipulation, acupuncture, and Yoga, all of which have a long history and a large following. Manipulation is the mainstay of chiropractic care and osteopathy. Acupuncture and Yoga, both foreign imports, have stood time's test, worldwide, over *hundreds* of centuries.

Several hundred of the US Arthritis Survey participants and nearly half of the UK survey participants tried these treatments and many found the help they were looking for. Others were disappointed, and a few were actually injured. In this chapter, you can share their experiences with manipulation manoeuvres, with acupuncture needles, and with Yoga positions – and discover their relative risks and benefits. You may be surprised to learn, for example, that acupuncture is *safer* than manipulation, in spite of the needles, and that Yoga is one of the most helpful approaches available.

Manipulation

Hands-on healing that sometimes gets rough

Chiropractors cite 1895 as the year their profession was officially introduced to the world. They created their 'natural method of health care' in reaction to what they saw as an overuse of drug treatments by medical doctors of the day, and an overemphasis on *curing diseases*, as opposed to *maintaining health*. The name *chiropractic* comes from the Greek word for hand, and the hand of the practitioner is the primary healing instrument. The hand manipulates and adjusts errant vertebrae in the patient's spine, removing unwanted pressure on the nerves and thus restoring normal 'nerve supply' to keep all parts of the body functioning at peak performance.

Osteopaths practice manipulation, too, but they also use massage and are less focused on the spine. In a few cases, survey participants received manipulation treatments from a physiotherapist or a nurse. The manipulation techniques vary widely from one practitioner's hands to another's.

'The chiropractor worked on me while I lay face down on his table,' wrote a retired printer from Illinois. 'The osteopath manipulated my spine while I lay face up, and he put his hands *under* my back. I found I got more lasting results that way.' A homemaker from Florida noted, 'The chiropractor helped to relieve pain with a new method of using pressure points instead of pushing on my body.'

No matter how it was performed, manipulation provided at least temporary relief for more than half of the US survey participants who tried it, and in the UK survey, 75 percent of participants experienced temporary relief or better. 'I went to a chiropractor when my back was so bad that I could not straighten up,' said a housewife from North Carolina with arthritis in her back, knees, wrists, and feet. 'He used a sound-wave treatment, applied heat and ice, and manipulated my back – and I walked out of his office standing straight.' 'Regular visits to the chiropractor has been the single most effective treatment for me,' reported one participant from Surrey.

Despite all the good reports, we endorse this technique with *caution*, since the 'Made participant feel worse' rate was higher for manipulation than for most other types of hands-on treatments, including surgical procedures. Only traction, at 22 percent in the US survey, caused relatively more misery. The reasons our survey participants give for feeling worse after manipulation include one broken bone and episodes of increased pain that lasted for weeks or months in some cases.

	US Survey	US Percentage	UK Survey	UK Percentage
Number of participants who tried manipulation	190		78	
Outcome:				
Temporary or lasting relief	116	(61%)	58	(75%)
No relief (ineffective)	22	(12%)	9	(11%)
Made participant feel worse	22	(12%)	11	(14%)
No rating (too soon to tell)	30	(15%)	0	0

Most of the participants who benefitted from manipulation noted that they had to go for regular treatments to keep up the improvement. 'Spinal manipulation has helped a great deal in allowing me to keep my mobility,' said an amateur musician from Michigan. 'I see the chiropractor three times a week. If I miss a treatment, I start having difficulty walking.' A retired engineer from New York reported, 'Manipulation helps me get through the acute attacks of shoulder pain I suffer every one to three months, but it does not prevent the *next* acute attack.'

Acupuncture

Ancient medicine, still practised and still promising

The origins of acupuncture are buried in myth and mystery going back thousands of years, at least to the time of China's Yellow Emperor in the fifth century B.C. One often-told story is that acupuncture was discovered accidentally in battle, when warriors pierced by arrows felt a sudden release from long-standing pain or illness. But no one can verify the story, *or* explain how that chance observation got translated into a complex philosophy of medicine, based on universal harmony, with a whole new view of anatomy. For acupuncture goes beyond the body as Western science knows it. East and West both see the musculoskeletal system, the digestive system, as well as the reproductive, respiratory, and circulatory systems. Acupuncture also recognizes a grand independent network of channels called 'meridians' that unite all those other systems, and unite mind with body, too. A vital energy courses through these meridians, acupuncturists say, and they can tap into it by stimulating one or more of the 360 distinct acupuncture points charted along the meridian pathways. Inserting needles into these precise points restores energy imbalances, breaks up energy blockages, and charges the body to heal itself.

Even before acupuncture followed President Richard Nixon home from China in the early 1970s, modern medical scientists began trying to explain *how* it works, in their terms, because they simply couldn't live with the concept of 'vital energy' moving inside *invisible* anatomic structures.* Electricity makes more sense to them, since the nerves are known to carry electrical impulses, and acupuncture points lie near peripheral nerve endings. Based on their experiments with animals, they suggest that acupuncture electrifies the nerve endings, which then signal the brain and spinal cord to release their own internal pain-blockers and painkillers. Other chemicals that may shower into the blood-stream in reaction to acupuncture are the body's own *anti-inflammatory* agents, and this may further explain why acupuncture sometimes helps people with arthritis.

'I've found that acupuncture in conjunction with the various medication I take can provide me with really effective short-term pain relief,' reported a thirty-one year old woman from Birmingham. 'It always helps to relax me and I come away from sessions feeling in less pain than when I arrived. This pain relief can last anything from a few days to two weeks. I wish this treatment was readily available on the NHS.'

Another thirty-one-year-old woman from Sandbach reported, 'I've found that a combination of acupuncture, red raspberry, Vitex, evening primrose oil and flaxseed oil plus a good multivitamin is helping my arthritis tremendously.'

'I was treated in a hospital by a Korean acupuncturist who was also an M.D.,' wrote a forty-four-year-old bookkeeper from

* The ancient Chinese, it is said, did not dissect human bodies, and no modern-day autopsy or surgical procedure has ever revealed any sign of the meridians. The only evidence for their existence comes from French scientists who spent ten years injecting radioactive tracers into the acupuncture points of human volunteers and following the tracers' migrations through the body with detectors called 'gamma cameras.' Their slides, presented at the World Research Foundation's Congress of Bio-Energetic Medicine in Sherman Oaks, California, in 1986, showed the tracers aligned along the classical acupuncture meridians.

upstate New York. (She kept up her orthodox treatments, too, which have included Indocin, prednisone, gold shots, Ridaura, and penicillamine.) 'He told me right up front that he could *not* cure my rheumatoid arthritis, but he felt he could help relieve pain. At the time, I was in excruciating pain, and had been for quite a while. So I tried it, and it did indeed help. I went from barely being able to get out of a chair alone – or walk, or use my hands – to feeling enough relief to begin a careful joint-exercise program that helped me become more flexible.'

	US Survey	US Percentage	UK Survey	UK Percentage
Number of participants who tried acupuncture	104		92	
Outcome:				
Temporary or lasting relief	39	(37%)	58	(63%)
No relief (ineffective)	36	(35%)	30	(33%)
Made participant feel worse	6	(6%)	4	(4%)
No rating (too soon to tell)	23	(22%)	0	0

The US statistics above are not encouraging. In fact, the 37-percent relief rate looks like nothing more than the one-third improvement we might expect from the placebo effect (the good feeling one gets from a treatment one *thinks* is helping). But the ho-hum success rate changes dramatically when we look at what happened to those US participants who got acupuncture treatments from bona fide acupuncturists, and not from a chiropractor or an M.D. who was dabbling with the technique (see next page). This distinction was not made in the UK survey, however the UK results were much stronger for acupuncture with an impressive 63% reporting temporary or lasting relief.

If you are going to try acupuncture, then look for a well-versed practitioner. (See Chapter 4 for more information about acupuncturists.)

'When I started seeing the acupuncturist,' recalled a sixty-six-year-old retired inventor from Washington, 'I couldn't drive, and my wife had to take me to and from his office. After about two months of receiving treatments three times a week, I was doing all the driving on the seventy-mile round trip. I continued

	US Survey	US Percentage
Number of acupuncturists (M.D. or non-M.D.)	37	
Outcome:		
Gave temporary or lasting relief	27	(73%)
Gave no relief (ineffective)	8	(22%)
Made participant feel worse	2	(5%)

taking acupuncture treatments for three years, and it helped a great deal.' Aside from the pain relief, he noticed one other benefit: 'Soon after I was stricken with rheumatoid arthritis in 1966, I had a terrible flare-up, and couldn't even stand to be touched because I felt like I was being skinned alive. My doctor put me in the hospital and shot me full of cortisone and painkillers for a *month*. The cortisone made my skin as thin as wet tissue paper, with about as much strength, and for years I continued to get sores that took up to twelve months to heal. But after three years of acupuncture, my skin cleared up and my sores healed.'

For reasons they cannot explain, some participants who enjoyed acupuncture found that it helped some joints but not others. 'Acupuncture helped my back pain and related leg pain tremendously,' reported a fifty-year-old executive secretary from South Carolina, 'but I've relied on physiotherapy and exercise for my hands, shoulders, and elbows.' A thirty-nine-year-old company vice-president from Minnesota told a similar story: 'Physiotherapy helps my hands, wrists, shoulders, and knees, but the arthritis in the ball of my foot went away completely with acupuncture.' The sixty-two-year-old owner of a yarn shop in Massachusetts said: 'Acupuncture was great for my shoulders but didn't do any good for my hands or feet.'

The risk of acupuncture is minor. If the needles are sterile,* there is scant possibility of infection, and there are no other known physical side effects. Although six of the US participants and four UK participants noted that they felt worse after acupuncture, no one complained of any injury to the joints. For example, a retired

---

* Check to see that the acupuncturist sterilizes the needles before each use, or uses disposable needles for each patient.

machinist from California recalled, 'Acupuncture sometimes helped a lot. At other times, I felt worse, but I was never injured.'

A few participants did complain about the cost of the treatment, though. 'Acupuncture helped for about three or four days after my weekly treatment,' wrote a forty-six-year-old legal assistant from Oregon, 'but I couldn't justify the expense for only a little relief.' A fifty-eight-year-old seamstress from Minnesota observed, 'Acupuncture helps the most to relieve pain, but I can't afford it often enough.'

Traditional acupuncture is practised with very fine needles, which may be inserted in places fairly far removed from your painful parts. The acupuncturist may then twirl the needles in place, for added effect, or burn moxa (an herb) in a small cup atop the needle. Some practitioners prefer to attach electrodes to the needles and turn on the juice. Modern acupuncture can even be performed by beaming laser light on the acupuncture points instead of needling them. Another needleless variation, called acupressure, or Shiatsu, substitutes fingertips for the fine needles. The practitioner prods the spot, or spots, or shows you where they are so you can treat yourself. 'Acupressure made some difference!' said a heavy-equipment operator from Washington state. 'Because it's basically pressure on various nerves, you can do it yourself. I get seven to eight hours of reduced pain this way.'

Yoga

A way of exercise, a way of life

Yoga is the living heritage of ancient India. Its philosophy may seem mystical and remote, based as it is on a belief in the unity of all that is. The same energy, or consciousness, exists everywhere and unites everything with everyone. Mind and body, especially, are united. Indeed the word *Yoga* means unity.

But many of the Yoga postures, or positions, which students of Yoga use to attain relaxation and open themselves to the flow of universal energy, also have a very mundane aspect. They stretch and strengthen the muscles. And they may look *exactly* like the range of motion exercises you received from your doctor or physiotherapist. The names have been changed, naturally, from

Sanskrit images to modern descriptions. And the movements prescribed for people with arthritis stop far short of the goals in some Yoga texts, which leave you marvelling at the way a man can sit with his legs crossed in front of him and his arms crossed in back of him, holding his toes in his fingers! Several of the exercises based on survey participants' advice (see Section 10), such as the Head Roll, for example, have their counterparts in *simple* Yoga movements.

'I do light Hatha Yoga for the lower spinal pain,' wrote an electrician from Florida. 'I feel it really lessens the pain, as long as I am gentle and very, very self-aware. I never do forceful, stressful exercise.' Yoga differs substantially from most aerobic exercises in this regard. The emphasis is on slow motions, awareness of your own physical limits, relaxation, and deep and even breathing. There's no bouncing, no panting, no thought of any given number of repetitions of a movement. Still, injuries can and do occur.

'I tried a few Yoga postures that were too advanced,' conceded a secretary from California, 'and pushed my body too far. I overdid, causing a lot of pain.' Usually, novices do better learning Yoga from an instructor instead of a book, so they can have expert guidance on safe positions, but this participant was taking instruction when she was injured. Not all teachers, unfortunately, have the ability to work with people in pain. If you decide to try Yoga, explain your condition to the instructor and find out how much experience he or she has in teaching people with arthritis. An anatomy professor from Missouri recommended, 'Find a good Yoga instructor who is easygoing and is not primarily gung ho for Hinduism.'

'I stumbled into a course in Hatha Yoga to fulfil a physical-education requirement when I went back to school to finish college,' reported a sixty-one-year-old freelance writer from Ohio. 'I took it for three years, from 1974 to 1977, then kept it up by following Yoga programs on television, and I enjoyed a total remission of my arthritis that lasted until 1986. The experience with Hatha Yoga carries over into all my everyday activities, which I do at my *own* easy, comfortable pace. I also find I get relief from using good posture, whether I'm standing, sitting, or lying down.'

We are concentrating here on Yoga as a form of *exercise*, but it had other benefits for some participants. 'I do believe that

	US Survey	US Percentage	UK Survey	UK Percentage
Number of participants who tried Yoga	41		40	
Outcome:				
Temporary or lasting relief	36	(88%)	27	(68%)
No relief (ineffective)	2	(5%)	11	(28%)
Made participant feel worse	3	(7%)	2	(5%)

Yoga has been *extremely* beneficial for me,' wrote a childcare worker from South Dakota who began taking Yoga instruction twenty years ago when she lived in a big city. 'I have seven sisters, but I am the only Yoga practitioner in my family. At forty-five, I'm third from the oldest, but more limber than all but the 'baby' of thirty. If nothing else, daily Yoga keeps one *thinking* healthy and spry.'

Summary of Unconventional Treatments

Manipulation – Is a technique for adjusting the spine so as to remove pressure from the spinal nerves, and thereby maintain health.

Is practised most often by chiropractors and osteopaths.

Is performed in different styles by different practitioners.

Provided at least temporary relief for about 60 percent of the US participants those who try it, and 75 percent of UK survey participants.

Carries a relatively high risk of injury.

Needs to be repeated frequently to maintain its effect.

Acupuncture – Is a technique for correcting energy imbalances or blockages in the body by inserting fine needles along the energy pathways.

May bring relief by stimulating the brain and spinal cord to release the body's own internal painkillers.

Provides relief to nearly 40 percent of those who try it, according to the US survey findings and 63 percent in the UK survey.

Is more effective when practised by well-trained acupuncturists, whether or not they are medical doctors.

May bring more relief to one joint than another.

Carries a negligible risk of injury.

Yoga – Is an ancient philosophy of life that includes beneficial exercises.

Differs from aerobic exercises in pace, goal, and physiological effects.

Provides temporary or lasting relief to 88 percent of those who try it, according to the US survey and 68 percent according to the UK survey.

Carries a risk for those who attempt advanced positions too soon.

Section 5
Nutrition and Arthritis

What rheumatologist has not been asked about the role of diet in the treatment of rheumatoid arthritis? Who among us has not responded that there is no evidence that diet treatment works?

— Nathan J. Zvaifler, M.D., from an editorial in *Arthritis and Rheumatism*, April 1983

Surprisingly, despite the fervour of advocates and scepticism of rheumatologists, little objective information exists about nutritional therapy for rheumatic diseases, and virtually all conclusions have been based on inadequate data or improper study design.

— Richard S. Panush, M.D., from an editorial in *Annals of Internal Medicine*, April 1987

The doctor said what I eat doesn't affect arthritis, but I know better.

— Survey Participant #664, a carpenter from Texas

Chapter 11
A Revolution in Medical Thinking about Nutrition and Arthritis

• Diets for arthritis • Supplements that control symptoms • Fasting for periodic relief • Food allergies that aggravate arthritis

Is There an Arthritis Diet?

There are *hundreds* of arthritis diets, and up until quite recently, rheumatologists have been content to brand them all 'quack therapy' and pay no attention to their individual differences. But in 1981, Dr. Richard S. Panush and his colleagues at the University of Florida College of Medicine decided to put one popular arthritis diet to the test. They chose the diet laid out in two books by Dr. Collin H. Dong and Jane Banks – *The Arthritic's Cookbook* and *New Hope for the Arthritic*, published by Thomas Y. Crowell in 1973 and 1975, respectively. It was a strict diet that ruled out all dairy products, all fruits, all meats, all alcoholic beverages, and all preservatives, among other things. They selected it, they said, because it had won tremendous media attention, and not for any particular promise they could see in it. In fact, they judged the diet deficient in certain vitamins and minerals, and they beefed it up with a daily vitamin-plus-iron supplement.

Having chosen a diet plan, the researchers had to devise a way to study its effectiveness. They decided to test it against a mock diet of their own creation that ruled out certain foods arbitrarily – sour cream, turkey, bananas, cornflakes, and others – while allowing red meat and white wine. They would ask half the people in their study to follow one diet, half to follow the other, and they would watch and see what happened. But first they had to round up a group of volunteers who all had arthritis and who would all promise to follow a strict diet to the letter – for ten full weeks – in the interest of science.

Luckily for the doctors, the average person with arthritis is so open to the idea of diet therapy that they were able to attract thirty-three highly motivated men and women who had rheumatoid arthritis and were willing to give nutrition a whirl. Importantly, none of these people had read the Dong-Banks books or heard about the diet. Experimental science, like justice, is blind. Volunteer subjects must have *no idea* whether the pill or the diet they ingest is the real object of study or some sham or placebo pill that is tested for the sake of comparison. All these volunteers knew was that they were following a diet different from their usual one and that it might help. And the doctors who periodically examined them every two weeks over the course of the experiment were likewise blind as to which diet which patient was on.

Only the dietitian knew who was eating what. The dietitian, after all, was the one who gave each participant detailed personalized instructions, including menu plans and recipes, who telephoned all the participants several times a week to encourage them in their efforts, and who dropped in at their homes, unannounced, *eighty-seven times* at lunch or dinner hour, just to make sure they weren't cheating. But the dietitian was blind as to which individuals showed signs of improvement in terms of their blood-sedimentation rate, for example, or the strength of their grip. (They had all been in pretty much the same shape, on these and other measures, when the study began, and every subject's medical treatment continued unchanged throughout.)

Partway through the study, seven of the original thirty-three volunteers dropped out. It was too dull or too difficult to follow the diet, or too hard to keep track of what they ate in their food diaries, as the experiment demanded. The other twenty-six stuck it out the whole ten weeks. And here's how it ended up.

Five of the eleven patients on the experimental diet got better during the study. But so did *six* of the fifteen patients on the placebo diet. What was going on here? Was there some feature common to both diets that could have been responsible? The researchers say they couldn't identify one. More likely, the participants were having a remission for some other reason. Maybe their hopes were buoying them, making them feel better and appear better on examination. If the diet were *really* therapeutic, scientific thinking holds, then it would have had obvious benefit compared to the placebo diet; and it did not.

But one man and one woman on the experimental diet completed this study feeling so greatly improved that they chose to stay on the diet indefinitely. Nine months later, when the researchers completed their report for the April 1983 issue of *Arthritis and Rheumatism*, these two individuals were *still* following the diet. Every time they went off it – she for an ice cream or a candy bar, he for a spicy meat dish or a beer – their arthritis symptoms flared. 'Without further study,' the researchers said of them, 'it is uncertain whether their course was indeed modified by diet or merely reflected the natural history of disease.'

It is hard to imagine how a months-long trend of well-being, interrupted only by an occasional binge on a forbidden food item, could reflect 'the natural history of disease.' Why won't the researchers admit that the diet scored two cures? Because the standards of scientific proof are rigorous, and two out of eleven is a scientific bust. If five or six of the people on the experimental diet had gotten better, and one or none on the placebo, then the scientists might have had something approaching preliminary proof. As it is, we are left with two isolated cases, interesting to be sure, that 'support, but do not prove, the suggestion that individualized dietary manipulations may be beneficial for selected patients.'

Diet Instead of Drugs

More 'observation' and 'support' were soon to follow, when doctors in Surrey, England, tested a diet as *sole therapy* for rheumatoid arthritis. They took the fifty-three patients in their study off their regular medications for two weeks before even starting them on the diet. During this pre-diet period, the volunteers got placebo pills, although they didn't know what they were, of course, along with two tablets of a non-aspirin painkiller (acetaminophen, which you may know as **Tylenol**) four times a day.

In the next step, half the group began to follow the special diet, which consisted of excluding various foods that might aggravate arthritis. Then, after one week, the foods were gradually reintroduced, a few at a time, beginning with those least likely to offend. Any food that fomented the symptoms of arthritis was quickly eliminated again. Thus, each volunteer's treatment became unique over the six weeks of diet therapy.

Meanwhile, the other half of the volunteers continued, without any change in their normal diet, on placebos and non-prescription painkillers for six more weeks – a total of *two months* away from their standard treatment. (This proved too difficult for some, and in all, eight people dropped out of the study before its completion.) Only then did they begin their six weeks of diet therapy – identical to what the first half of the subjects had tried. The researchers designed the study this way so they could compare people on diet therapy to people on placebo therapy for six weeks, and compare some people to themselves in two different situations, to see whether and how they changed when they made the switch from placebo pills to diet.

No matter how the researchers looked at it, the diet wrought improvements that were swift and dramatic. Within the first week of diet therapy, the first group of participants had less pain, shorter periods of morning stiffness, fewer painful joints, and a stronger grip. Over the next five weeks, they enjoyed continued relief. The second group, too, despite their longer wait before starting the therapy, responded to the diet with markedly reduced pain and stiffness. On all comparisons, diet therapy proved superior to placebo therapy, from group to group and within the same individuals over time. What's more, nearly everybody in the study lost weight and felt the better for it.

Reporting their results in the *Lancet* of February 1, 1986, Dr. L. G. Darlington and his co-authors wrote, 'It is one thing to describe improvement with dietary therapy in patients with rheumatoid arthritis and quite another to explain how it may work.' They had a few ideas, though.

- The people may have had genuine *food intolerances*, so that not eating certain food(s) brought relief.
- The *weight loss* alone might have changed the course of the disease.

- Taking the people off their *prescription medications* may have solved some drug-related intestinal problems and made them better able to keep irritants from entering the bloodstream through the gut.
- Eating more of some foods containing certain *fatty acids* (more about these later) may have reduced joint inflammation.
- The *power of suggestion* from being involved in a dietary experiment could have produced the very real improvement seen.
- Perhaps a combination of two or more of these factors was at work.

'For some physicians the use of diet in rheumatoid disease has a disturbing flavour of fringe medicine,' they conceded, and they suggested that 'perhaps the greatest need now is for more careful and well-designed research so that preconceptions may be put aside and any role of diet . . . may be determined.'

In other words, caution is crucial, for the scientist who uses anything short of the most exacting standards in diet studies will undermine the revolution and wind up being dismissed as just another quack.

Do Certain Foods Aggravate Arthritis? And If So, Which Ones?

That's what Dr. Deepa Beri and fellow researchers at the All India Institute of Medical Sciences in New Delhi sought to learn in 1987. On the road to discovery, they asked their research subjects to stop taking their non-steroidal anti-inflammatory drugs (NSAIDs) and try to get by on acetaminophen. Under the circumstances, nearly half the group — thirteen people out of twenty-seven — were unable to make it through even the first phase of the study, which put them on a two-week diet of nothing but fruit, vegetables, sugar, and refined oil. (Later on, a fourteenth person dropped out. Despite the fact that he had moved on to a slightly less stringent diet *and* was doing well, he simply stopped going to the clinic, and the doctors couldn't find him.)

The study stretched out over ten months and required the patients to persevere through six variations of the diet. Their first two weeks on fruits and vegetables excluded all the foods that the researchers suspected might be arthritis-aggravating, such as milk, wheat, and meat. By the end of this period, ten of the fourteen subjects (71 percent) showed significant signs of improvement. Now they were ready to add on one of the staples of the Indian diet – pulses, which are the edible seeds of certain plants, such as peas, beans, and lentils. Almost immediately, one patient suffered a rapid flare of arthritis symptoms, and two others also grew worse.

On to the third phase and the introduction of wheat and wheat products. Again, there were instant reactions to the foods from some of the volunteers. This pattern repeated itself through each successive stage, in which each added food item decked one or more of the participants. Some could tolerate no rice, others no milk. Unfortunately, some of them proved to be so sensitive to so many foods that the researchers had no choice but to start them on drug therapy, since it seemed impossible to restrict their diets as severely as their symptoms suggested.

'The results showed that a high proportion of patients improved on dietary manipulations,' the doctors concluded in 1988 in *Annals of the Rheumatic Diseases*, 'and that there was marked individual variation in response to the elimination of different dietary items.' Yes, certain foods clearly do aggravate arthritis. But the 'certain foods' change from one person to the next. (See Chapter 12 for a list of foods that our survey participants found most likely to be arthritis-aggravating.)

What About Not Eating at All?

Diet studies that include a period of fasting show that arthritis almost always improves in the absence of food. This may sound like a sick joke, since starvation is hardly the way to health, but the finding is a strong argument for the existence of some aggravating factor in food.

'About five years ago,' wrote a retired industrial designer from Florida who participated in the US survey of 1,051 people with arthritis, 'I tried a one-month fast from solid foods. I had only vegetable and fruit juices, with vitamins, and enemas to clean out my system. I lost forty pounds in ten days. After being very weak for the first seven days, I began to feel better. After another ten days, I felt cured and even the rheumatoid nodules were disappearing. As the weight returned, so did the arthritis. But I was afraid of damage to my heart if I continued fasting, and I didn't have a doctor who would agree to supervise me, so I stopped.'

Unlike this survey participant, the twenty Swedish men and women who fasted for science in 1982 *were* under a doctor's supervision *and* inside a hospital during their two-week fast. Then they stayed for another three weeks, following a strict vegetarian (vegan) diet with no eggs or dairy products. The researchers observing them modelled this experimental fast and diet after popular programs at Swedish health resorts, which were promoted as being particularly helpful for people with arthritis and other diseases.*

Of the ten people in this study who had arthritis, eight said they felt much better while fasting. For eleven days, they had nothing but vegetarian broths, juices made from vegetables or berries, and herbal teas every two or three hours, and their symptoms seemed to wash away.

Fasting studies are not blind, obviously, since there is no way to keep people from knowing that they're not eating; but not everyone had the same reaction to the fast. Two members of the group grew *worse*, even though they continued taking their regular medications all through the experiment.

After the Fast Is Over

No sooner did the subjects start to eat solid food again than their symptoms began to creep back. Even so, they finished the study feeling slightly better than they had at the outset, and one person felt considerably better.

The doctors observed that 'fasting seems to have a fairly potent anti-inflammatory effect,' (*Acta Dermato-Venereologica*, 1983), although they could not explain why. A few years later, however, other Swedish scientists watched fourteen women with arthritis

---

* These 'health farm' treatments, involving fasting and vegetarian diets, spurred doctors in Sweden to conduct, by our count, at least a half-dozen separate scientific investigations between 1979 and 1986 – several of them aimed at answering patients' questions about nutrition and arthritis.

improve during a one-week total fast, and they began to piece together the reasons.

The fact that the women in the study felt better while fasting was obvious from the degree of pain relief they enjoyed – despite having dropped their drug treatments (NSAIDs) two weeks before entering the study. But the *explanation* for their well-being came from intensive analysis of their blood before, during, and after their week of consuming nothing but water.

As Dr. Ingiäld Hafström and others pointed out in May 1988 in *Arthritis and Rheumatism*, fasting changes the blood chemistry of people with arthritis. It slows the action of certain enzymes and blocks key steps in the chain of events leading to painful inflammation. Although aspirin and other anti-inflammatory drugs also block these events, they don't create quite the same changes as fasting does.

No one in the study suffered any kind of side effects from fasting, except for a little passing weakness, weight loss, and light-headedness. This is light stuff compared to the side effects of the majority of arthritis treatments, even over-the-counter ones, which often cause nausea, vomiting, indigestion, ulcers, and diarrhoea or constipation.

'Thus,' the researchers concluded, 'fasting is one possible way to induce rapid improvement in rheumatoid arthritis.' And although fasting could never be used, of course, for any appreciable length of time, volunteers who fast so that others may learn are revealing the healing processes involved.

The UK Arthritis Research Campaign states that fasting for a week can improve rheumatoid arthritis but that the evidence is that arthritis quickly returns after you resume a normal diet. It does not recommend fasting as a treatment for arthritis and if you are interested in this approach you should definitely consult your doctor before attempting it.

A Fish Tale

One promising possibility for gaining some of the advantages of fasting without forgoing food is by supplementing the diet with fish oil – or rather, the omega-3 fatty acids that fish-oil supplements contain, especially eicosapentaenoic acid, or EPA. Dr. Joel M. Kremer and other scientists at Albany Medical

College have looked long and hard at this possibility, as have Drs. Richard Sperling, Michael Weinblatt, and K. Frank Austen at Harvard Medical School.

Inspired by a long line of animal and human experiments, Dr. Kremer's group set out to discover whether changing the source of fat in the diet could change the course of inflammation in arthritis.

Their subjects were thirty-eight willing and able patients, who followed dietitians' orders and took special supplements for twelve weeks. And as you know, *they* did *not* know who among them followed the experimental diet and took fish-oil supplements or who followed the sham diet and took placebo pills.

The experimental diet in this case was specially tailored to deliver a high ratio of polyunsaturated fat (the kind found in many types of fish) to saturated fat (the kind you find in butter). Volunteers on the experimental diet were told to eat fish wherever and whenever possible. They could eat red meat twice a week at most, and only if they stuck to lean cuts with *all* visible fat removed. Chicken was okay, too, provided they took the skin off. Under no circumstances could they indulge in sausage, bacon, hot dogs, or other lunch meats. Other no-nos included whole milk, butter, and cheese. If they cheated, they had to say so in the food diaries they kept, where they entered everything they ate all day. On top of all that, they had to take ten MaxEPA capsules daily.

The volunteers in the control group had dietary restrictions, too, which turned their mealtimes, likewise, into assignments of sorts. For example, they were told to avoid foods high in polyunsaturates, such as corn oil and safflower oil, and they also took ten capsules a day (all duds, however, made of non-digestible paraffin wax). Both groups had to balance their diets and try not to gain or lose any weight, and both groups continued their regular drug regimens, which ranged from NSAIDs and steroids to the more potent 'second-line' treatments such as gold, penicillamine, and hydroxychloroquine.

The kinds of changes the researchers could hope to see in their subjects would take at least six weeks to emerge on the changed diet, and the experiment lasted twice that long. By the twelve-week point, there were indeed differences between the two groups in terms of morning stiffness and the number of painful joints they had. The people in the experimental group were better off. But when the follow-up exams came around a month or two after the study ended, the people in the experimental group had lost all the ground they'd gained, while those in the control group felt improved.

The researchers saw these after-effects as further proof of their theory. In other words, the experimental group grew worse when they went off the diet and stopped taking fish oil because they were no longer getting the combination's anti-inflammatory effect. As for the control group, the rebound relief they enjoyed in the weeks after the experiment was probably the result of dropping the diet high in saturated fat and returning to a more healthful way of eating. Just going back to a polyunsaturated cooking oil, which they had been told to avoid during the study, could have made an appreciable difference, the researchers said (*Lancet*, January 26, 1985), as too much saturated fat may affect the immune system and aggravate arthritis symptoms.

For more information on fish oil see Chapter 14 on supplements.

Was It Something I Ate?

A thirty-eight-year-old mother of three made medical history when her severe chronic rheumatoid arthritis – which could not be controlled with aspirin, with NSAIDs, with gold, with penicillamine, with prednisone, or even with the immunosuppressive drug azathioprine – responded to a simple change in diet. Eleven years of suffering ended abruptly when she stopped eating milk, cheese, and butter.

The strange thing about this pale sickly looking woman, according to doctors at the Royal Postgraduate Medical School in London who treated her and reported her case history in the *British Medical Journal*, was that she had none of the usual symptoms of food allergy. No foods upset her stomach, gave her diarrhoea, made her skin break out, or brought on a headache. She had no reason to believe that her passion for cheese – she often ate as much as a pound of it in a day – was fanning the flame in her joints. However, she had been through so many medical treatments with so many toxic reactions that she willingly agreed to try the doctors' suggestion to stop eating dairy products.

After three weeks on her new diet, she began to feel better, with less pain and swelling and a shorter period of stiffness in the mornings. As the months passed, most of her symptoms completely disappeared.

The doctors were delighted, but they couldn't let it go at that. They had to show that her case was truly an example of food-induced arthritis. And so they invited her to check into the clinic, where they fed her three pounds of Hammersmith Hospital cheddar cheese in as many days, along with seven pints of milk. The effect was awful. Within twenty-four hours her old stiffness was back, she could barely make a fist, and her fingers swelled until some of them were two whole ring sizes larger.

There was no question that she met two of the most important criteria for food allergy: Her symptoms went away when she stopped eating certain foods and came back with a vengeance when she ate them again. The results of the allergy tests the doctors gave her weren't so clear-cut, however. In fact, such tests may be inadequate to discover food sensitivities in people with arthritis. There seem to be no good shortcuts – yet – around the difficult but definite route of excluding this or that from the diet for weeks at a time and watching for signs of improvement.

This woman's case is not the only documented case of food-aggravated arthritis on record, but it is one of very few. Swiss rheumatologists recently tried to raise the number of cases by mailing a food-allergy questionnaire to three hundred of their patients with arthritis. Only 158 people filled out and returned the form, however, and only 52 of them believed that certain foods increased their symptoms. When the doctors examined six of these people in person, testing them and challenging their symptoms to flare by feeding them the foods they avoided, *nothing happened.*

'It seems, therefore,' the researchers concluded in a 1987 report in *Clinical Rheumatology*, 'that true allergic reactions in joints of rheumatoid arthritis patients are rare.' Maybe so. Or maybe, as the London doctors suggested, allergies that cause arthritis symptoms work in ways that are not yet fully understood.

Mystery Capsules

Dr. Panush of the University of Florida, who tested a popular diet on a group of his patients (see pages 169–171), looked into the question of food allergy in an ingenious way. He solicited people who noticed that their symptoms got worse after eating certain foods, and then, instead of openly offering them the foods they feared, he disguised various foodstuffs in capsules, with no telltale aromas or appearances. Some of the capsules contained the aggravating items, but some of them contained foods that had never caused these people a lick of trouble. Would the people react to the foods if they were 'blind' as to what they were eating?

Dr. Panush and his colleagues began their investigations with a middle-aged woman who couldn't eat milk, milk products, red meat, or dry beans. Her rheumatoid arthritis flared from these foods, she had found, and so she limited herself to fish, chicken, vegetables, and fruits. Her arthritis and her certainty that food affected it made her just the person Dr. Panush and his colleagues were looking for.

After examining her twice and getting her enthusiastic consent to go along with a rather taxing sort of study, they took her out to lunch at a nearby restaurant, where they ordered her the house specialty, containing milk *and* beef *and* beans. Before the afternoon was over, the poor woman literally lost her grip. Her grip strength weakened by 40 percent from the morning's measurement, and she felt much worse. Several of her joints became tender, while other joints swelled. And her walking slowed way down. The luncheon had been a success, and three months later the woman checked into the clinic to go through the rest of the study as an inpatient.

About a week into her hospital stay, the doctors asked her to fast for three days. Within twenty-four hours of starting the fast, she felt worlds better. Her morning stiffness, for example, which usually lasted about half an hour, disappeared altogether while fasting. Then, for the next *month*, she lived on Vivonex, a liquid diet, only marginally more appetizing and satisfying than being fed intravenously. But Vivonex was not the least bit arthritis-aggravating, and she continued to feel and function almost as well as she had while fasting. She was a great good sport about all of this, too, the doctors reported in *Arthritis and Rheumatism* (February 1986), describing her as 'extremely cooperative and motivated.' She was also a model subject because she proved to the scientists' satisfaction that her arthritis was most definitely aggravated by food. She even passed the mystery challenge test.

At most of her 'mealtimes,' she drank her Vivonex with a capsule that contained some disguised food item. Some of the capsules contained milk, others had chicken, beef, rice, lettuce, carrot, or nothing (placebo). She didn't know what was in them, of course, but her body reacted unerringly to the milk every time – with tender joints, with swollen joints, with morning stiffness, and with weakening grip.

Buoyed by this experience, the researchers went on to work with several other people in a similar fashion. Out of fifteen subjects who were tested this way, three felt their symptoms flare every time the capsule delivered one of the offending food items, which included milk, shrimp, and nitrates. Another two people reacted some of the time, and ten didn't react at all. Dr. Panush suspects that only about 5 to 10 percent of people with arthritis have true food sensitivities. However, he wrote in a commentary in *Annals of Internal Medicine* (April 1987), 'The notion that food or food-related environmental antigens induce or perpetuate symptoms, at least for some patients, is novel, logical, and potentially enlightening.'

More Questions Than Answers

Some of these studies raise more questions than they answer, but they have broken new ground, at last, making nutrition a reasonable and respectable field of inquiry for rheumatologists and other scientists interested in arthritis.

We salute the scientists who stuck their necks out to initiate studies in this area, putting their reputations on the line. We also salute the people who helped them carry out their investigations – the subjects in their research.

Over and over in the reports of these studies, we've seen people willingly give up their freedom of choice in matters of food, staying on highly restricted diets for weeks, even months at a time. Sustained by the encouragement of researchers and by the hope that their efforts will help themselves and others, they are the army of the revolution. And it is an all-volunteer army.

Early nutrition studies, by comparison, such as the ones at the beginning of this century that started to define minimal daily requirements for certain nutrients, didn't have to rely on volunteers. In those days, before research subjects were protected by the doctrine of informed consent, doctors were free to experiment on captive populations in hospitals, asylums, reformatories, and prisons.

Today, doctors know they can expect a certain number of people to drop out of a diet study, and this makes their job harder. To take Dr. Kremer's earlier trial, for example, in which the participants had to change their diet *and* take ten capsules a day, three people dropped out because they couldn't stick to the diet, two quit because they couldn't swallow the capsules, another two left when their arthritis got worse, and one suddenly required chemotherapy for cancer. On top of these problems, Dr. Kremer found that six more people, who weren't voicing any particular complaints, were simply *not taking* the capsules as they were supposed to. He was forced to drop them.

In one report we reviewed of a study on food allergy and arthritis, the researchers got openly disgusted with the people who had promised to be their subjects. 'The most noteworthy point of this trial,' they said, 'has been the frequency with which patients have abandoned their declared interest in dietary management once faced with a controlled and demanding protocol of this kind. . . . The self discipline demanded by the trial comes as a harsh antidote to the facile optimism of so many glib theories about food allergy and arthritis.'

Nutrition studies make demands of people that most scientific studies do not. If you're asked to take a new drug in the interest of science, then you take it, or you take the placebo, and you let the doctors chart your symptoms for a time. But if you agree to take a diet as treatment, you either consent to being hospitalized so the researchers can control exactly what you eat, or you're stuck keeping a written record of every mouthful. From personal experience as a volunteer research subject, I can say that it is sometimes *easier*, in these situations, to go a little hungry than to start taking tests or making notes every time you want a snack.

Chapter 12
Expert, Experienced Advice About Nutrition and Arthritis

• What doctors won't tell you • What weight loss can accomplish
• What foods are most likely to aggravate arthritis pain

Every day, the following scene is acted out in countless doctors' offices. Maybe you've played a role in it yourself.

Patient: Tell me, Doctor, is there any special diet I should follow, or any particular foods that would make my arthritis better or worse?

Doctor: No, there is no known connection between nutrition and arthritis.

The trouble with the doctor's part in the drama is that it is unconvincing. Most people with arthritis find it simply incredible that nutrition could have nothing to do with the disease – especially when they are bombarded with messages about nutrition's importance in other common illnesses, such as diabetes, heart disease, hypertension, cancer, and osteoporosis. It is even more unbelievable if their own experiences show them that diet *does* make a difference in the amount of pain they feel.

'Most of the rheumatologists I have seen,' wrote a twenty-nine-year-old teacher from Texas who's had rheumatoid arthritis for ten years, 'dismiss nutrition, other than to say it is important to eat balanced meals and not to become over-weight. But personally, I find that whenever I eat a lot of sugar products I will feel pain in one or more joints. So I try not to indulge my sweet tooth too often. And although I believe it is important to follow a doctor's advice, ultimately I am the judge of what is best for my body, because I know my body better than anyone else does.' Her doctor is helping her dramatically, she told us, through a very effective treatment combining the anti-cancer drug Methotrexate with prednisone and Naprosyn. Excluding certain foods from her diet is something helpful that she can do for herself.

Nearly half of the 1,051 US participants in the Arthritis Survey – 495 individuals, or 47 percent of the group – said they had changed the way they eat because of arthritis. A few others made a change because of some other health problem. 'After my heart attack,' reported a retired executive from Michigan with a twenty-year history of osteoarthritis, 'I lowered my cholesterol and fat intake. I eat less red meat, more fish and chicken. This seems to have helped the arthritis, too.'

Does nutrition play a role in arthritis care? The short answer is: *Yes, it does*. But the full answer – the one that addresses your surprise or pleasure or disgust at the very idea of a nutritional approach to arthritis; the one that explores the issue with awareness of the hundreds of 'arthritis diets' laying false claim to a cure; and the one that serves up the fruits of survey participants' experience as specific information for your use – that answer will take the rest of this chapter to explain.

Nutrition's Role in Arthritis

The word *nutrition* is a shorthand way of saying many different things. When we state that nutrition plays a role in arthritis care, we have three definitions in mind: (1) your *general approach* to diet, whether you are extremely health-conscious or an avowed 'junk food junkie'; (2) the *amount* you eat, whether that makes you overweight or undernourished; and (3) the *specific food items* you may try to avoid or consume in quantity, because they either aggravate or ameliorate your arthritis pain. As you will see, some survey participants have succeeded in making themselves feel better by adopting a more healthful, well-balanced diet, by losing weight, by identifying certain foods as friend or foe, and by combining two or three of these approaches. Overall, the changes in their eating habits add up to a more healthful, sensible diet that their families can enjoy with them.

The participants who have eased their arthritis pain by changing their food habits include people with osteoarthritis and rheumatoid arthritis, many of whom had been seriously afflicted for years and had already undergone a wide variety of advanced treatments, from 'second-line' drugs such as penicillamine and gold injections to joint-replacement surgery.

It is more than likely that you, too, can benefit from a change in diet.

Conflicting, Confusing Claims

If doctors have been taciturn on the subject of nutrition (and they have), self-styled experts have more than made up for medicine's silence by generating dozens of diets and dietary theories about arthritis. The result, survey participants reported, is mass confusion. Even those participants who were *receptive* to the help nutrition may bring were frustrated by the welter of conflicting opinions. 'I have tried to put the suggestions on diet and nutrition which abound in the books and magazines into practice,' wrote a housewife from New York. 'But because much of this information is so contradictory, it is hard to know what is valid and what is not. For just about every group of foods, there is a practitioner who will approve its use, and on the other side of the issue, one who will suggest that it be avoided or eliminated completely.

'Some nutritionists,' she continued, 'stress the importance of the acid-alkaline or the calcium-phosphorus balance, or balancing the complete body chemistry. Others stress proper food-combining or a raw foods diet. And most nutritionists advise gradually eliminating medications once nutrition therapy is started. I once wanted to try a combination of zinc and manganese supplements I had read about that was supposed to have the same effect as the penicillamine I was taking. But when I described the plan to my doctor, he called the idea quackery and said he could not be responsible for my condition if I went ahead with it, and I did not. As for the diets, I have kept notebooks and charts for myself so I could follow the effects of various ones without losing my mind.'

Her perseverance paid off: 'Over the years I have worked out a diet plan for myself through trial and error that seems to keep my severe rheumatoid arthritis from getting worse.'

What the Doctor Ordered

Although about half of the US survey participants heard nothing from their doctors about nutrition, several hundred did get *some* advice, even if it was just a casual suggestion to lose weight, or to try to eat more fibre or less salt. Here's a summary of what our participants were told.

US Survey Advice	Number of Participants Given This Advice
Nothing (no advice) / 'There is no connection.'	583*
'Avoid fats.' / 'Eat more greens.' / Other specific dos and don'ts	146
'Eat a well balanced diet.' / 'Get proper nourishment.'	112
'Lose weight.' / 'Don't gain weight.'	95

* These are numbers of participants, not the numbers of doctors who advised them. Many participants heard the same advice (or lack of it) from several doctors. Thus, the 583 participants who report that their doctors told them nothing about nutrition may be referring to several thousand physicians.

It's not hard to understand why the most common advice is no advice. Most medical doctors have little or no training in nutrition and are hard put to offer such counsel. They could, of course, refer their patients to experts on nutrition, and some of them do, but most medical doctors don't see any reason to refer – because they don't see any connection between nutrition and arthritis. Some of them are prejudiced against nutritional approaches as a result of watching their patients try faddish and even exploitative diets, to no avail. And, since medical research has ignored the role of nutrition in arthritis until very recently (see Chapter 11), doctors have felt justified in ignoring it, too. Doctors' no-comment stance on nutrition evoked lots of comments from participants, however. Here's a sample.

A retired graphic artist from Florida: 'Doctors avoid talking about nutrition, and very often, when questioned, will just snicker.'

A naval officer from California: 'Doctors don't give such information. One has to beg or force this data.'

A retired college professor from Minnesota: 'I have learned that rarely does an M.D. know much about nutrition.'

An archaeologist from Tennessee: 'Most know less about this than I do.'

A former research chemist from Pennsylvania: 'I don't think there is enough known about the relationship between nutrition and arthritis. Most doctors seem to know very little about nutrition. I would like to know what foods are hurting me and what foods would help my condition.'

The bulk of the specific dietary advice from doctors, such as it was, did not relate to arthritis per se, but to improving the participants' general health or to applying a nutritional solution to some other health problem they had, whether it was high cholesterol ('Eat fewer eggs') or high blood pressure ('Stay away from salt').

The Importance of a Well-Balanced Diet

Many survey participants and the doctors who advised them stressed the importance of a well-balanced diet. But *well-balanced diet*, like *proper nutrition*, is a vague term that leaves too much unsaid. After all, the diet that was long synonymous with good living in the United States – full of meats, whole milk, and lavish desserts – was well balanced. But now it turns up unhealthy on several counts, and gets blamed for a variety of unwanted conditions that are all too prevalent in this country, such as obesity and clogged arteries.

While it seems obvious that anyone stands to benefit from a well-balanced diet, people with arthritis need to take extra care to eat well, because the illness creates its own special obstacles to good nutrition. For example, you may find, as nearly two hundred of the US participants reported, that pain often interferes with your food shopping or cooking. Nausea and other gut reactions to medications may kill your appetite, while *requiring* you to eat something each time you take a pill. And there is evidence that arthritis, especially rheumatoid arthritis, interferes with the way your body absorbs nutrients from foods. Indeed, doctors at the University of Alabama's Spain Rehabilitation Centre found that twenty-seven of thirty-eight hospitalized patients with rheumatoid arthritis were malnourished, and that the malnutrition *alone* made these individuals fare worse in the long run than their peers who also had rheumatoid arthritis.

What's more, several arthritis medications can rob your body of one or more vitamins and minerals. (See Chapter 14 for specific drug-nutrient interactions.)

The details of a healthful well-balanced diet are spelled out in our Arthritis Survey Diet and Thirty-Day Meal Plan (see Chapter 13). A registered dietitian worked with us to create this diet. It combines participants' successful strategies with the best available medical wisdom on general nutrition, and it translates the information into tasteful menus that you can prepare easily – with the least amount of peeling or dicing and the shortest possible time at the stove.

'I can't prove that nutrition directly helps or relieves arthritis,' conceded a homesteader from Wisconsin. 'I simply believe a healthy dietary program has given me a basis for good health – even with some arthritis.'

There are several other benefits of healthful eating that our participants enjoyed. 'I get a better sense of well-being from eating fresh, well-balanced meals,' said the coordinator of an antipoverty agency in Maryland, 'and this helps to counteract the depression and anger that often accompany arthritis.' A former manager and lecturer for Weight Watchers in Delaware wrote, 'A light diet of fruits, vegetables, and seafood, chicken, turkey, or veal makes me feel more alert and in control.' And a librarian from West Virginia found, 'When I eat well-balanced meals low in salt and full of vegetables, fruit, and fibre, I feel much more active and happy.'

The (Relative) Value of Weight Loss

Excess body weight undoubtedly puts an extra burden on joints already stressed by arthritis. Most participants who adopted a weight-loss diet to take the load off their joints were extremely pleased with the outcome. 'My doctor told me to lose thirty-five pounds or there was no sense in my seeing him for treatment,' said a thirty-seven-year-old insurance agent from New York. 'He encouraged me along the difficult road, and I have managed to keep my weight down because I know I am being helped. Diet and weight maintenance go hand in hand with my arthritis. When I was heavier, I felt more uncomfortable. I did not realize then how the extra weight was pulling on my spine.' 'It is essential to keep weight under control – carrying more hurts, whether it's shopping or body fat,' said one woman from London.

A few participants bemoaned the fact that they had been unable to shed excess weight, and even wonder what's the use of trying. 'My doctor insists I lose weight,' wrote a lab technician from New Jersey. 'This is easier said than done, because if I could, I would. Nobody likes to be fat. It makes sense to take the pressure off my knees by losing weight, but there is no such pressure on my finger joints – and look how they ache.'

True, there is a limit to what weight loss can do for arthritis pain.* It seems most helpful for the weight-bearing joints – the spine, legs, and feet. But weight loss has also improved conditions in the *non*-weight-bearing joints of some of our participants. This may have come about because the dietary changes they made to cut calories removed some offending foods from their dinner plates and replaced them with others that may have had positive effects. A case in point is the substitution of fish for red meat.

Foods to Avoid

Food allergies are sometimes at the root of arthritis. The fire in the joints turns out to be an allergic reaction to some food – milk, for example – and cutting the food out of the diet amounts to curing the disease. The arthritis goes away, but the allergy remains, and drinking milk again will bring the arthritis back. Although true food allergies can masquerade as arthritis, such cases are thought to be quite rare. A more common phenomenon, observed by roughly 10 percent of the US survey group, is food *intolerance* or *sensitivity*. If you are sensitive to certain foods, they may trigger pain when you eat them, even though your body does not mount an allergic reaction to them. It would be great to avoid pain by avoiding those foods, but how do you learn which ones are the culprits?

One way is to seek them out systematically – by keeping a food diary, in which you write down everything that goes down,

---

* *Before* the fact, avoiding excess weight may help people avoid osteoarthritis of the knees, according to doctors at the Boston University Arthritis Centre who studied the connection between obesity and arthritis.

and a pain diary, where you track the course of your arthritis pain. By comparing the two records, you may be able to discover telling patterns. Suppose, for instance, that you are sensitive to tomatoes. Then each mention of tomatoes in the food diary should match up with a note about extra discomfort in the pain diary. But, as you might imagine, this kind of record keeping is a lot of work. And even if you are meticulous with your notes, you may be stymied by other factors that blur the relationships between food and pain. Was it the tomato salad on Tuesday that gave you grief on Wednesday? Or was it the fact that you exercised too vigorously? And wasn't that the night you didn't get enough rest?

Another way is to take advantage of the US participants' findings. Since many of them agreed on the identity of certain food troublemakers, we can post a 'most *un*wanted' list of items. You could start by avoiding or cutting down on your consumption of one or more of these and see how you feel as a result. It will likely take several weeks for you to notice any difference in the way you feel. In scientific studies of dietary changes for people with arthritis, results have followed within one to six weeks, depending on the kind of changes made.

Beef and Other Red Meat

More people in the US survey avoided red meat than any other single staple. It's not that all 155 of these individuals are vegetarians, since most of them do eat fish and fowl. Some avoid red meat simply because cutting out the beef enables them to cut down on calories and consume less fat and cholesterol. Others have found that eating meat aggravates their pain. 'Red meat seems to increase pain and stiffness,' wrote a homemaker from Michigan, 'so I have virtually eliminated it from my diet. I eat more fruits and vegetables, and have increased my intake of calcium-rich foods, such as low-fat milk. I wish more research were being done into the relationship between diet (especially the chemicals used in growing and processing foods, the hormones given to animals, etc.) and the level of pain and crippling. I don't think these things cause arthritis, but they may exacerbate the symptoms.'

Some participants discovered the aggravating effect of meat by accident. 'My daughters are vegetarians,' said an accounting clerk from New York. 'This past year I've followed a mainly vegetarian diet, and I find I feel better and seem to have less arthritis pain.'

'I decreased my red meat intake at the suggestion of a nurse,' reported a program secretary from Florida. 'I have less swelling of my knees and toes since that time.'

A photojournalist from Massachusetts said her medicines made her give up meat: 'Since I started taking anti-inflammatories, I have been unable to eat meat. My idea of bliss used to be a totally fatless, medium-rare roast beef sandwich on super caraway rye. When I threw up seven times after eating one, I began to catch on that something had changed in my system.'

Switching to a strict vegetarian, or vegan, diet proved helpful to a group of Swedish men and women with rheumatoid arthritis who took part in a diet study. They learned how to cook vegetarian cuisine from Dr. Lars Sköldstam and his staff at Sweden's Sundsvalls Hospital, and they stayed on the diet for four months. After that many weeks without meat, twelve of the twenty patients said they felt better, although by Dr. Skoldstam's more rigid criteria, only eleven (55 percent) had really improved. 'Many patients with mild or moderate rheumatoid arthritis benefit from eating the vegan diet,' Dr. Skoldstam concluded in the *Scandinavian Journal of Rheumatology* (1986), 'in that they will feel subjectively better. However, the diet does not seem to significantly suppress the rheumatoid disease. . . .' This is high praise for vegetarianism, since most prescription drugs for arthritis also make people feel better without squelching the disease.

In the UK survey 52 people out of 462 participants said they avoided red meat – that's 11 per cent of the survey group.

Sugar . . . and sweets in general

A sweet tooth is an added handicap for a person with arthritis, claimed 148 of the US survey participants. 'When my arthritis was at its worst,' recalled a twenty-eight-year-old registered nurse from Texas, 'the main thing that aggravated it was sugar.' Many others echoed the same theme, including this magazine editor from New Jersey: 'I avoid processed sugar in high concentration because it seems to make me flare.' And a retired teacher from California said, 'I changed my eating habits many years ago because of high cholesterol. Now I find that if I go off my diet and eat sweets, my fingers become swollen and inflamed.'

In the UK survey 59 people, or 13 per cent of the survey group said they avoided sugar.

Fat and Fried Foods

Public enemy number three in the US survey participants' estimation was fat, forsworn by 135 of them. 'After seeing a rheumatologist and an internist, I went to a nutritionist who changed my diet and eased the pain,' wrote an aluminium welder from upstate New York. 'I eat nothing fried. I cook vegetables in a wok with a small amount of oil. My fish is baked or broiled.'

Please be sure not to throw out the good fats with the bad. Tuna and salmon, for example, are fatty fish, but theirs is the good kind, or highly unsaturated fat, which has been shown in scientific studies to help control joint inflammation for some people with arthritis. Bad fat is the saturated kind found in butter, palm oil, and untrimmed meat – the fat condemned by the 1988 Surgeon General's Report on Nutrition and Health.

To find out about the amount of fat in many of the foods you eat, just read the labels. It takes a little time to get familiar with the format, but food labelling is the most accessible and reliable source of information about what's in what you eat. The label tells you, among other things, the number of calories per serving and the amount of protein, carbohydrate, and fat in the food. These amounts are given in 'grams per serving,' and the fewer grams of fat, the better. (A gram is the metric system's equivalent of ½₈ of an ounce.)*

---

* Food labels let you calculate the number of calories from fat in any food, if you remember that fat gives you 9 calories per gram. The label on a quart of skim milk, a very low-fat food, shows that it contains 1 gram of fat per serving. That's 9 calories worth of fat in each glass of skim milk. Whole milk, by comparison, contains 8 grams of fat per serving, or 72 calories' worth of fat. And the fat is what gives a glass of whole milk almost twice as many calories as there are in a glass of skim milk.

Salt

Salt aggravates pain or swelling for ninety-eight US survey participants. 'Salt is one of the worst things for arthritis,' maintained a corporate vice-president from Iowa. To cut it down or out of your diet, you not only have to stop using the saltshaker at the table but leave this ingredient out of your cooking, and avoid it when you shop, the way this masonry contractor from Pennsylvania does. 'I eat low-sodium-chloride foods, low- or no-fat foods, low sugar. I buy low-sodium, low-fat cheese. When my knee is most inflamed, eating foods that are high in salt or refined sugar will intensify the arthritis and prolong the pain.'

A Pennsylvania researcher found that salt exacerbated the side effects of her medication. 'I avoid salt because prednisone encourages water retention and swelling, and the low-sodium diet reduces the swelling.' Since it is the sodium in salt that causes most salt-related problems, look for the sodium content in foods when you read labels.

In the UK survey 69 participants or 15 percent of the survey group avoided salt.

Caffeine

Of the fifty-six US participants who avoided caffeine, twelve mentioned coffee in particular, and eight singled out tea. Other sources of caffeine are cola-type sodas and chocolate. If you are really sensitive to caffeine, watch your pharmacy purchases, too, since several over-the-counter medicines contain caffeine. A retired aerospace engineer from New York, who once drank seven to ten cups of coffee a day, made several helpful changes in his diet: 'I quit drinking so much coffee and began avoiding the nightshades [see pages 196–197] as much as possible. After I started on this diet, the pain diminished and has mostly disappeared. But two or three cups of coffee will bring the pain back to my hips within twelve hours.

'My younger brother has arthritis in his hips, knees, and hands,' the engineer continued. 'He was in the same environment and business as I was. He usually spends a month with us each summer on board our boat, eating our diet, and feels and acts much better. But I can't convince him to change his diet.'

Scientists at Washington State University found that caffeine makes people lose calcium in their urine faster than they usually do. Since the health of your bones may already be threatened by arthritis itself or some of the drugs used to treat it, *losing* calcium is a bad idea. This study suggests a rationale for switching to decaffeinated brews.

In the UK survey 59 participants or 13 per cent of the survey group avoided caffeine.

Dairy Products

Adding the number of US participants who avoided dairy products altogether (nineteen), or milk alone (sixteen), or cheese alone (fifteen), gave a total of fifty individuals. One, a student and math tutor from Washington, was forced off milk by her inability to digest milk sugar – a condition known as lactose intolerance. But several participants blamed dairy products for arthritis pain. A California waitress found, 'If I eat any dairy product or calcium-rich food, I become immobile! My fingers and ankles swell and I cannot walk. I worry about osteoporosis, but the arthritis pain is too great if I eat these foods. I never noticed any milk sensitivity before four years ago. And as long as I don't drink it, I remain fairly pain free and mobile.' The same is true for a few people whose stories have been told in the medical literature because their severe chronic arthritis all but vanished when they banished milk from their diet. (See Chapter 11.)

Cheese avoidance often has as much to do with the fat and salt in cheese as the milk it contains. Likewise, the four additional participants who avoided ice cream may be offended by the fat, the sugar, the cream/milk, or all three.

In the UK survey 13 people or 4 per cent of the group avoided dairy products altogether, 19 or 4 per cent avoided milk, 33 or 7 per cent avoided cheese and 19 or 4 per cent avoided ice cream. Adding the dairy products, milk and cheese avoiders gives a total of 65 people.

Nightshade Vegetables

Although hundreds of survey participants advocate eating more vegetables, forty-eight US participants steered clear of one or all vegetables in the family known as the nightshades – tomatoes, white potatoes, eggplant, and bell peppers of all colours. The black pepper used for seasoning is not part of this problematic family, but paprika is.

'I do not eat any of the nightshade vegetables,' wrote a retired dressmaker from New York. 'If I do, I get red hot and swollen knuckles on both hands. It takes a week or two for this to clear up.' Some participants sacrificed these foods willingly, while others mention how much they miss eating the produce from their summer gardens. 'I eliminated the nightshade vegetables, which helped relieve the discomfort,' reported a sales associate from New Jersey, 'but it is very difficult cooking for my Italian family without tomatoes, peppers, and eggplant.'

The 48 people in the US survey who avoided nightshades accounted for about 5 percent of the entire group of 1,051 participants. This statistic is in line with the estimate made by Dr. Norman Childers, who first observed the irritating effect of nightshades on his own arthritis and later concluded that only 5 to 10 percent of all people with arthritis could be helped by dropping these foods from their diet. If you are one, you must be especially careful to read labels on prepared foods, from soup to chips, because flakes of tomatoes, starch from potatoes, and pieces of peppers can crop up *anywhere*. It may take six weeks for you to notice an improvement on a no-nightshades diet. And remember that tobacco is also a nightshade, or solanaceous plant, so you can't smoke it or chew it.

In the UK survey 23 people or 5 per cent of the survey group avoided nightshade vegetables.

Pork and Smoked or Processed Meats

Whether they mention pork by name or make a blanket rejection of smoked or processed meats such as bacon and bologna, thirty-seven US survey participants stayed away from them. Pork is a pain-inducer for some, while others find it too fatty. Smoking and processing add carcinogens to these insults. Nitrates, which often show up on lunch-meat labels as preservatives, were found to aggravate some people's arthritis in a food-allergy study at the University of Florida. In the UK survey 26 people or 6 per cent of the survey group avoided pork, while 32 or 7 per cent avoided smoked or processed meat.

Alcohol

Several of the thirty-four US participants who curtailed or cut out alcohol consumption said they understood the temptation to drown out pain by having a few drinks. The irony, they said, is that the alcohol can actually make things worse. 'Alcohol makes my joints swell,' wrote a visiting nurse from New Hampshire. 'I avoid alcohol and foods that will upset my stomach, since the medicines do enough damage.'

Another reason to avoid alcohol is that heavy drinking (more than two drinks per day) can weaken your bones. Indeed, the Arthritis Foundation now warns that alcohol may contribute to osteoporosis.

In the UK survey 69 participants or 15 per cent avoided alcohol.

Junk Food

With deference to those who believe a balanced meal is a fast-food special in each hand, thirty-two US participants gave up junk food for more healthful diets featuring lots of fresh fruits and vegetables. The UK survey group actively avoided junk food in greater numbers – 148 participants or 32 per cent avoided junk food.

Starches

Highly processed starches such as white bread, white flour, and white rice fell by the way for thirty-one US participants, who replaced them with whole-wheat bread and flour and brown rice. Most of them were after the fibre that whole-grain products preserve. Some find that the fibre works better than taking a laxative for the constipating effects of various arthritis medications.

An additional sixteen US participants avoided any and all wheat products, including cereals and pasta, because they find these foods aggravate pain and inflammation.

In the UK survey 35 participants or 8 per cent avoided refined starches; 16 or 4 per cent avoided wheat.

Additives and Preservatives

Do you ever feel you need to study chemistry to understand the ingredients in foods? Twenty-nine of the US participants studiously avoided the chemicals put in foods to give them longer shelf lives. Colourings were also suspect for some. 'U.S. yellow #4 makes my joints swell,' said a receptionist from Washington. 'I avoid all medicines coloured with this. I eat a high-protein, high-fibre diet, avoiding grease and saturated fats, and find this gives me increased general health and enhanced response to pain medications and anti-inflammatories.' In the UK survey 66 participants or 14 per cent avoided additives and preservatives.

Acid Foods

Twenty-three US survey participants avoided foods with a high acid content, such as tomatoes and vinegar. 'I find acid-heavy foods produce a reaction and increase my pain level,' wrote the manager of an automobile dealership in Massachusetts, 'so I try to monitor my acid intake.'

Another seventeen US participants specified citrus fruits, high in citric acid, as items to avoid. 'By trial and error, by eliminating certain foods over a period of more than two years,' reported a retired bookkeeper from Florida, 'I have found that I must avoid members of the nightshade family, as well as wheat and citrus.'

Seventy-three UK participants or 16 percent of the survey group avoided acid foods. A further 60 participants or 13 percent avoided citrus fruits.

Chocolate

Chocolate stands in a class by itself. In addition to the 148 US participants who avoided sweets in general, 21 made it a point to turn down chocolate. Chocolate is not only sweet but high in fat, and also contains caffeine, so it's hard to say which element is the offending one. 'I try to avoid an overload of chocolate,' said a homemaker from Michigan, 'which I've found tends to make my hands and fingers feel stiff and achy.' By contrast chocolate didn't present as a major food to be avoided by our UK participants.

Purines

If you've ever been told that diet plays no role in arthritis, you've probably also heard the tag line, 'except for gout.' Gout is the one form of arthritis that everyone knows can be controlled by diet. The pain of gout is caused by crystals that accumulate inside the joints. The crystals come from uric acid, and much uric acid comes from eating certain foods, such as liver and kidney, and drinking certain drinks, such as beer and wine. If you have gout, you can help keep the crystals from lodging in your joints – and protect yourself from painful attacks – by avoiding foods that contain *purines*, which break down to form uric acid in your body. Thirteen of the US survey participants had gout in addition to rheumatoid or osteoarthritis, and sixteen said they avoided foods with a high purine content. It is ironic that anchovies, herring, and sardines, which may be so beneficial for people with other forms of arthritis, can actually aggravate gout because of their high purine content. Other types of fish, however, have no more purines than equivalent portions of chicken, turkey, or non-organ meats. Purines were avoided by 19 people or 4 percent of the UK survey group.

US Survey

Item	Number of Participants Who Avoid it
Red meat	155
Sugar	148
Fats	135
Salt	98
Caffeine	56
Nightshades	48
Alcohol	34
Junk food	32
Starches:	
Refined (white) flour and rice	31
All wheat products from cereal to pasta	16
Additives and preservatives	29
Acid foods	23
Citrus	17
Pork	20
Smoked or processed meats	17
Dairy products:	
All	19
Milk	16

Cheese	15
Ice cream	4
Soda (colas/carbonated beverages)	16
Purines (liver, etc.)	16
Mixes, prepared or processed foods	20
Canned vegetables	11
Spices	14
Eggs	13
Yeast or fermented foods	6

UK Survey

Type of food	No. of participants avoiding it
Junk foods	148
Acid foods	73
Alcohol	69
Salt	69
Additives and preservatives	66
Citrus	60
Sugar	59
Caffeine	59
Carbonated drinks	55
Red meat	52
Refined flour	35
Smoked or processed meat	32
Cheese	33
Pork	26
Nightshade vegetables	23
Milk	19
Ice cream	19
Purines	19
Wheat	16
All dairy	13

Having listed the foods most likely to offend, let us reiterate that these sensitivities are a personal matter. 'I do believe in my case that there is a correlation between food allergy and a flare-up of pain with my rheumatoid arthritis,' wrote a thirty-two-year-old registered nurse from South Dakota who saw an allergy specialist because she also had asthma. 'But even if arthritis is food-related for everyone, not everyone is allergic to the same food substances. Milk, eggs, and chocolate cause my problem. Someone else could be allergic to peanuts!'

Foods to Favour

Just as they have learned to avoid certain substances, many of the US participants sought out other foods for their good features, from high-fibre and low-calorie content to extra bounties of vitamins, minerals, and essential fatty acids. They chose some items as more healthful substitutes for others they must avoid, such as eating chicken or turkey instead of red meat. Perhaps even more interesting are the foods they pile in because they saw them as a form of treatment, whether it's calcium disguised as a glass of skim milk or an anti-inflammatory that looks like fillet of sole. Here are the items our participants ate more of, and the reasons why.

Vegetables

Green, leafy, raw and *fresh* were the words most commonly used by the 204 US survey participants who added more vegetables to their diet. 'My doctor told me that nutrition *can* help with arthritis,' reported a retired accountant from California whose rheumatologist was treating her with a combination of experimental and standard treatments. 'I eat more leafy green vegetables, more fruit, and fewer dairy products. After paying more attention to my eating habits, I find a marked difference in the inflammation of my joints.'

Fruit

Fresh fruits follow right behind the vegetables in the US survey, with 174 participants eating more of them, or drinking more fruit juice, or both. 'I notice a lot of what I eat depends on how I feel on certain days,' said an Idaho homemaker who cut out fats, curtailed sugar, and now eats more raw vegetables and fresh fruit. 'The fresh fruits are so refreshing when you don't feel so perky.'

Fruits, like vegetables, are also a good source of dietary fibre. An additional forty-two US participants said they ate more high-fibre foods now, including fruits, vegetables, and whole grains.

Fish

'I try to eat more fish,' wrote a personnel specialist from Illinois, one of eighty-nine US survey participants who made this change. Why? 'I read an article that suggested the oils from cold-water fish have a beneficial effect on some forms of arthritis.' There is indeed a great deal of research interest now in fish-heavy diets and in dietary supplements of fish oil. (See Chapter 12 for research on diets, and Chapter 11 for studies regarding fish-oil supplements for arthritis.)

'My husband and I are vegetarians,' said an executive secretary from California, 'but we have recently added fish to our diet because of current information.'

Although fish has always been a healthful alternative to meat protein, the big news in fish now is the high content of omega-3 fatty acids in certain cold-water varieties, such as Norway sardines, Atlantic mackerel, herring, salmon, and Greenland halibut. One of the US participants, a retired airplane pilot from Alaska, reported that he had been following this hot new trend for more than thirty-five years: 'I got off sugar and salt in 1953,' he wrote. 'As a bush pilot I often had trouble getting green or fresh vegetables, but I ate a high percentage of fish, heavy on omega-3 – lots of king salmon – and the red meat of wild game like moose and caribou.' Omega-3 fatty acids, which are thought to protect the heart and relieve inflamed joints, can also be found in the wild-growing green vegetable called purslane, and in several kinds of beans, as well as walnuts and chestnuts. Two participants said they had begun to eat more tofu, or soybean curd, which is yet another omega-3 source.

Chicken and Turkey

Fowl is a fine low-fat alternative to beef and other meats, particularly if you remove its skin before cooking. Sixty-one survey participants said they ate more chicken and turkey now.

Milk

Milk, especially low-fat milk, was the favourite way of getting more calcium for thirty-seven US participants. It's also the best drink to take with many medications, including aspirin, because it can protect your stomach from some drug side effects. Another five participants ate more yoghurt, and seven prefered to get their calcium from cheese.

Calcium-rich Foods

Not counting the more-milk drinkers, another twenty-two US participants told us that they sought out calcium-rich foods to ward off osteoporosis. Participants who took prednisone and other steroids were particularly worried about thinning bones as a side effect of the drugs. And arthritis alone can do a fair degree of bone damage at selected sites.

We tend to think of dairy products as the prime providers of calcium, and most of them are, but sardines or salmon (eaten with the bones), and oysters are also rich sources. So are selected vegetables, such as spinach, collard greens, and broccoli.

Water

Whether it comes from the tap or an imported bottle, twenty-two US participants advocated drinking more water because it performs so many vital functions, from aiding digestion to helping the kidneys eliminate the end products of various arthritis drugs.

A List of Foods
US Participants Favour

Item	Number of Participants Who Eat More of It
Vegetables	204
Fruit	174
Fish	89
Fowl	61
Fibre	42
Milk	37
Whole grains	34
Calcium-rich foods	22
Water	22
Protein, including lean meats	14
Garlic	7

Summary of Nutrition Advice from Survey Participants

Although opinions vary widely on the subject of nutrition and arthritis, survey participants' experience supports these ten recommendations.

1. At the very least, you may improve your overall health by re-evaluating your eating habits and trying to improve your diet to make it more nutritious.

2. Take care to avoid faddish or extreme diets that may leave you open to vitamin deficiencies or other nutrition problems.

3. Question any diet or any advisor who urges you to stop taking your prescribed medications.

4. Don't expect a lot of nutrition advice from your doctors, but do inform them of any significant change in diet that you plan to make.

5. If you are overweight and are troubled by arthritis in your weight-bearing joints, you can likely gain mobility and comfort by losing the extra pounds.

6. If you decide to lose weight, do it slowly, by adopting a more healthful style of eating, rather than following a 'crash' diet for a quick loss.

7. Try to discover your own food sensitivities by eliminating some of the food items voted by participants as the most likely to be irritating. The top five offenders are red meat, sugar, fat, salt, and caffeine.

8. Try eating more of the foods participants find the most beneficial. The five top favourites are vegetables, fruits, fish, fowl, and high-fibre foods such as whole-grain breads and brown rice.

9. Choose fresh foods over prepared items that are smoked, canned, or highly processed.

10. Read all you can, think it over carefully, experiment cautiously, and observe yourself to prove the value of any dietary measures you take.

Chapter 13
The Arthritis Survey™ Diet and Thirty-Day Meal Plan

• A sensible new diet based on participants' experience and current research
• General dietary guidelines • Specific thirty-day menu plan with recipes

The healthful diet laid out in this chapter is a blending of the survey participants' successful experiments with nutrition and the exciting new research that indicates an important role for dietary changes in the treatment of arthritis. If you follow the plan, you can be sure that you're heeding your doctor's advice to 'Eat well balanced meals.' You'll also have the kind of low-fat diet that is endorsed by researchers and physicians for the prevention or control of heart disease, diabetes, and certain forms of cancer. You'll be getting a rich supply of the fish oils that have been shown to control arthritis symptoms. And, although the diet is not a calorie-counting, weight-loss program, you'll find that you can indeed lose excess weight by following it.

Nutritionist Kathleen Pratt, M.S., R.D., of Olympia, Washington, worked with us to translate the survey findings on nutrition into the meal plans you see here. The recipes she created are all designed for ease of preparation, too, so that you don't have to stand and fuss for long, or do a lot of peeling, chopping, or other activities that might strain your hands.

The Arthritis Survey Diet is presented in two forms – guidelines and specifics. The guidelines sketch the basic principles and give suggestions for putting them into practice. The specifics are just that – thirty days' worth of detailed menus and recipes that you can follow to the letter or modify to meet your own particular needs.

General Guidelines

Eat less fat. Foods that are low in fat generally have fewer calories and are more healthful and nutritious. Fruits, for example, contain almost no fat. Choose naturally low-fat items over fatty foods and snacks. If you drink milk, make it skim milk. Always look for low-fat alternatives to things you normally eat, such as light margarine, light sour cream, low-calorie mayonnaise, and tuna fish packed in water instead of oil. Try to reduce the amount of fat (oil, shortening, butter, or margarine) that you use in cooking.

Cook smart. Broiling, baking, poaching, and grilling are all low-fat cooking techniques. Even stir-frying uses less fat than pan-frying. And a microwave oven, if you have one, can cook many items in a fat-free way. If you must fry, try using a non-stick pan or a cooking spray instead of butter or oil. To keep as many vitamins in your vegetables as possible, steam or microwave them instead of boiling in water. You can also sauté vegetables in a small amount of water and oil, or in a low-salt broth.

Eat more vegetables. Eat fresh ones especially, and raw vegetables in salads. Try to eat at least one meatless, vegetable/pasta dinner per week. If you wash carrots carefully, you can save yourself the aggravation of peeling them.

Eat less red meat. Substitute poultry and fish for meat as often as possible. When you do prepare red meat, select the leanest cuts and remove the visible fat before you cook it. Avoid pork altogether, if possible.

Eat more fish. Aim for a minimum of three fish dinners per week and at least two fish lunches. If you can't get fresh fish, look for frozen fish without breading. Pick the varieties that have the highest content of omega-3 fatty acids, such as Norway sardines, Atlantic mackerel, lake trout, Atlantic herring, albacore tuna, anchovies, Atlantic salmon, bluefish, pink salmon, and Greenland halibut. When you buy canned tuna, choose water-packed, as the oil used in canning is vegetable oil, which contains no omega-3 fatty acids.

Eat more poultry. When you prepare chicken for cooking, remove the skin from the individual pieces, since the skin contains much of the fat. Then prevent the meat from drying out by cooking in a covered dish or using a sauce for basting. If you roast chicken, remove the skin as you carve.

Cut down on sodium in general, and salt in particular. You can drastically reduce your sodium intake by cutting down on lunch meats, salty snacks, and prepared processed soups and sauces. In your own cooking, try substituting various herbs and spices for salt, such as rosemary on chicken, sage on cooked carrots, nutmeg on spinach, basil on peas or green beans, and fresh-squeezed lemon juice on broccoli. When you shop, look for low-salt alternatives to foods you usually buy, including low-sodium or low-salt cheeses, snack crackers, soy sauce, tomato sauce, and tomato paste.

Use sugar in moderation. You can reduce the amount of sugar in most dessert recipes without hurting the taste at all. Sugar substitutes are easily obtained, if you crave them, but you may find that you enjoy the taste of low-sugar or no-sugar-added jams and jellies, and canned fruit packed in its own juice instead of heavy syrup.

Eat lots of fibre. The complex carbohydrates that have a high-fibre content, as well as important vitamins and minerals, are whole-grain breads and cereals, fruits, vegetables, and dried beans and peas.

Don't skip breakfast. Your first meal of the day, ideally, should supply about one-quarter of your daily requirement for calories and nutrients. If you take medication with meals, a good breakfast may help you minimize some of the drug's side effects.

Learn your own food sensitivities. Many people with arthritis find that certain foods aggravate their symptoms. Chocolate is the culprit for some, while others avoid citrus fruits or the nightshade vegetables – tomatoes, white potatoes, green peppers, and eggplant. Try to determine whether you have a food sensitivity (Chapter 12 tells you how), and then avoid that food at all costs. The recipes in this section offer alternatives for most ingredients that participants singled out as problem foods.

Read labels. Let the rich trove of information on food-package labels lead you to the most nutritious items. Since ingredients are always listed in order of their concentration, with the most abundant ones first, you'd do well to pass up foods that list sugar or salt among the top three. You can also rely on the labels to alert you to hidden enemies in prepared or processed foods. Potato starch, for example, shows up in more items than you would imagine. Also check the protein, carbohydrate, and fat contents, which are listed as grams per serving, and select items that have the least fat. Low-fat foods are lower in calories, too, because fat contains more than twice as many calories per gram as protein or carbohydrate.

Make it easy on yourself. Look through the frozen foods at your grocery for nutritious convenience items that you can store for a day when you are unable to cook. Frozen vegetables are almost as good as fresh, and come to you already washed, peeled, and diced. If you can't comfortably crush a clove of garlic, by all means buy a jar of peeled, chopped garlic or use one-eighth of a teaspoon of garlic powder for each clove mentioned in a recipe.

Drink lots of water, milk, and juice. Everyone needs about eight glasses of water a day, and medications may require you to drink even more than that. Milk (skim) is generally considered the best chaser for many arthritis drugs because of its stomach-coating action. Try to have at least two glasses a day for the calcium milk provides – provided, of course, that dairy products sit well with you. If citrus is your enemy, you can still drink other fruit juices such as apple, grape, apricot, and pear. If you find caffeine irritating, stick to decaffeinated coffee and herbal tea. Postum (made from bran, wheat, and molasses) is another caffeine-free alternative in the hot-beverage department. As for alcohol, several participants report they must avoid it altogether. Alcohol's effect on the stomach is reason enough to skip it if you take aspirin or related anti-inflammatory drugs, not to mention the many other problems associated with drinking. A couple of our recipes call for small amounts of sherry or wine in sauces, but these are added before heating, so that the alcohol cooks away.

Enjoy your meals. This is neither a starvation diet nor a fad diet. For example, although we say whole-wheat bread is the best choice for toast or sandwiches, breakfast suggestions include English muffins, bagels, and biscuits. You need to eat nutritious foods, but you also need to have some variety and enjoy your meals within sensible guidelines. A very strict limited diet is impossible to stick with for long, and our goal is to give you a lifetime plan.

The Arthritis Survey Diet: Thirty-Day Meal Plan

Recipes for each day's specials (marked with an asterisk) are included right below the meal suggestions. If you read through the whole plan, you'll see we've tried to anticipate and use up leftovers where possible. Snack and dessert items are listed at the end of the chapter. Unless otherwise stated, the recipes serve four – so your family or friends can enjoy sharing these meals with you.

Day 1

Breakfast Oatmeal with raisins; whole-wheat toast with no-sugar-added jam; skim milk; fruit juice

Lunch Wild rice and chicken salad*; whole-wheat roll; melon slices; skim milk (juice)

Dinner Poached fish with snow peas*; Steamed broccoli, carrots, and onions; baked (sweet) potato with light margarine, plain yoghurt, or light sour cream

Wild rice and chicken salad

⅔ cup light mayonnaise	3 cups cooked wild rice
⅓ cup skim milk	1 (8 oz.) can sliced water
2 T lemon juice (optional)	chestnuts, drained
¼ t dried tarragon	½ t pepper
3 cups cooked cubed chicken	1 cup seedless green grapes, halved
⅓ cup finely sliced spring onions	1 cup unsalted cashews

Blend mayonnaise, milk, lemon juice, and tarragon, and set aside.
In large bowl, combine chicken, spring onions, wild rice, water chestnuts, and pepper.
Stir in mayonnaise mixture until blended.
Cover and refrigerate for two to three hours.
Just before serving, fold in grapes and cashews.

Poached fish with snow peas

2 T dry sherry	2 spring onions, split and cut into
2 T light (low-salt) soy sauce	2-inch sections
½ t grated fresh ginger	16 snow peas (mangetout)
1½ lb. fish fillets	1½ T toasted sesame seeds†

Prepare sauce by combining sherry, soy sauce, and ginger in small bowl.

Place fish in 10-inch fry pan, cover with spring onions, snow peas, and sauce.

Cover and cook over medium heat for 10 minutes, or until fish flakes.

Garnish with sesame seeds.

† To toast sesame seeds, spread them in a pan and bake at 350°F. for 10–12 mins, shaking the pan often to prevent burning.

Day 2

Breakfast   English muffin with jam; berries (fresh, or frozen ones defrosted and warmed slightly) served over vanilla yoghurt; skim milk (juice)

Lunch   Tuna with pineapple salad*, served on lettuce leaf as salad, or in pocket (pita) bread as sandwich; celery and carrot sticks; skim milk (juice)

Dinner   Spaghetti with lean ground beef and tomato sauce or white clam sauce; tossed green salad with creamy vinaigrette dressing*; (whole-wheat) Italian bread

Tuna with pineapple salad

1 can (20 oz.) crushed, unsweetened pineapple, well drained†	*1 medium red pepper, chopped (optional)*
1 can (12 ½ oz.) water-pack tuna, drained‡	*¼ cup light mayonnaise*
½ cup sliced spring onions	*¼ cup light sour cream*
	1¼ t lemon juice (optional)

In large bowl, combine pineapple, tuna, spring onions, and red pepper.

In small bowl, combine remaining ingredients, stirring until smooth.

Add dressing to tuna mixture and toss until well mixed.

Cover and refrigerate at least one hour before serving.

† If you cannot eat citrus fruits, substitute seedless green grapes.

‡ Rinsing tuna in a sieve under cold water, then pressing it dry, removes much of the salt added in packing.

Creamy vinaigrette dressing

1 T olive oil	*1 T water*
1 T red wine vinegar	*1 clove garlic, crushed (or 1 t prepared*
1 T fresh lemon juice (optional)	*garlic, or r ⅛ t garlic salt)*
1 T plain yoghurt	*¼ t pepper*

Combine all ingredients in a jar with a tight-fitting lid.
Shake well, and refrigerate until ready to serve.
(The oil may harden when chilled, so shake the jar or stir the dressing before you serve it.)

Day 3

Breakfast   Frozen waffle with light syrup or pureed fruit; skim milk; fruit juice

Lunch   Vegetable and lentil soup*; unsalted wheat crackers; apple or other fresh fruit; skim milk (juice)

Dinner   Sliced turkey breast; rice pilaf; steamed carrots; fresh fruit salad

Vegetable and lentil soup

2 cups lentils	*1 clove garlic, minced*
1 cup chopped onion†	*½ t pepper*
1 cup chopped celery†	*½ t dried oregano*
1 cup chopped carrots†	*1 can (1 lb.) or 2 cups tomato puree‡*
3 T parsley	*2 T vinegar*

Rinse lentils, drain, and place in soup kettle with 8 cups of water.
Add remaining ingredients except tomato and vinegar.
Simmer, covered, for 1½ hours.
Add tomato puree and vinegar, and cook 30 minutes longer.

   † If chopping is difficult, use frozen diced vegetables.
   ‡ If you avoid nightshades, substitute chicken broth.

Day 4

Breakfast   Shredded-wheat cereal with blueberries; bagel with cream cheese; skim milk (juice)

Lunch   Tuna salad on whole-wheat bread; celery and carrot sticks; canned peaches (in juice); skim milk (juice)

Dinner   Shrimp with lemon and garlic*; baked (sweet) potato wedges; steamed broccoli, cauliflower, and carrots

Prawns with lemon and garlic

2 lbs. raw, peeled, deveined prawns
½ cup light margarine
2 cloves garlic, chopped

¼ t pepper
1 T chopped fresh parsley (or flakes)
¼ cup fresh lemon juice (optional)

Bring 6 cups water to boiling, add prawns, bring to boil again, then lower heat and simmer about 1 to 3 minutes until prawns turn pink. Drain.

Melt the margarine in a frying pan, add garlic, and sauté a minute or two.

Add the prawns, lemon juice, and pepper; sauté about 5 minutes.

Sprinkle with parsley just before serving.

If you have a *microwave oven*, try preparing the dish this way:

In small bowl, cook garlic in margarine on HIGH for 30 seconds.

Stir in lemon juice and pepper.

Arrange prawns in a single layer in a flat baking dish.

Pour sauce over prawns and cover with wax paper.

Microwave on HIGH for 6 minutes, stopping once to stir and baste prawns.

Let stand for 2 minutes. Sprinkle with parsley.

Day 5

Breakfast Bran muffin with honey; soft-boiled egg; canned pears packed in fruit juice; skim milk

Lunch Minestrone soup; crackers with unsalted tops; bagel with light cream cheese; orange or other fresh fruit; skim milk

Dinner Baked fish fillets*; stir-fried rice*; steamed green peas; Waldorf salad prepared with low-calorie salad dressing

Baked fish fillets

2 T light margarine
½ cup slivered almonds
1 ½ T lemon juice (optional)
½ t onion powder (or powdered mustard)

Dash of pepper
1 t paprika (optional)
1 lb. fish fillets

Melt the margarine in a baking dish, stir in the almonds, and toast them in the margarine in a 350°F. oven until almonds are golden brown.

Add the lemon juice, onion powder, pepper, and paprika.
Arrange fish fillets in the mixture, turning to coat each side.
Bake in 350°F. oven for about 25 minutes, or until fish flakes.

Stir-fried rice

1 onion, chopped†
1 green pepper, chopped
2 cloves garlic, pressed
⅓ cup bouillon or broth
1 egg, slightly beaten
2 cups cooked brown rice (can be made the day before and refrigerated)

1 cup frozen peas and carrots
2 T light (low-salt) soy sauce

In a work or large fry pan, stir-fry the fresh vegetables in the bouillon until tender.
Push the fresh vegetables aside, add the egg, stirring as it cooks.
Add remaining ingredients.
Heat until peas and carrots are hot.

Day 6

Breakfast Cream of Wheat, or Wheatena, with raisins; whole-wheat toast with jam; fruit juice; skim milk

Lunch Turkey with lettuce on whole-wheat bread; skim milk (juice); banana or other fresh fruit

Dinner Vegetable linguine*; fruit salad; French bread

Vegetable linguine

8 oz. linguine or other pasta, uncooked
4 cups vegetables in bite-size pieces
(peas, broccoli, snow peas (mangetout),
zucchini (courgettes), mushrooms)
1½ t light margarine
¼ t minced garlic

1 cup low-fat ricotta cheese
2 T grated Parmesan cheese
2 T skim milk
1 egg yolk
½ t oregano, crushed
⅛ t pepper

Cook pasta according to package directions, drain, and place in large serving bowl.
Blanch vegetables in boiling water until crisp-tender (2 to 3 minutes).
Drain vegetables, add to pasta, toss gently, and cover to keep warm.
In small sauce pan, melt margarine.

Add garlic and sauté until golden. Remove from heat.

Stir in ricotta, Parmesan, milk, egg yolk, oregano, and pepper.

Cook, stirring, over low heat until hot (about 3 minutes).

Do not boil.

Blend until smooth and creamy, pour over pasta mixture, and toss gently.

Day 7

Breakfast Biscuits with no-sugar-added jam; canned peaches in their juice; low-fat cottage cheese; skim milk

Lunch Chicken and vegetable soup; whole-wheat toast; grapes or other fresh fruit; skim milk (juice)

Dinner Fish fillets with stir-fried broccoli*; brown rice pilaf; shredded apple, carrot, and raisin salad (store-bought, if the preparation taxes your hands too much)

Fish fillets with stir-fried broccoli

1 T vegetable oil
1 (16 oz.) package frozen broccoli
1 small onion, sliced
½ cup celery
1 clove garlic, minced (or ⅛ t garlic powder)

½ t oregano
1 lb. fish fillets dash of pepper
2 t lemon juice (optional)
Lemon slices, for garnish (optional)

Put oil in 10-inch fry pan, add vegetables, garlic (powder), and oregano.

Cook, stirring frequently, over medium-high heat until vegetables are crisp-tender (about 5 minutes).

Remove from heat.

Add fish to fry pan with ¼ cup water, pepper, and lemon juice.

Bring to a boil over high heat.

Reduce heat to low, cover, and simmer 5 to 10 minutes until fish flakes.

Garnish with lemon.

Day 8

Breakfast Oatmeal with nectarines; English muffin with jam; fruit juice; skim milk

Lunch Toasted cheese on whole-wheat bread; cucumber spears; fresh or frozen melon balls; skim milk (juice)

Dinner   Fish and apple kebabs*; whole-wheat noodles; steamed peas and carrots

Fish and apple kebabs

1 green pepper, cut in 1½-inch squares†
1 Golden Delicious apple, thickly sliced
½ lb. fish steak, cut in 1½-inch cubes

6 cherry tomatoes†
2 t lemon juice (optional)
1 T light margarine, melted
dash of pepper
dash of thyme

On 6 skewers, alternate green pepper, apple, fish, and tomato. Combine remaining ingredients and brush over all surfaces of kebabs.

Grill 3 to 4 inches from heat, 2 minutes per side (8 minutes total), or until fish flakes easily with fork.

Day 9

Breakfast   Whole-wheat pancakes with strawberries; fruit juice; skim milk

Lunch   Sardines on whole-wheat bread; tossed green salad; fresh fruit cup

Dinner   Poached chicken breast with fresh vegetables*; baked (sweet) potato; fresh fruit salad with yoghurt dressing*; skim milk

Poached chicken breast with fresh vegetables

4 chicken breasts
2 cloves of garlic, minced
Dash of pepper
Dash of onion powder
2 medium tomatoes, chopped‡

1 medium onion, chopped
1 large green pepper, chopped‡
2 cups mushrooms, quartered

In 10-inch fry pan, bring 1 cup of water to the boil.
Add chicken and spices.
Cover and reduce heat; simmer for 15 to 20 minutes, until chicken is partially cooked, adding more water if needed.
Add vegetables; simmer 10 to 15 minutes, until vegetables are cooked.

Fruit salad with yoghurt dressing

Apples	*Blueberries*
Bananas	*Strawberries*
Seedless grapes	*Vanilla yoghurt*
Oranges (optional)	*Shredded coconut (unsweetened)*
Raisins	
Kiwi fruit	

Use any combination of fruits you like.

Wash and prepare fruit by cubing, slicing, or separating into sections. Leave grapes, raisins, and small berries whole. Combine them in large serving bowl, cover, and refrigerate until ready to serve.

Spoon yoghurt over fruit at last moment. Sprinkle with coconut.

Day 10

Breakfast Puffed-rice cereal with banana; English muffin with jam; fruit juice; skim milk

Lunch Pasta vegetable salad; whole-wheat roll; melon slices; skim milk (juice)

Dinner Baked salmon; steamed asparagus; baked (sweet) potato wedges; marinated cucumbers; cinnamon apple ring

Day 11

Breakfast Oat'n'fruit muffin*; scrambled egg; cantaloupe; skim milk

Lunch Tuna salad in pocket (pita) bread; vegetable soup; unsalted crackers; skim milk (juice)

Dinner Beef (or chicken) and vegetable kebab; rice pilaf; fruit salad with yoghurt dressing

Oat'n'fruit muffin

1 cup whole-wheat flour	*2 eggs, beaten*
1 cup rolled oats	*2 T honey*
½ cup bran flakes	*2 T molasses*
2 t baking powder	*1 cup chopped apples, pears, or nectarines, or use prepared chopped dates, or raisins.*

1 t cinnamon
½ t nutmeg
½ t salt (optional)
1 cup skim milk
¼ cup light margarine, melted

In large bowl, combine dry ingredients. Preheat oven to 375°F.
Combine milk, margarine, eggs, honey, and molasses; stir into
dry ingredients, along with fruit, until flour is moistened.
Fill baking cups in muffin pan ⅔ full.
Bake at 375°F. for 25 minutes, or until muffins test done.
Remove to wire rack to cool. (Leftover muffins freeze well.)

Day 12
Breakfast   Cooked wheat cereal; bagel with jam; skim milk; fruit
juice; applesauce
Lunch   Herring salad plate; whole-wheat roll; melon slices
Dinner   Fast turkey pie*; tossed green salad; fruit cup; skim milk
(juice)

Fast turkey pie

2 cups cooked turkey or chicken pieces
1 (4½ oz.) can sliced mushrooms, drained
½ cup sliced spring onions

1 cup shredded Swiss cheese
1½ cups skim milk
¾ cup Bisquick
3 eggs

Layer turkey, mushrooms, spring onions, and cheese in pie plate.
Beat remaining ingredients until smooth (about 15 seconds
in blender at high speed) and pour into pie plate over turkey
combination.
Bake at 400°F. for 30 to 35 minutes, until golden brown and
knife inserted into pie comes out clean.
Let stand 5 minutes before cutting.

Day 13
Breakfast   Low-fat cottage cheese; canned peaches (in fruit
juice); raisin toast; fruit juice; skim milk
Lunch   Turkey in pita; celery and carrot sticks; kiwi or other
fresh fruit; skim milk (juice)

Dinner Poached fish fillets*; whole-wheat pasta; steamed asparagus; fruit salad

Poached fish fillets

4 cups water
1½ t salt

1½ lbs. fresh fish fillets, or frozen ones, thawed

In a 10-inch fry pan, bring water to a boil.
Add salt and place fish in a single layer in the hot water.
Cover, reduce heat, and simmer for 8 to 10 minutes, or until fish flakes easily with fork.
Drain fish before serving.

Day 14

Breakfast Apple oatmeal*; whole-wheat toast with jam; fruit juice; skim milk
Lunch Vegetable and lentil soup; rice and spinach salad*; pear or other fresh fruit; skim milk (juice)
Dinner Broiled salmon with mustard dill sauce*; steamed cauliflower; whole-wheat roll; fresh fruit salad

Apple oatmeal

½ cup diced Golden Delicious apple
⅓ cup apple juice
⅓ cup water

Dash of cinnamon
Dash of nutmeg
⅓ cup quick oats, uncooked

Combine apples, juice, water, and seasonings, and bring to a boil.
Stir in oatmeal and cook for one minute.
Cover and let stand several minutes before serving.

Rice and spinach salad

1 cup brown rice, uncooked
½ cup low-calorie Italian dressing
1 T light (low-salt) soy sauce

2 cups fresh spinach
½ cup sliced celery
½ cup sliced spring onions
Fried bacon, chopped (optional)

Cook rice according to package directions.
Transfer cooked rice to bowl and cool slightly.
Combine dressing and soy sauce, and stir into warm rice.

Cover and chill. Fold in remaining ingredients just before serving.

Grilled salmon with mustard dill sauce

1½ lb. salmon steaks (1-inch thick)	*2 T Dijon mustard*
1 cup plain low-fat yoghurt	*½ t dried dill weed*

Preheat grill.

Remove skin from salmon steaks.

Mix together yoghurt, mustard, and dill weed.

Place steaks on grill rack and brush each with sauce.

Grill 6 inches from heat for 8 to 10 minutes, brushing with more sauce as needed.

Turn steaks, brush other side with sauce, and grill 8 minutes, or until fish flakes easily with fork.

Day 15

Breakfast   Fruit and nut muffin*; poached egg; fruit juice; skim milk

Lunch   Sardine salad plate; crackers or rice cakes; kiwi or other fresh fruit

Dinner   Fast vegetable pie*; tossed green salad with dressing; fresh or frozen melon balls; skim milk

Fruit and nut muffin

2 cups flour	*1 cup grated apple*
½ cup sugar	*½ cup raisins*
2 t baking soda	*½ cup chopped pecans*
½ t salt (optional)	*3 eggs, slightly beaten*
1 t cinnamon	*½ cup vegetable oil*
1 t nutmeg	*2 t vanilla*
1 cup grated carrots	

Combine flour, sugar, soda, salt, cinnamon, and nutmeg.

Stir in carrots, apple, raisins, and pecans.

Combine eggs, oil, and vanilla until blended; add to flour-fruit mixture, and stir until blended.

Spoon into baking cups in muffin pan.

Bake in preheated 350°F. oven for 20 to 25 minutes, or until muffins test done with a wooden toothpick.

Let muffins cool in pan on wire rack for 5 minutes. (Freeze the extras.)

Fast vegetable pie

3 cups vegetables (A cauliflower-broccoli-carrot mixture works well.)
1 (4½ oz.) can sliced mushrooms, drained
½ cup sliced spring onions

1 cup shredded Swiss cheese
1½ cups skim milk
¾ cup Bisquick
3 eggs

Steam the vegetables briefly.

Layer vegetables, mushrooms, spring onions, and cheese in pie plate.

Beat remaining ingredients until smooth (about 15 seconds in blender at high speed) and pour into pie plate over vegetable combination.

Bake at 400°F. for 30 to 35 minutes, until golden brown and knife inserted into pie comes out clean. Let stand 5 minutes before cutting.

Day 16

Breakfast Whole-wheat toast with apple butter; canned peaches (in fruit juice) with low-fat, low-salt cottage cheese; fruit juice; skim milk

Lunch Clam chowder; cheese melt on bagel; celery and carrot sticks; juice

Dinner Turkey broccoli bake*; cooked noodles; tossed salad; whole-wheat roll; skim milk

Turkey broccoli bake

1 (16 oz.) package frozen broccoli
1½ lbs. cubed cooked turkey
4 T light margarine
1 medium onion, diced
4 T flour

2 cups skim milk
1½ T lemon juice (optional)
½ t curry powder
¼ cup cheddar cheese, shredded

Steam broccoli, drain, and place in baking dish. Arrange turkey on top.

Melt margarine in small saucepan over medium heat.

Add onion and cook until tender, stirring occasionally.

Reduce heat; blend in flour.

Add milk all at once. Add lemon juice and curry powder.

Cook quickly, stirring constantly, until mixture thickens and bubbles.

Pour sauce over turkey and broccoli. Sprinkle with cheese.

Bake in preheated 375°F. oven for 30 to 40 minutes.

Day 17

Breakfast   Cream of Wheat, or Wheatena, with raisins; bagel with jam; fruit juice; skim milk

Lunch   Tuna and apple salad*; whole-wheat toast with light margarine; raw vegetables (broccoli, carrots, zucchini (courgette)); skim milk (juice)

Dinner   Beef (or chicken) Stroganoff prepared with lean meat and yoghurt; noodles or rice; steamed green beans; sliced tomatoes or cucumbers

Tuna and apple salad

1 red or Golden Delicious apple, cored
1 can (6½ oz.) water-pack tuna, rinsed and drained
¼ cup sliced water chestnuts
¼ cup chopped spring onions
Lettuce leaves
4 t lemon juice (or water)
1½ t vegetable oil
2 t light (low-salt) soy sauce

Chop half the apple; slice the other half.

Combine chopped apple with tuna, water chestnuts, and spring onions.

Arrange apple slices on leaves; top with tuna mixture.

To make dressing, combine remaining ingredients and mix well.

Day 18

Breakfast   Frozen waffle with peaches; fruit juice; skim milk

Lunch   Peanut butter and banana on whole-wheat bread; apple or other fresh fruit; skim milk (juice)

Dinner   Stovetop fish steaks*; tossed green salad; corn on the cob; whole-wheat roll; cinnamon apple ring

Stovetop fish steaks

¼ cup light (low-salt) soy sauce

¼ cup rice-wine vinegar

1 clove garlic, crushed

2 T sesame oil

1 t grated fresh ginger (¼ t powdered)

1½ lb. fish steaks (fresh tuna, halibut, or other thick fish)

1 T margarine

Combine soy sauce, vinegar, garlic, sesame oil, and ginger.

Marinate fish in above mixture for 30 minutes at room temperature.

Melt margarine in skillet.

Add fish, with marinade, and cook about 8 minutes on each side, or until fish flakes easily.

Day 19

Breakfast   Puffed-rice cereal with banana; blueberry muffin; skim milk; fruit juice

Lunch   Potato soup (or corn chowder); turkey sandwich; pear or other fresh fruit; skim milk (juice)

Dinner   Grilled fish with tangy dressing*; brown rice; steamed broccoli and carrots; fruit salad with yoghurt dressing; whole-wheat roll

Grilled fish with tangy dressing

¼ cup light mayonnaise

2 T Dijon mustard

2 T white wine

2 T lemon juice (optional)

1 clove garlic, crushed

¼ t pepper

1 to 2 lbs. bluefish or other fresh fish

2 T chopped spring onions

Combine mayonnaise, mustard, wine, lemon juice, garlic, and pepper.

Preheat grill. Place fish, skin side down on the rack.

Spread dressing thickly over top of fish.

Grill 8 to 10 minutes, or until fish flakes easily with fork.

Top with spring onions.

Day 20

Breakfast   Low-fat, low-salt cottage cheese; canned pears (in fruit juice); raisin toast; fruit juice; skim milk

Lunch   Salmon salad plate; rice cakes; carrot/pineapple/raisin salad; banana or other fresh fruit; skim milk (juice)

Dinner   Broiled chicken; rice; steamed asparagus or zucchini (courgettes); orange wedges or grapes; apple sauce

Day 21

Breakfast   Pancakes with light syrup or pureed berries; cantaloupe; fruit juice; skim milk

Lunch   Crab and prawn salad; soft bread sticks; apple wedges; skim milk (juice)

Dinner   Grilled fish fillets with sauce*; tossed green salad; baked acorn squash; steamed green beans

Grilled fish fillets with sauce

4 mackerel fillets	or
Sauce #1	Sauce #2
1/3 cup lemon juice	1/3 cup light (low-salt) soy sauce
1/2 t garlic, minced	1 T rice vinegar
1 T olive oil	1/2 t garlic, minced
1/2 t dried basil, crumbled	2 t fresh ginger, minced (1/2 t powdered)

Rinse mackerel, pat dry with paper towels, and place in baking dish.

Prepare either one of the sauces and drizzle it over the fish.

Refrigerate, covered, for 1 hour.

Arrange fillets, skin down, on grill.

Sprinkle with pepper, if you like.

Grill 6 inches from heat until fish flakes easily with fork (about 5 to 7 minutes), basting once with marinade.

Day 22

Breakfast   Bagel with light cream cheese; cantaloupe; fruit juice; skim milk

Lunch   Turkey sandwich; raw vegetables (celery, etc.); nectarine or other fresh fruit; skim milk (juice)

Dinner   Spinach quiche*; whole-wheat roll; steamed broccoli, carrots, onions; fruit salad with yoghurt dressing

Spinach quiche

2 T shallots, onions, or spring onions, minced	*⅛ t nutmeg*
2 T light margarine	*1 cup low-fat cottage cheese*
1 (10 oz.) package frozen chopped	*3 eggs*
spinach, cooked and well drained	*¼ cup shredded Swiss cheese*
⅛ t pepper	*1 9-inch pie shell (unbaked)*

Sauté shallots in margarine.

Add spinach and stir over moderate heat until water is evaporated.

Remove from heat. Add spices.

Blend cottage cheese and eggs in electric blender.

Stir in spinach mixture and Swiss cheese. Pour into pie shell.

Bake at 425°F. for 12 minutes; reduce heat to 375°F. and bake another 25 to 30 minutes until set.

Day 23

Breakfast   Oatmeal with raisins; bran muffin; honeydew melon; skim milk (juice)

Lunch   Chicken salad sandwich; cucumber spears (and tomato slices); grapes or other fresh fruit; skim milk (juice)

Dinner   Seafood fettuccine*; steamed broccoli, cauliflower, carrots, and zucchini (courgettes); fruit salad with yoghurt dressing; whole-wheat roll

Seafood fettuccine

2 cups fresh or frozen scallops, prawns, and crab meat	*1½ t light margarine*
1 clove garlic, minced	*1 cup low-fat ricotta cheese*
¼ t white pepper	*1 egg yolk*
½ t nutmeg	*2 T skim milk*
1 T parsley, chopped (or flakes)	*2 T grated Parmesan cheese*
8 oz. fettuccine or other pasta (uncooked)	

Combine seafood and garlic in a bowl, sprinkle with pepper, nutmeg, and parsley; toss gently, cover, and refrigerate for 10 to 15 minutes.

Cook pasta according to package directions, drain, place in large serving bowl, and cover to keep warm.

In large sauce pan, melt margarine, then sauté seafood over medium heat for 3 to 4 minutes, stirring constantly.
Remove from heat.
Blend ricotta cheese, egg yolk, and milk in electric blender until smooth and creamy.
Add cheese mixture to seafood and cook until thoroughly heated.
Add to fettuccine and toss gently. Sprinkle with Parmesan cheese.

Day 24

Breakfast   Poached egg on whole-wheat toast; canned peaches (packed in fruit juice); skim milk (juice)

Lunch   Mushroom barley soup; toasted cheese sandwich; apple or other fresh fruit; skim milk (juice)

Dinner   Crispy baked fish fillets*; steamed green beans; baked (sweet) potato wedges; coleslaw

Crispy baked fish fillets

1 lb. fish fillets	2 T vegetable oil
Black pepper	⅓ cup cornflake crumbs

Wash and dry fillets.
Season, brush with oil, and coat with crumbs.
Arrange in a single layer in a lightly oiled shallow baking dish.
Bake at 500°F. for 10 minutes.

Day 25

Breakfast   Shredded-wheat cereal with banana; blueberry muffin; fruit juice; skim milk

Lunch   English muffin pizza; lettuce wedge with dressing; fresh fruit cup; skim milk (juice)

Dinner   Whole fish with vegetable stuffing*; three-bean salad; brown rice; melon slices

Whole fish with vegetable stuffing

1 T light margarine	¼ t pepper
1 small onion, minced	4 red snappers (1 lb. ea.),
	Coho salmon, or trout

½ stalk celery, minced   *1 small lemon, in 4 wedges (optional)*
2 medium zucchini (courgette), diced
1 T lemon juice (optional)

Melt margarine over medium heat in 2-quart saucepan.

Add onion and celery and cook for 5 minutes, stirring occasionally.

Add zucchini (courgettes), ¼ cup water, lemon juice, and pepper; heat to boiling.

Reduce heat to low; cover and simmer for 10 minutes until tender.

With slotted spoon, fill cavity of each fish with vegetable mixture, saving the vegetable liquid. Close each cavity and fasten with toothpicks.

Arrange stuffed fish in roasting pan; spoon remaining vegetable mixture around fish and pour vegetable liquid over fish.

Bake in preheated 350°F. oven for 30 to 40 minutes, basting occasionally with pan juices until fish flakes easily with fork.

Remove toothpicks and garnish with lemon wedges.

Day 26

Breakfast   Raisin toast; fresh or frozen blueberries with yoghurt; skim milk

Lunch   Sardine sandwich; spinach salad; orange or other fresh fruit

Dinner   Vegetable pasta; Waldorf salad; whole-wheat roll; skim milk (juice)

Day 27

Breakfast   Puffed-rice cereal with blueberries; English muffin with jam; fruit juice; skim milk

Lunch   Salmon sandwich*; tossed green salad; grapes or other fresh fruit; juice

Dinner   Grilled chicken; rice pilaf; steamed peas and carrots; applesauce; skim milk

Salmon sandwich

1 can (7½ oz.) salmon, rinsed   *1 t lemon juice (optional) thin*
and drained   *slices of cucumber or zucchini (courgettes)*

2 T chopped dill pickle   whole-wheat bread
2 T reduced-calorie salad dressing

Combine salmon, pickle, salad dressing, and lemon juice; mix well.
Spread salmon mixture on whole-wheat bread, top with cucumber or zucchini (courgettes).
Serve as open-face sandwich, or top with another slice of bread.

Day 28

Breakfast   Oatmeal; biscuit with jam; fruit juice; skim milk
Lunch   Chicken salad with nuts*; whole-wheat toast;
    cantaloupe or other fruit; skim milk (juice)
Dinner   Broccoli and fish bake*; brown rice; steamed peas and
    carrots; grapes or other fresh fruit

Chicken salad with nuts

2 cups cubed cooked chicken breast   Dressing
¾ cup seedless green grapes, halved   ½ cup low-calorie salad dressing
¾ cup sliced celery   ¼ cup light sour cream
½ cup chopped pecans   ½ t grated fresh ginger (or ⅛ t powdered)
                                          ⅛ t pepper

Combine chicken, grapes, celery, and pecans in bowl and set
aside.
In another bowl, combine ingredients to make dressing.
Mix well.
Stir dressing into chicken mixture; cover and refrigerate 1 to 2
hours before serving.

Broccoli and fish bake

1 (10 oz.) package frozen broccoli   2 T flour
1 lb. fish fillets   ¾ t dried dill weed
1 T lemon juice (optional)   ⅛ t pepper
2 T light margarine   1 cup skim milk
                                          1 T grated Parmesan cheese

Cook broccoli according to package directions; drain.
Place fish fillets in baking dish; top with lemon juice and
broccoli.

Melt margarine in saucepan over low heat; add flour, dill weed, and pepper, stirring constantly over low heat until smooth.
Whisk in milk and bring to a boil, stirring constantly.
Boil and stir one minute, pour sauce over broccoli.
Sprinkle with cheese. Bake at 350°F. for 25 minutes, or until fish flakes.

Day 29

Breakfast Cream of Wheat with raisins; bagel with jam; fruit juice; skim milk

Lunch Meat loaf or tuna sandwich; tossed green salad; grapefruit or other fresh fruit; skim milk (juice)

Dinner Prawn and vegetable stir fry*; rice; Waldorf salad; melon or papaya slices

Prawn and vegetable stir fry

1 lb. fresh or frozen prawns, washed and deveined
½ t cornstarch
½ t light (low-salt) soy sauce
⅛ t sesame oil
dash of white pepper
4 oz fresh or frozen snow pea pods (mangetout)
1 T cornstarch
1 T cold water
1 T vegetable oil
1 clove garlic, finely chopped

1 t ginger root, minced (¼ t ground)
2 T vegetable oil
8 oz. bok choy (4 or 5 stalks), sliced diagonally
1 cup fresh mushrooms, quartered
2 T light (low-salt) soy sauce
¼ cup chicken broth
3 spring onions, cut in 2-inch pieces

Combine first five ingredients; cover and refrigerate for 30 minutes.
For fresh pea pods, remove strings, then cook, covered, in boiling water for 1 minute; drain. Rinse immediately under cold water, drain, and set aside.
Mix 1 T cornstarch and 1 T cold water, and set aside.
Heat work or large fry pan. Add 1 T vegetable oil, then garlic and ginger, and stir fry until garlic is light brown.
Add prawns and stir fry until prawns are pink. Remove prawns.

Add 2 T vegetable oil to wok; add bok choy and mushrooms and stir fry for one minute.

Stir in 2 T soy sauce and the chicken broth, and heat to boiling.

Stir in cornstarch/water mixture; cook and stir about 10 seconds until thickened.

Add prawns and pea pods; cook and stir for another 30 seconds.

Garnish with spring onions.

Day 30

Breakfast   Banana-bran muffin*; soft-boiled egg; orange or other fresh fruit; skim milk

Lunch   Turkey soup; spinach-avocado salad; apple or other fresh fruit; skim milk (juice)

Dinner   Chicken chow mein; rice; fresh fruit salad

Banana-bran muffins

1¼ cup whole-wheat flour	¾ cup skim milk
¼ cup sugar	1 cup mashed ripe banana
3 t baking powder	1 egg
1½ cup whole-bran cereal or bran	¼ cup vegetable oil

Sift together flour, sugar, and baking powder. Set aside.

Combine bran cereal, milk, and banana in bowl and set aside to soften.

Add flour mixture, egg, and oil to cereal mixture; mix until all ingredients are moist.

Spoon into baking cups in muffin pan.

Bake in preheated 400°F. oven for 25 minutes or until muffins test done with a toothpick.

Cool on wire rack for 5 minutes before removing muffins from pan.

Snack Items

Fresh fruit; dried fruit; low-salt crackers (with low-salt, low-fat cheese); fruit drink*; raw vegetables – plain, with creamy cottage dip,* or yoghurt and dill dip* (celery, carrots, broccoli, cauliflower, cucumber, zucchini (courgettes), snow peas, etc.); unsalted nuts; air-popped popcorn; mineral water or seltzer

Fruit drink

1 cup unsweetened strawberries or raspberries   1 banana
1 cup orange (or apple) juice

Blend fruits and juice until smooth in electric blender.
If your blender can crush ice, add a few ice cubes for a frothier drink.

Fruit shake

1 banana   Ice cubes (if blender can crush ice)
½ cup low-fat yoghurt
½ cup skim milk
1 cup fresh fruit (peaches, berries,
crushed pineapple)

Blend all ingredients until smooth in electric blender.

Creamy cottage dip

1 (12 oz.) container low-fat, low-salt   1½ T minced onion
cottage cheese   1 T chopped pimento
6 T skim milk   1 T chopped parsley

Combine cottage cheese, milk, and onion in a bowl; blend with electric mixer.
Stir in pimento and parsley.
Cover and refrigerate.

Yoghurt and dill dip

1 cup plain low-fat yoghurt   2 T chopped fresh chives (or 1 t dried)
1 t dried dill weed   Dash of pepper
1 clove garlic, pressed (¼ t powder)

Combine all ingredients and blend thoroughly.
Cover and refrigerate.

Dessert Suggestions

Ginger snaps (2); vanilla wafers (up to 5); angel food cake (thin
   slice) with fruit; arrowroot cookies (up to 3); fresh fruit (apple,

orange, grapes, banana, kiwi, melon, berries, peach, etc.); fresh fruit with yoghurt dip*; graham crackers (1 whole, or 4 small sections)

Yoghurt dip for fruit

1 cup peach- or raspberry-flavoured yoghurt   *coconut topping (unsweetened)*
⅛ t almond extract

Combine all ingredients.
Cover and refrigerate.

‡ To avoid nightshades, substitute zucchini, yellow squash, celery, onions, pineapple chunks, and sweet-potato wedges for tomatoes and green peppers.

Chapter 14
How and When to Supplement Your Diet with Vitamins and Minerals

• Countering the effects of arthritis itself
• Countering the effects of the drugs used to treat arthritis

What could be more appealing than a cheap bottle of pills – made from the same natural ingredients found in good food – that promises pain relief or overall better health, with hardly any risk of side effects? That is the inimitable appeal of dietary supplements, from vitamins and minerals to yeast, amino acids, and herbal essences such as ginseng or black cohosh root, all of which have been tried by survey participants.

In all, 777 of the 1051 participants in the US Arthritis Survey, or 73 percent of the group, and 310 of the 456 participants of the UK survey, or 68 percent of the group, take supplements of some kind. Most rely on the shotgun approach of a multivitamin and mineral tablet manufactured by a reputable company. But many seek out a single nutrient for its particular virtues, or combine a few carefully chosen correctives in a regimen tailored to meet their own special needs.

In this chapter, we'll examine all these strategies, giving you the participants' winning combinations, with support, where possible, from medical research on the value of nutritional supplements for people with arthritis. We'll translate these ideas into specific recommendations that you can discuss with your doctor.

'My rheumatologist sent me to a nearby medical school for a vitamin assay,' reported a writer from New Jersey who had osteoarthritis in her hands, ankles, and knees. 'Despite my lust for grapefruit, I turned out to be low in vitamin C, as well as several of the B vitamins. Adding supplements has been most helpful. The rheumatologist increased my C to a minimum of 1,000 milligrams daily, and double or triple that for flare-ups.'

Others have received no professional counsel, and they try this or that supplement because of its rumoured benefits, with varying degrees of success.

What Survey Participants Say About Supplements

Although close to three-quarters of the US survey participants use one or more supplements regularly, only 160 of them chose to comment on the advantages of doing so. Here's a summary of what they said.

Comment	Number of Participants Saying So
I feel supplements help/seem to help my arthritis	77
I take them for help with a specific problem, not necessarily arthritis related, such as C for colds	32
They give me more energy	26
I feel my general health is better as a result of taking them	26

Several of the 280 US participants who take no supplements say that they rely on a good nutritious diet for the vitamins and minerals they need. This may be the safest, surest course for people enjoying perfect health, but the fact that you have arthritis makes it *likely* that you might need some kind of supplement – especially if any of the following statements could have come from your lips.

- I use aspirin or other NSAIDs daily to control pain and inflammation.
- I find that arthritis drugs upset my stomach.
- I have taken lots of prednisone or other steroid drugs.
- I take penicillamine or immunosuppressive drugs for rheumatoid arthritis.
- I am about to have (or have just had) surgery.
- I am over sixty-five.

- I bruise easily.
- I frequently skip meals because of pain, and just get by on snacks.
- I am on a restricted diet.

All of these statements applied to at least some participants, and here are the supplements the US participants relied on, beginning with the most popular ones.

Supplement	Number of US Participants Taking It
Daily multivitamin with minerals	429
Vitamin C (including rose hips, bioflavonoids, and rutin)	279
Calcium	270
Vitamin E	191
Vitamin B complex	113
Vitamin A	62
Zinc	61
Vitamin D	55
Cod Liver Oil	55
Vitamin B_6 (pyridoxine)	51
Iron	43
Vitamin B_{12} (cobalamin)	40
Magnesium	39
Potassium	38
Fish Oil (such as MaxEPA)	33
Lecithin	31
Alfalfa	30
Garlic Capsules	28
Herbal Teas (including nettle, comfrey, and willow)	20
Selenium	19
Bee Pollen	17
Beta Carotene	14
Brewer's Yeast or Yeast Tablets	14
Vitamin B_3 (niacin, nicotinamide, or nicotinic acid)	12
Multiminerals	12

Kelp	10
Lysine	10
Yucca	8
Vitamin B$_1$ (thiamin)	7
Pantothenic Acid	7
Ginseng	6
Vitamin B$_2$ (riboflavin)	5
DLPA (DL-phenylalanine)	5
Folacin (folic acid)	5
Tryptophan	5
Wheat Germ Oil Capsules	5
Chromium	4
Evening Primrose Oil	4
Aloe Capsules	3
Manganese	3
PABA (Para-aminobenzoic acid)	3
Protein Powder	3
S.O.D. (Superoxide Dismutase)	3
Anti-Oxidants	2
Barley Green	2
Black Cohosh	2
Chapparal	2
Copper	2
Co-Enzyme Q10	2
Horsetail Grass	2
Iodine	2
Liver	2
Royal Jelly	2
Safflower Oil	2
Wood Betony	2
Ammonium Molybdate	1
Arginine	1
Biotin	1
Choline	1
Vitamin K	1
Ornithine	1
Phosphorus	1
Tyrosine	1

And here are the results of the UK survey. As you can see glucosamine has emerged as the leading supplement with cod liver oil and chondroitin not far behind.

Supplement	No of UK participants taking for mobility	No of UK participants taking for pain
Glucosamine sulphate	179	163
Cod liver oil	120	113
Chondroitin	92	84
Omega 3 fish oil	58	45
Evening primrose oil	36	30
Daily multivitamin	35	37
Calcium	32	35
Vitamin C	31	26
Folic acid	31	27
Selenium	28	19
Garlic capsules	27	25
Folic acid	31	27

Glucosamine

Glucosamine occurs naturally in the body and is an essential building block of complex structures called glycosaminoglycans, which are in turn essential for the growth and repair of cartilage and synovial fluid. In osteoarthritis, the cartilage roughens and the bone becomes thickened. Bony spurs form and the body tries to repair itself by producing more synovial fluid and more cartilage. Glucosamine supplements can provide the nutritional base to encourage this process.

Evidence is building to support the use of glucosamine for arthritis. The results of a major trial were reported in the *Lancet* in 2001. Professor Jean Reginster and colleagues from CHU Centre Ville, Belgium, gave patients with osteoarthritis a daily 1500 mg dose of glucosamine or a placebo over a period of three years. The researchers took radiograph images of the patients' knees while lifting a weight after one and three years. They found that those patients who completed the full course of treatment showed a 20–25 percent improvement in their symptoms compared with a slight worsening of symptoms in the placebo group.

One practical point that emerges from several studies is that glucosamine takes about a month to exert its full effects. And there is no help, as yet, in choosing which of the many different preparations available is best (if any). The cheapest might be a good place to start. No undesired side effects have been reported.

In the UK survey over 150 participants were taking glucosamine sulphate. The results look impressive for both mobility and pain relief. Sixty-eight percent reported some degree of improvement in mobility, while 58 percent reported at least some reduction in pain.

	UK Survey	UK Percentage
Number of people taking glucosamine sulphate	179	
Outcome for mobility:		
Improved mobility	55	(31%)
Somewhat improved mobility	66	(37%)
Made no difference to mobility	58	(32%)

	UK Survey	UK Percentage
Number of people taking glucosamine sulphate	163	
Outcome for pain relief:		
Greatly reduced arthritic pain	43	(26%)
Somewhat reduced pain	52	(32%)
Made no difference to pain	68	(42%)

The source material for making glucosamine products is the shells of shrimps, prawns and other shellfish, therefore making it unsuitable for vegetarians; however a vegetarian glucosamine supplement is now available produced from corn during a fermentation process.

Fish Oil

Oil from fish contains omega-3 fatty acids (EPA and DHA) which have anti-inflammatory activity. Omega-3 fatty acids are needed for prostaglandin formation, hormone-like substances within the body that regulate dilation of blood vessels. There is now good evidence to support the effectiveness of fish oil in the treatment of arthritis. In a study conducted at Albany (NY) Medical College for example, doctors gave fish-oil capsules to forty men and women.* As usual, the participants were divided into two groups, but instead of giving fish oil to one group and placebo pills to the other, *everyone* got equal time on each. Half the participants took fish oil for the first fourteen weeks, while the other half took an identical-looking pill, made by the same manufacturer but containing no fish oil. Then, for a period of four weeks, everyone took placebos, although the participants were not told when they were being switched from one type of pill to the other. In the next stage, the group that had taken fish oil for fourteen weeks started fourteen weeks of placebo capsules, and those who had taken placebos all along received fourteen weeks of fish-oil capsules. The experiment ended with another four-week period when everyone took the placebo version.

If you're wondering what it would be like to swallow fifteen pills a day in addition to your other medication(s), as these individuals had to do, you may be interested to learn that five of the original forty participants dropped out of the study because of the inconvenience of it all – downing handfuls of capsules and making regular visits to the clinic for tests. Two more were kicked out by the experimenters because blood tests showed they were not really taking the pills. Research is hard work for everyone involved – subjects and scientists alike.

At the end of the thirty-six weeks, after averaging the experiences of the thirty-three volunteers who completed the study, the researchers found that fish oil had helped the participants a lot. On the whole, they felt less pain while taking it; they had fewer tender joints; and they didn't get tired until later in the day. What's more, these benefits stuck with them for weeks after they stopped taking the fish oil. Reporting their work in *The Annals of Internal Medicine*, the researchers allowed that higher doses of fish oil, given over a longer period of time, might have done even more good. (A later study, conducted in Australia and reported in the October 1988 *Journal of Rheumatology*, supported this idea.)

Dr. Joel M. Kremer, who headed this research project as well as an earlier study that also showed rheumatoid arthritis could be improved with fish-oil supplements, recommended more fish on the dinner plate. 'The doses of fish oil given,' *Prevention* magazine quoted him, 'were roughly equal to a salmon dinner or a can of sardines.' In *Medical Tribune*, a weekly newspaper for health professionals, Dr. Kremer said, 'It is very, very interesting. Just the fact that diet can change anything, I think, is fascinating.'

Experts estimate that because of changes in our dietary habits over the past few decades 85 percent or more of people in the Western world are deficient in omega-3 fatty acids. The recommended intake of EPA plus DHA is 650 mg rising to 1000 mg per day during pregnancy and lactation.

A fifty-one-year-old Missouri waitress wrote: 'Fish oil is a wonder drug – or should I say a wonder food? The medicines the rheumatologist gave me all helped my rheumatoid arthritis, but the side effects nearly killed me. I took aspirin, Motrin, and Disalcid, and I lost twelve pounds and wound up in the hospital for five weeks with an ulcer, liver problems, heavy periods, and ringing in my ears to the point of deafness. He was about to put me on gold when I found out about fish oil *on my own*. I started taking fifteen capsules a day two years ago, and I can live again. I can move. I work five days a week as a waitress, with no stiffness, even. I get around like a sixteen-year-old.'

The Arthritis Research Campaign recommends eating oily fish, especially mackerel, sardines, pilchard and salmon, three to four times a week, and notes that apart from its benefits in helping with arthritis and rheumatism, it can also help protect you against heart disease.

Cod Liver Oil versus Fish Oil

As its name makes plain, cod liver oil comes from the liver of a cold-water fish. And some brands contain the omega-3-type essential fatty acids found in fish-oil capsules. There are important differences between the two fish oils, however. Fish oil supplements are derived from the flesh of oily fish, not the liver. The liver origin is what gives cod liver oil its store of vitamins A and D. Fish oil supplements contains very low levels of these vitamins. And so, while volunteers in research studies have taken as many as fifteen or twenty capsules of fish oil capsules every day for weeks on end – with no known ill effects – an equivalent number of cod liver oil capsules could deliver a *toxic dose* of vitamins A and D. Cod liver oil also contains more cholesterol. 'I started taking cod liver oil (my own idea to grease my joints!),' wrote a retired NASA secretary from Texas, 'and was relieved so much, but when my doctor discovered during an annual physical that my cholesterol level was three points below heart-attack level, I had to stop taking the cod liver oil.'

Vitamin A is dangerous in large amounts and in particular should not be taken by pregnant women or women who might become pregnant, as vitamin A can harm the unborn baby. Other adults should not take more than 9000 micrograms of vitamin A per day for men and 7500 per day for women. Check the amount of vitamin A listed on the packaging of your supplement.

In the UK survey 120 people took cod liver oil , while 58 said they took an Omega 3 fish oil supplement. Participants were asked to rate the supplement in terms of improved mobility and pain relief. Here are the results:

	UK Survey	UK Percentage
Number of people taking cod liver oil	120	
Outcome for mobility:		
Improved mobility	29	(24%)
Somewhat improved mobility	60	(50%)
Made no difference to mobility	31	(26%)

As you can see, an impressive 74 percent of participants found cod liver oil improved or somewhat improved their mobility.

	UK Survey	UK Percentage
Number of people taking cod liver oil	113	
Outcome for pain relief:		
Greatly reduced arthritic pain	19	(17%)
Somewhat reduced pain	45	(40%)
Made no difference to pain	49	(43%)

While the results aren't quite as impressive as for mobility, a nonetheless creditable 57 percent of participants found cod liver oil reduced their pain to some degree.

We also asked people to rate a general Omega 3 Fish Oil supplement. The results for mobility were virtually identical to those for cod liver oil:

	UK Survey	UK Percentage
Number of people taking Omega 3 fish oil supplement	58	
Outcome for mobility:		
Improved mobility	14	(24%)
Somewhat improved mobility	29	(50%)
Made no difference to mobility	15	(26%)

The results for pain relief were also very similar.

	UK Survey	UK Percentage
Number of people taking Omega 3 fish oil supplement	45	
Outcome for pain relief:		
Greatly reduced arthritic pain	8	(18%)
Somewhat reduced pain	21	(47%)
Made no difference to pain	16	(35%)

Chondroitin

Chondroitin sulfate is another natural substance found in the body. It prevents other body enzymes from degrading the building blocks of joint cartilage. The type sold in health-food stores and pharmacies is derived from animal products. Three recent clinical trials found evidence for the effectiveness of chondroitin in the treatment of osteoarthritis. In a study conducted by Ghent University Hospital, Belgium, a total of 119 patients suffering osteoarthritis in the finger joints were included in a placebo-controlled trial conducted over a three-year period. The group took 400 mg of chondrotin sulfate three times a day. The trial found that the group taking chondroitin had a significant decrease in the number of patients with new 'erosive' osteoarthritis finger joints compared to the control group. The study showed that chondroitin can modify cartilage erosion and may prevent osteoarthritis in the finger joints. Chondroitin is safe and relatively free of side effects when used at the recommended daily dosage at least for short periods of time. Unfortunately, few studies have investigated the safety and effectiveness of chondroitin when used for long periods of time. Until the long-term use of chondroitin is deemed safe, it is best to consult a healthcare practitioner before taking chondroitin supplements. Mild side effects of chondroitin reported in recent studies include diarrhoea, constipation, and abdominal pain. There have been rare reports of swelling and accumulation of fluid in the eyelids and lower limbs, irregular heartbeats, and alopecia (hair loss) after taking the supplement.

In the UK survey 92 participants were taking chondroitin for mobility and 84 for pain relief. The results again look impressive with 72 percent reporting some improvement in mobility and 64 percent reporting some degree of pain relief.

	UK Survey	UK Percentage
Number of people taking chondroitin	92	
Outcome for mobility:		
Improved mobility	27	(30%)
Somewhat improved mobility	39	(42%)
Made no difference to mobility	26	(28%)

	UK Survey	UK Percentage
Number of people taking chondroitin	84	
Outcome for pain relief:		
Greatly reduced arthritic pain	17	(20%)
Somewhat reduced pain	37	(44%)
Made no difference to pain	30	(36%)

Evening Primrose Oil

The evening primrose, whose yellow flowers open at nightfall, yields an oil from its seeds that is the plant world's answer to fish oil. Evening primrose oil, like fish oil, contains an essential fatty acid that can fight against inflammation. It is called gamma-linolenic acid, or GLA. Indeed, some researchers suspect that the combination of fish oil and evening primrose oil could be potent enough to replace NSAIDs in treating people with arthritis. Doctors at the Royal Infirmary in Glasgow tried to do just that. They enrolled forty-nine patients with mild rheumatoid arthritis in a study that lasted more than a year, and they watched many of their subjects decrease or altogether drop their drugs, while controlling their arthritis symptoms with evening primrose oil alone, or a combination of evening primrose oil and fish oil.

For the first three months of the experiment, the participants stayed on whatever NSAID they had been taking, and began swallowing an extra twelve capsules a day. Unbeknownst to them, only sixteen of the volunteers were receiving evening primrose oil in these capsules. Fifteen got identical-looking pills that contained a mixture of evening primrose oil and fish oil, while eighteen took yet another look-alike that was a placebo.*

After the first three months, the patients all tried to cut down on their drugs. (Actually, four of them had stopped taking their NSAIDs by themselves, even before the study began, because they were suffering more drug-induced stomach upset than they could bear.) The doctors' orders were to take less of the drugs, or none at all – but *only* if they could do so without making their symptoms worse. Here's what happened.

- Twenty-eight people in the study were able to reduce or stop their NSAIDs.
- Eleven of these people were taking evening primrose oil at the time.
- Twelve were taking the evening primrose/fish oil combination.
- Five were taking the placebo, although these five didn't reduce their drug dose as markedly as the others.

During this phase of the study, which lasted nine months, thirteen patients dropped out because their arthritis grew worse. And ten of them turned out to be on the placebo pills. Of the other three, one was taking evening primrose oil, one was taking the combination, and one wasn't taking anything! Routine blood tests given as part of the experiment proved that he was cheating by not using the capsules he'd been given, and he was dropped from the study.

At year's end, all the remaining patients spent three more months trying to maintain themselves on their new low dose (or no dose) of NSAIDs. Meanwhile, their daily dozen capsules were all changed to placebos (containing no vitamin E), although the subjects didn't know that this had happened. Gradually, everybody who had been doing fine on evening primrose oil began to feel worse, as did most of those who had been taking the combination capsules. By comparison, the group that had been on placebos all along continued about the same.

'In conclusion, therefore,' the doctors wrote in 1988 in *Annals of the Rheumatic Diseases*, 'we have shown that it is possible to decrease or stop NSAIDs in some patients with rheumatoid arthritis by introducing evening primrose oil or evening primrose/fish oil treatment.' They added that the best use of the oils might be for patients who couldn't take NSAIDs because of ulcers or kidney problems that would only be aggravated by the drugs.

They didn't make the next leap, though, and suggest that the oils replace the drugs generally. After all, the patients in the study didn't do *better* on the oils than on the drugs. They simply did as well.

In the UK survey fewer participants took evening primrose oil than fish oil for mobility and pain relief, but fortunately sufficient numbers did to allow us to rate their responses. The results are very similar to those for fish oil in terms of improved mobility: 70 percent found their mobility improved to some degree.

	UK Survey	UK Percentage
Number of people taking evening primrose oil	36	
Outcome for mobility:		
Improved mobility	10	(28%)
Somewhat improved mobility	15	(42%)
Made no difference to mobility	11	(30%)

Interestingly evening primrose oil scores significantly higher for pain relief than fish oil, with 70 percent saying it greatly or somewhat reduced their pain.

	UK Survey	UK Percentage
Number of people taking evening primrose oil	40	
Outcome for pain relief:		
Greatly reduced arthritic pain	13	(32.5%)
Somewhat reduced pain	15	(37.5%)
Made no difference to pain	12	(30%)

The UK participants took a number of other supplements but none in as great a number and none recorded as impressive a set of results as fish oil, evening primrose oil, glucosamine or chondroitin. However, the results did highlight some interesting tendencies. Here are the results for mobility in order of effectiveness:

Supplement	Number of people taking for mobility	Improved or somewhat improved mobility	Made no difference to mobility
Selenium	28	19 (68%)	9 (32%)
Daily multivitamin	35	21 (60%)	14 (40%)
Garlic capsules	27	15 (56%)	12 (44%)
Vitamin C	31	16 (52%)	15 (49%)
Calcium	32	13 (40.5%)	19 (59.5%)

And here are the results for pain relief.

Supplement	Number of people taking for pain relief	Reduced or somewhat reduced pain	Made no difference to pain
Daily multivitamin	37	18 (49%)	19 (51%)
Selenium	19	7 (37%)	12 (63%)
Garlic capsules	25	9 (36%)	16 (64%)
Vitamin C	26	9 (35%)	17 (65%)
Calcium	35	9 (26%)	26 (74%)

Selenium

Selenium is a trace mineral mainly found in plant foods. The content of selenium in food depends on the selenium content of the soil where plants are grown or animals are raised. Selenium levels are lower in Europe than in the United States, for example. Selenium has antioxidant properties which help prevent cellular damage from free radicals. Free radicals are natural by-products of oxygen metabolism that may contribute to the development of chronic diseases such as cancer and heart disease. Other seleno-proteins help regulate thyroid function and play a role in the immune system. Selenium, as an antioxidant, may help to relieve symptoms of arthritis by controlling levels of free radicals.

According to the US National Institute of Health, surveys indicate that people with rheumatoid arthritis have reduced selenium levels in their blood and some people with arthritis have a low selenium intake. Current findings are considered preliminary, and further research is needed before selenium supplements can be recommended for individuals with arthritis. Judging by the results of our survey, however, taking selenium supplements can help improve both mobility and reduce pain.

Multivitamins

Taking a multivitamin and mineral supplement is surely the simplest solution to deficiency worries for most people.

A housewife from Utah: 'I take Theragran (a US multivitamin) and I seem to have more energy.'

A foster grandparent from Oklahoma: 'I take Theragran and I think it helps.'

A high-school English teacher from South Dakota: 'I have taken Theragran-M for twenty-five years, and I'm experiencing arthritis at a much older age, and less severely than my grandmother, mother, and younger sister.'

A retired production vice-president from Pennsylvania: 'I take Theragran on the advice of my neurosurgeon, but I don't notice any difference if I stop taking it.'

Based on participants' experience and our reading of the medical literature, it is highly recommend that you take a multivitamin and mineral supplement that provides 100 percent of the U.S. Recommended Daily Allowances (U.S. RDA). Although it is no substitute for a healthy diet, the supplement can fill in some of the gaps for you. It is a well-documented fact that many people with arthritis are at least marginally malnourished, with deficiencies in one or more nutrients, according to studies in the United States and Europe. For some, the disease itself is to blame. You yourself may have experienced pain and swelling in your hands that make cooking difficult, or jaw pain that turns eating into a chore. Arthritis also seems to interfere with the way your body utilizes some of the nutrients from foods, so that you may need supplements as a safety net, even though you eat well. Other people find that the drugs they take for arthritis treatment can rob the body of one or more essential nutrients (more about this later), or affect the gut in such a way that it can't properly absorb the nutrients from food.

Although you can buy a multivitamin over the counter (or through the mail), it's a good idea to talk to your doctor before starting any new supplement regimen. Unpleasant side effects from taking multivitamins according to package directions are extremely rare, but a California social worker in our survey, for example, was advised *not* to take vitamins since her stomach haemorrhage. A retired mechanical engineer from Florida noted that vitamins caused his mouth and lips to break out in blisters.

Taking extremely large quantities, or megadoses, of vitamins and minerals, on the other hand, is risky business. This is especially true of the fat-soluble vitamins A and D, which can build up in your body and lead to assorted horrors. Megadoses of vitamin A have been known to *cause* joint pain in some people, and too much vitamin D, ironically, can weaken your bones.

Vitamin C

Of the 270 US participants who used vitamin C (ascorbic acid), 24 explained why: 13 found that it helped relieve pain or swelling; another 7 cited prevention of colds and infections as their rationale; 2 took it for general well-being; and 1 said it kept him from bruising. Two British physicians documented this anti-bruising effect while trying to treat the spontaneous skin bruises that often accompany rheumatoid arthritis. They gave 500 milligrams of vitamin C a day to three of their patients who had been troubled with this problem, and all three stopped getting bruises. Writing in the *British Journal of Rheumatology*, the authors explain that the three elderly women in the trial were poorly nourished and actually deficient in vitamin C, and, further, that inflammation reduces the body's store of this vitamin.

According to data from the Framingham Heart Study – an ongoing study of the diet and lifestyle of more than 5,000 men and women from Framingham, Massachussetts that started in 1948 – people with more vitamin C in their diets had higher bone density. Low bone density is a major risk factor for fractures. Higher bone density means stronger bones, as well as a reduced risk of osteoarthritis progression and even prevention of knee pain.

Vitamin C is needed to make collagen, which makes up cartilage. Cartilage cushions bones, and not having enough leads to deterioration and osteoarthritis. Vitamin C is thought to play a role in treating rheumatoid arthritis because it battles free radicals that injure cartilage.

The fact that people with rheumatoid arthritis have lower-than-normal levels of vitamin C in their joints and in their blood has been known since the 1930s. However, the (few) studies conducted in the past fifty years have failed to set an amount of vitamin C that might produce improvement.

Dr. Richard S. Panush, working with colleagues at the University of Florida College of Medicine, has shown that vitamin C can enhance the immune response for people with rheumatoid arthritis, although he isn't convinced it really helps their arthritis.

Vitamin C may also boost the effectiveness of aspirin in your body. This action has not been shown in human subjects, but there is some test-tube evidence from researchers at Simon Fraser University in British Columbia. Another aspect of the aspirin–C interaction is that aspirin may literally dump C out of your system, causing you to excrete it much faster than people who don't take the drug regularly.

The recommended dose of vitamin C varies from 60 milligrams a day, as the U.S. government advises for average adults,*

* A 60-milligram dose of vitamin C is the Recommended Dietary Allowance (RDA) for healthy adults. RDAs are determined by the Food and Nutrition Board of the National Academy of Sciences-National Research Council. The RDAs specify the necessary amounts of certain nutrients for groups of people at different age levels (from under six months to over fifty-one years) and life stages (adolescent boys, for example, or pregnant women). In turn, the Food and Drug Administration uses this information to construct the more general U.S. Recommended Daily Allowances (U.S. RDA) that appear on food labels.

to three hundred times that much, or 18 grams, which is what Dr. Linus Pauling recommends for life extension and general disease prevention. We suspect that 500 milligrams – the most popular amount mentioned in the survey – is adequate for most people with arthritis. More may be required for those undergoing the physical stress of surgery, since vitamin C helps the body heal. Some people can't tolerate a C supplement at all, however, because it upsets their stomachs. Vitamin manufacturers have tried to meet this challenge with buffered C tablets, but there is always the natural vitamin C in citrus fruit, if you can eat it, in papaya and other melons, and in dark-green vegetables. Several members of the nightshade family – tomatoes, peppers, and potatoes – are good C sources for those who can enjoy them.

Calcium

In the wake of the furore over osteoporosis, calcium has become one of the most popular dietary supplements of all time, particularly among women, who are especially prone to the disease after menopause. But most people with arthritis – men and women alike – need lots of calcium anyway. It helps keep the bones strong, along with vitamin D, and may ward off the bone damage from steroid drugs. A New Zealand study tested the value of calcium supplements for people taking these drugs, and the researchers were gratified to discover that 1,000 milligrams of calcium a day (200 milligrams more than the RDA of 800 milligrams) seemed to slow down and even *reverse* the process of bone loss. 'The dose of calcium used and its timing require further study, as do its effects on bone density,' they report in the *American Journal of Clinical Nutrition*. 'Until such information is available, the use of calcium supplements in steroid-treated subjects would appear to have a reasonable basis.'

If you are over sixty-five, your ability to absorb calcium from foods is not what it used to be, making it even more unlikely that a healthy diet could fulfil your calcium needs.

In the US survey 270 of the participants used from 250 to 1,500 milligrams daily. The advantages, they said, included relief of leg cramps for nine of them and relief of arthritis pain or swelling for another fifteen. 'I once ran out of calcium tablets and had to wait three or four weeks before my order arrived,' said a retired legal assistant who now lives in rural Wisconsin. 'After several days of missing my calcium supplement, my hands became very sore. After nearly two weeks without calcium I could hardly use my hands and would awaken in pain and stiff every morning. Once back on calcium, it took a few days, but all symptoms disappeared and have not returned. My daily calcium intake, including the calcium in food I eat, is between 1,500 and 2,000 milligrams.'

Very few participants mentioned the brand of calcium supplements they use, but a study reported in 1987 in *American Pharmacy* showed vast differences in the way these products disintegrate and dissolve in the gut. For example, Potent Calcium 600 mg from General Nutrition Centres took over an hour to disintegrate when tested, so that only 5 percent of the tablet had dissolved after thirty minutes, while Calcium Carbonate from Roxane Labs, Inc., disintegrated in just two minutes and was 100-percent dissolved after thirty minutes. Your best assurance of getting the full dose of calcium in any product is to swallow it with a meal, so that the tablet stays in your stomach long enough to dissolve completely. Splitting up your dosage – 500 milligrams with two meals instead of 1,000 milligrams all at once – offers still more assurance of absorbing the nutrient.

Ask your doctor about taking 1,000 milligrams of calcium a day, or 1,500 milligrams if you are a woman past menopause. You need to take vitamin D along with the calcium to give your body the best chance of putting the calcium to good use. Also remember that what you *do* is as important as anything you take. For no amount of calcium supplements can undo the bone loss caused by inactivity. In other words, exercise is essential. (See Chapter 17.)

The UK Arthritis Research Campaign recommends a daily intake of calcium of 1000 milligrams (mg) or 1500 mg if you are over 60.

Other Vitamins and Minerals

The last of the thirteen known vitamins was identified more than forty years ago, yet various ones come to the forefront of attention from time to time, like changing fashions, as more of their actions are understood – vitamin C for colds in the 1970s, vitamin A for cancer prevention in the 1980s. Although no vitamin has yet been scientifically proven to alter the course of arthritis, some of our participants say they have found pain relief from taking vitamin E, or one or more of the B vitamins.

Vitamin E

Vitamin E was taken regularly by 191 of the US participants, for several different reasons, two of which had to do with side effects from arthritis drugs. 'I have cornea damage in both eyes as a result of taking Butazolidin thirteen years ago,' wrote a housewife from New Jersey. 'Vitamin E seems to improve my vision.'

'My skin condition has gone downhill since I started gold treatments about a year ago,' reported a draftsperson from Pennsylvania. 'Vitamin E seems to help it.' A plumber from Wisconsin also took vitamin E for his skin, although not for any specified drug reaction.

Two participants increased their E intake because of concern for their heart and circulation. Two more found it heightened their energy and sense of well-being. One believed it boosted her body's natural cortisone, and eight said it helped, or seemed to help, their arthritis. How might it accomplish this feat? No one knows for sure, but in animals, vitamin E shows promise of keeping the immune system operating at peak performance. One theory about the way vitamin E may boost immunity is by interfering with the action of the prostaglandin called E_2, or PGE_2, which can curtail immune function. But PGE_2 is also a known inflammatory agent. So it is just possible that the vitamin exerts an anti-inflammatory effect by blocking PGE_2.

Scientists in Israel, who tested vitamin E on a group of twenty-nine people with osteoarthritis, concluded their report in the *Journal of the American Geriatrics Society* by suggesting a possible anti-inflammatory role for E. Without that possibility, they were at a loss to explain the good results of their experiment. Fifteen people – more than half the group – had significant pain relief while taking vitamin E.

Most adults are thought to need 30 international units of vitamin E every day. Most survey participants who specified the amount they use took 400 international units, although a few took 800 or more – amounts that threaten to bring on headaches, blurred vision, and extreme fatigue.

No arthritis drugs are known to deplete the body of vitamin E, but diet can increase your need for it. If you follow a diet that is high in polyunsaturated fats – such as the Arthritis Survey Diet and Thirty-Day Meal Plan (see Chapter 13) and other experimental diets that have been shown to help reduce some symptoms of arthritis – your vitamin E requirement rises accordingly. The amount of vitamin E in most multivitamin and mineral tablets should be sufficient. If you want to test the effects of an extra measure, talk to your doctor about a daily supplement of 400 to 600 international units.

The B Vitamins

The B complex is a family of eight vitamins, some numbered, some not: B_1 or thiamin, B_2 or riboflavin, B_3 or niacin (or nicotinamide or nicotinic acid), B_6 or pyridoxine, B_{12} or cobalamin, folacin or folic acid, pantothenic acid, and biotin. B-complex tablets vary widely, from formulas that contain a few milligrams of each B vitamin to high-potency pills that deliver at least 100 milligrams of each. The formulas balance the B vitamins, which work together in such a way that taking an excess of one may cause a deficiency of another. Although 113 of the US participants took the B complex, too few of them specified any dosage formulation for us to make a recommendation. Their reasons for taking the whole complex include relief of pain or swelling (four participants), less fatigue (two participants), physical flexibility (one participant), diabetes (one participant), and a vegetarian diet (one participant).

B vitamins often come up short in the diets of people with arthritis, according to researchers at the University of Florida who made an in-depth study in 1983 of the way their patients normally ate. As a group, the twenty-four people with rheumatoid arthritis and twelve others with osteoarthritis were consuming far less than the RDA for folacin, vitamin B_6, and pantothenic acid, as well as these other nutrients: magnesium, zinc, and vitamin E. Some of the foods that are richest in B vitamins, such as liver and kidney, are forbidden for certain people with arthritis. Others that abound in them, however, are whole-grain cereals and breads, fish, and green leafy vegetables. These, incidentally, are some of our survey participants' most highly recommended food items. (See Chapter 13.)

In a later dietary assessment study at Albany Medical College, reported in 1987, a group of fifty-two people with rheumatoid arthritis were found to follow diets generally deficient in the B vitamins folic acid and pyridoxine. Some of them were also low in magnesium. The twenty-one women in the study group were getting too little zinc. Interestingly, the researchers found that most of the twenty-four patients who were taking food supplements were successfully correcting the deficits in their diets.

Methotrexate, an immunosuppressive drug used to treat rheumatoid arthritis, can cause a deficiency of folacin. This is a main action of the drug, not a side effect. In fact, some physicians believe that trying to correct the deficiency with folic-acid supplements will undermine the drug's usefulness. Four participants in the survey, however, were taking therapeutic doses (1 milligram) of folic acid on doctor's orders *because* of their methotrexate therapy – to help chase the nausea and other side effects caused by the drug. Practitioners are divided on this question at present; however, studies are under way to settle the issue. Meanwhile, if you are taking Rheumatrex or Methotrexate, you'll want to discuss your vitamin choices with your doctor, since many multivitamin supplements contain folic acid. The salicylates – aspirin, diflunisal (Dolobid), and salsalate (Disalcid and Monogesic) – can also create a folic-acid deficiency, and your doctor may want you to counteract it by taking at least the RDA of 400 micrograms that are included in most multivitamins and B-complex preparations.

Vitamin B_6

Vitamin B_6, or pyridoxine, has a long history as a popular lay treatment for a form of arthritis called carpal tunnel syndrome – a debilitating wrist problem that necessitated surgery for eleven US participants. Now there is scientific acceptance of the idea as well. In 1986, the American Chemical Society gave its highest award, the Priestley Medal, to Dr. Karl Folkers, director of the Institute for Biomedical Research at the University of Texas in Austin, for his painstaking efforts to prove that carpal tunnel syndrome can be treated with daily doses of 100 milligrams of vitamin B_6. There's a catch, though. Not *all* cases of carpal tunnel syndrome can be laid to B_6 deficiency.

Of the fifty-one US survey participants taking supplemental B_6, one used it as an antidote for stress, and five noted that it eased their pain. 'If I didn't take my 200 milligrams of vitamin B_6 every day,' said a sixty-year-old housewife from Indiana, 'I would not be able to write, draw, or raise my arms over my head.' The RDA for B_6 is just 2 milligrams, but many doctors believe that up to 200 milligrams a day (the amount often used to treat premenstrual syndrome) is a safe dose. More than that can lead to nerve damage.

Vitamin B_{12}

Vitamin B_{12} (cobalamin) was the second most popular B vitamin among US participants. Forty took it, but only four told why: for more energy (three participants), or because it helps arthritis (one participant). B_{12}, which is not found in any fruit or vegetable, is the one vitamin that strict (vegan) vegetarians can't get from their diets, and so they must rely on a supplement. The RDA for most adults is 3 micrograms. (Vegetarians take note that brewer's yeast contains no B_{12}.)

Vitamin B_3

Vitamin B_3 eased pain for at least one of the twelve US participants who took it, and imparted a healthy feeling to one other. It has three names – niacin, nicotinamide, and nicotinic acid. Niacin, a student teacher from Utah reports, makes her dizzy. And niacinamide (another form of niacin) is the treatment used for forty-odd years by internist Dr. William Kaufman of Stratford, Connecticut, to relieve arthritis pain and stiffness. The medical establishment rejected Dr. Kaufman's reports of success, however, and balked at the high doses he gave his patients. These ranged from 900 to 4,000 milligrams a day, while the RDA is less than 2 milligrams. Dr. Kaufman has been cited frequently in *Prevention* magazine and in books also published by Rodale Press, *Prevention*'s parent. To his credit, Dr. Kaufman always emphasized the fact that high doses of B_3 were not for self-treatment, and must be supervised by a doctor, though it would probably prove quite difficult to find one willing to do so.

Vitamin A

Vitamin A is drawing attention these days as a possible cancer preventive and as an important nutrient for proper immune-system functioning. Only one of the sixty-two US survey participants who took it, however, mentioned any special benefit as far as arthritis was concerned. Another fourteen took beta-carotene, a vegetable extract that your body can convert to the active form of vitamin A. Like vitamin C, A can make a healthy contribution to your recovery from surgery. The RDA is 4,000 international units a day for women and 5,000 for men.

Vitamin D

Do you now or have you ever taken corticosteroids? These drugs include prednisone, prednisolone, and cortisone acetate. They are all powerful anti-inflammatories, but they all contribute to bone deterioration, such as osteoporosis (thinning of the bones), osteomalacia (softening of the bones), and osteopenia (loss of bone substance). Rheumatoid arthritis alone – even if you've never had so much as a single dose of any steroid drug – may predispose you to thinning, weakening bones that break easily, and increase your need for vitamin D and calcium. Fifty-five of the US survey participants took vitamin D supplements, including a forty-four-year-old office manager from New York, whose rheumatologist has her take 50,000 international units per week, plus calcium.

Doctors at the Royal National Hospital for Rheumatic Diseases in Bath, England, examined a group of elderly women with rheumatoid arthritis. Five of the women had suffered fractures in the long bones of their legs, while the other twelve women had had no such bad breaks. When the doctors interviewed all the women at length about their diets, they discovered that the ones with broken bones were getting far less vitamin D than the other women. (They ate less margarine, for example, and fewer eggs, which are good sources of the vitamin.) 'This suggests,' the physicians wrote in the *British Medical Journal* (November 23, 1974), 'that dietary vitamin-D deficiency was an important cause of the fractures . . .'

They also noted that the women were poor, and perhaps could not afford to buy foods rich in vitamin D, so they prescribed an inexpensive supplement containing 300 international units (less than the RDA of 400) a day. Because these particular women were housebound, too, they weren't even getting the vitamin D that comes free for the asking by spending twenty minutes in the sunshine every day.

Zinc

Zinc was used successfully to treat arthritis in an experiment that involved twenty-four people with rheumatoid arthritis at the University of Washington in Seattle. In one part of the study, half the volunteers took zinc supplements three times a day for twelve weeks, while the other half took placebos. Those on zinc had less swelling, less morning stiffness, and an overall better sense of well-being, according to Dr. Peter A. Simkin's report in the British medical journal the *Lancet* in 1976. Since then, other studies have documented zinc deficiencies in the diets of people with arthritis, but there have been no formal attempts to treat the disease with large doses of zinc. (Volunteers in the Washington study took about ten times the RDA for this mineral.) Sixty-one of US participants took zinc regularly, perhaps because news of the zinc-arthritis study was reported in the popular press.

Nutritionists and physicians at Albany Medical College, Cornell University, and New York University, among others, have investigated the effects of arthritis drugs on various essential minerals. The drug penicillamine, for example, which is often used to treat rheumatoid arthritis, is supposed to make your body excrete copper, but it can also cause you to lose zinc.

Iron

Every time you take an aspirin or other NSAID, you may lose a tiny bit of blood. Over time, these little losses can mount into iron-deficiency conditions, and forty-three of survey participants are offsetting them with an iron supplement. (People with rheumatoid arthritis are often anaemic, regardless of their drug therapy, since the disease itself can *cause* anaemia.) The RDA for iron is 10 milligrams for men and 18 milligrams for women ages eighteen to fifty (to make up for the blood lost during menstruation). These quantities of iron are more than many people get in their diets, but the amount included in your multivitamin tablet is probably sufficient to make up the difference. If medications and upcoming surgery drive your personal iron needs even higher, though, ask your doctor about an appropriate supplement.

Summary of Vitamins and Minerals

- There is growing evidence for the benefits of taking fish oil, glucosamine, chondroitin and evening primrose oil supplements for improvements in both mobility and pain relief.
- A daily multivitamin and mineral supplement seems essential to fill the gaps in your diet and make up for some of the nutritional problems arthritis causes, from decreased appetite or cooking ability to incomplete absorption of some nutrients.
- If you have specific vitamin deficiencies, addressing the problem with the proper supplements can help you feel better.
- Surgery may drive up your need for certain nutrients, such as vitamin C, vitamin A, and iron.
- Many arthritis drugs create deficiencies of certain nutrients, by interfering with their absorption, for example, or by hastening them out of your body. The drugs include aspirin (vitamin C), methotrexate (folic acid), penicillamine (copper and zinc), and steroid drugs (calcium).
- Blood loss from chronic use of aspirin and other non-steroidal anti-inflammatory drugs can lead to iron deficiency.
- Some vitamins apparently play specific roles in relieving arthritis-related problems, such as vitamin C for the bruising common to rheumatoid arthritis, vitamin E for its possible anti-inflammatory action and relief of drug-caused tissue damage, and vitamin B6 for relief of some cases of carpal tunnel syndrome. Many other possibilities exist but have not been proven scientifically.

Section 6

How the Collective Wisdom of Survey Participants can Help you on a Daily Basis

My personal experience was a real crisis at first. Even though I had faith in my doctors, I still had a lot of unanswered questions that doctors don't have time for.

Survey Participant #610, a county sheriff from Kansas

Other people with arthritis are really helpful because they know from experience what works and what does not.

Survey Participant #232, an accounting clerk from Texas

I think you can learn to help yourself more than anyone else can help you.

Survey Participant #471, a homemaker from Utah

Chapter 15
How and *Why* to Build a Positive Outlook in Spite of Arthritis

• How arthritis affects emotions • How attitude affects arthritis
• How survey participants control stress • How they lift their spirits

No matter what medications they took or other kinds of help they received, many of the 1,051 US participants in the Arthritis Survey counted their own positive outlook on life among their most potent weapons against arthritis. They complained little, although they have suffereded much, and they believed that their attitude helped them feel and function far better than they otherwise might.

For although arthritis is a malady of the joints, it can also inflame anger, depression, and rob people of their self-esteem.

Arthritis is not *caused* by emotional problems, to be sure, but it kicks up a lot of strong feelings, and it can respond to feelings, too. Stress, for example, often makes arthritis symptoms flare, while the relief of stress may drive those symptoms into remission. Even when it comes to medical care, emotional factors seem to tip the odds in favour of benefiting from certain drugs or procedures. For it sometimes happens that two people with the same kind of arthritis, whose X rays reveal identical degrees of joint damage, react quite differently to the same treatment – apparently because one has a positive mental outlook and the other feels beaten before beginning.

In this chapter, participants will tell you all about their personal struggles, speaking frankly of dreams dashed by arthritis – and new dreams they conjured to fight their way out of hopelessness. We'll add to their comments a few accounts of medical studies showing how important it is to feel in control of

your arthritis, instead of controlled by it, and suggesting ways
for you to gain that control.

Survey participants will also describe the relaxation techniques
they rely on, like imagery and self-hypnosis, to reduce stress and
thereby relieve pain. And they're happy to share the things they
love to do, from praying to playing piano, that lift their spirits and
may do the same for yours.

Emotional Fallout

It should be easy to understand, even from a healthy distance,
how losing the ability to do what you've always done could make
you furious, or sad, or both. Anyone should be able to see that
being in pain is reason enough to get depressed occasionally.
Yet people in the US survey noted that most of their friends
and family members do *not* appreciate their emotional turmoil,
and definitely do not want to hear about it. Worse, some of their
so-called friends implied that arthritis came about as the *result* of
their internal upset, instead of the other way around.

Doctors, too, have sometimes been guilty of blaming their
patients for bringing on arthritis by virtue of their personality
problems. Dr. Martin A. Shearn of the University of California
School of Medicine in San Francisco, who has studied and
written about the psychological aspects of arthritis, found
several early attempts to categorize people with rheumatoid
arthritis as being by turns masochistic, self-sacrificing, moralistic,
perfectionistic, and inhibited. It has also been said that people
develop arthritis because they are unable to express anger and
therefore harbour hostility or resentment. But there is no evidence to support these stone-casting ideas. Indeed, as more
recent studies have shown (and as you could have told the
researchers), there is no personality 'type' that distinguishes
people with arthritis from anyone else.

'You have to have a good attitude,' concluded a sixty-five-year-
old former telephone operator from North Carolina, 'and be
happy, or, believe me, you'll feel worse. I've always been a cheerful person. I try not to get down in the dumps, and find that
people like me a lot better for the effort. I try to forget about
'Old Arthur,' as I refer to my arthritis, and still go on trips, go
shopping, laugh with friends, and do not complain.'

It Couldn't Happen to Me

On first hearing that they had arthritis, some of the US survey participants simply could not believe the news. Younger people especially, who tend to think of arthritis as a disease of old age, may deny what is happening to them, as a way of dealing with the shock. 'When the doctor showed me my X rays compared to normal X rays of someone else's hands and feet,' said a twenty-two-year-old college student from California, 'I finally started to face the fact that I had a problem.'

Denying arthritis means denying its proper treatment as well, and actually making the condition worse as a result. 'I was fourteen when I learned I had arthritis,' wrote a forty-seven-year-old occupational therapist from Colorado. 'I did not accept my disease for years, and continued to do activities, including sports, that I had done before, even though I had to take pain medication to get through them. I did a lot of damage to my elbows and feet that way.'

Denial, anger, anxiety, and depression are most often normal reactions to the challenge of adjusting to living with arthritis. Their normalcy, however, doesn't make them any easier to bear; and some physicians believe that depression and anxiety actually *lower* your tolerance for pain.

Some fifty of the US participants sought the help of psychologists or psychiatrists to get them through emotional crises related to arthritis. The college student mentioned above, for example, undertook psychotherapy and found that it helped her face the fact of her arthritis and consequently take better care of herself. And the occupational therapist reported that a psychiatrist 'enabled me to vent my feelings and work on my self-image, as well as other problems. He also prescribed antidepressants that were helpful.'*

* Twenty-two survey participants took antidepressant medications, such as **Elavil** (amitriptyline) and **Tofranil** (imipramine). Some of them took the drugs for depression, and some for pain, since the family of tricyclic antidepressants, to which these drugs belong, has been shown to help relieve arthritis pain. These are not first-choice drugs for arthritis, however, and have their own set of problem side effects.

A Sense of Loss

The majority of the US survey participants did what they wanted to do in spite of arthritis, but some of them felt a tremendous sense of loss. 'I have wishes unfulfilled, and poverty due to living on social security and Medicare,' wrote a forty-six-year-old former proof-reader from Oregon who was forced to leave her job in 1985 because of increasing pain and fatigue. 'I feel I'm always the watcher, never the participant, and it's sad. But I try to be cheerful because my arthritis also affects those who love me.'

Drs. John L. Black and Maurice J. Martin, two Mayo Clinic psychiatrists who wrote about depression and arthritis in *The Journal of Musculoskeletal Medicine*, explain that loss is a frequent cause of depression, and that people must have a chance to recognize and grieve the loss before they can pick up and carry on. The loss can take any form. One person loses sight of himself – becoming a patient instead of a person. Another loses a job, and with it her whole social network.

'I had a job I loved for twelve years,' said a sixty-one-year-old widow from Ontario. 'I ran the cafeteria for an import-export company. I did the ordering, cooking, and serving, and in general looked after my extended family every day. I even got to do special luncheons for out-of-town guests. When my knees became really bad three years ago, I had to stop work and go on a disability pension. It has taken me a long time to get it through my head that I cannot go back to work, even when I feel well, and stand for seven to ten hours at a stretch, then ride a highway bus home. But I am learning.'

One participant, a forty-five-year-old former insurance agent, not only lost her job because of arthritis but her marriage as well. 'As I became less able to be in control,' she recalled, 'our family life deteriorated. My son and middle daughter became unruly and involved in drugs. My husband would not face or acknowledge that I had rheumatoid arthritis. He called me a malingerer.

'On several occasions when I had severe flare-ups, I was unable to feed myself or the dog, as I could neither walk on the cold kitchen floor nor open a package or can. My husband would not change his lifestyle or buy devices or gadgets that would help me function. This was not because he was an ogre, but because he preferred to deny that I was ill and that I was no longer able to provide him with the services he was accustomed to having me provide. He renewed the lease on our two-storey condominium in San Diego in 1982, although I had obvious difficulty climbing the stairs, and by 1983 I could not climb them at all. I slept on the living room couch for the next year and a half.

'My eldest daughter, who was working as a nurse at a hospital, moved back home to become my help and chauffeur, since I could no longer drive a car. My youngest daughter was my cheerful friend. The other two children preferred denial.

'I was building a new way of thinking about life by 1984, and I was encouraged by finally winning the award of social security disability, retroactive to 1982. My twenty-fifth high school reunion came up that June, and with help from my daughter I was able to attend part of it.

'Then I acknowledged the final death of my hopes for my marriage. The social security settlement helped me have the funds, and reading helped me get the information on how to obtain a California divorce without an attorney or physically appearing in court. My daughter did the typing and legwork. The divorce, with alimony and child support, was granted in late December.

'My daughters helped me find things like kitchen gadgets and a hand-held shower attachment that helped me become more able to help myself. We three realized we couldn't afford to live in California any longer, so we made our lists of what we needed, did our research, and decided on a place in eastern Oklahoma. A Golden Retriever dog, a sick lady, a twenty-three-year-old lady, and a fifteen-year-old girl set out on a rainy April day from San Diego on a 1,500-mile, twelve-day adventure in an overloaded station wagon pulling an overloaded tent trailer. It was a *great* adventure.

'We've lived out here in the country for three years now. For beautiful imagery, I only have to look around me.'

How Powerful Is Positive Thinking?

The US survey files are full of stories from people who made up their minds, or made a pact with God, to win out over arthritis. There are hospital studies, too, showing that grit and guts are quite effective as pain-relievers.

To test the power of a positive attitude against the pain and disability of osteoarthritis, researchers at the University of Alabama gathered a group of sixty-five volunteers who had arthritis in at least one hip or one knee. They wanted to see whether these people's perception of pain and their ability to carry out everyday activities were influenced more by the extent of their actual joint damage – or by psychological factors such as depression, anxiety, and feelings of helplessness.

First they collected recent X rays from all the volunteers, and had two rheumatologists, who never saw the people in person, judge the severity of each one's arthritis on the basis of the joint damage alone. Then the researchers visited the volunteers at their homes, where they interviewed them about their daily lives and gave them a battery of psychological tests. At the end, they pooled all the information they had on each person to see what they could see. And they saw that joint damage alone does *not* account for the amount of pain a person feels, or for the amount of difficulty anyone has in getting dressed, getting around, or getting on at work. In fact, as the researchers reported in 1988 in *Arthritis and Rheumatism*, attitude and emotions may be more important. Depression, for example, is more likely than joint destruction to keep people from taking care of themselves. And those volunteers who scored the highest on tests of 'resourcefulness' (the feeling that they could cope with any curve life threw them) were the *least* disabled in terms of doing things, no matter what shape their joints were in.

We are painfully aware, in reporting the results of these kinds of studies, that you hardly need to be blamed for any difficulty you are having in controlling your symptoms or managing your daily activities. Having said that developing arthritis is not your fault, we are not about to claim that suffering from it *is* your fault because you aren't cheerful enough or resourceful enough to do better. Instead, these studies are presented because they validate participants' experiences, and because they suggest concrete measures anyone can take to try to improve the outcome of arthritis care. Anxiety and depression, for instance, are conditions that can be treated, whether in psychotherapy, with the help of support groups, or by other means. The elements of resourcefulness can be taught, psychologists have shown, by arming you with a series of positive statements you can repeat to yourself in times of need. Ideally, these learned 'coping statements' take the place of your old self-defeating beliefs, and give you the push you need to take control of your situation – even if you weren't born with a silver lining in your mental outlook.

A good all-around coping strategy is a combination of attitude and action. You use the positive ideas ('I *can* reduce my pain by staying calm and relaxed') along with specific self-care measures, which usually include taking medication on schedule, resting, applying heat or ice (or both), exercising, eating well, and practising a relaxation technique.

One woman from Stockton-on-Tees in the UK wrote, 'Try to keep positive at all times and try to keep happy (I have a five-year-old to look after and she keeps me busy). And cry if you have to – don't bottle it up!'

'For thirty-four years I have tried to look on the bright side of my problem,' said a retired automobile dealer from Massachusetts, who's had rheumatoid arthritis since age twenty-six, and diabetes, too. 'I can't run but I can walk and ride a bike. I can't ski, but I can watch. And when I hurt, I know I could hurt more. Attitude is my *best* doctor.'

Handicapped by Helplessness

Because arthritis may begin for no known reason and persist with no known cure, it often engenders a sense of helplessness. This is an understandable but counterproductive reaction – because helplessness can lead to depression and the inability, or unwillingness, to follow your prescribed treatment plan. Indeed, the feeling of helplessness is so common and so meaningful in arthritis that a group of psychologists developed a special test to measure it. Called the Arthritis Helplessness Index, it consists of a series of statements, ranging in outlook from 'Arthritis is controlling my life,' to 'I am coping effectively with my arthritis.' By agreeing or disagreeing with the various statements, you establish your score; and that score may well determine how you respond to medical care, according to a recent study at the Vanderbilt University Medical Centre in Nashville.

The point of the study was to see whether the Arthritis Helplessness Index could predict how well individuals would fare with their arthritis treatments over time. The researchers mailed the index to several hundred people who all had rheumatoid arthritis for seven years or less. In the course of the two-year study, the 368 volunteers filled out the index five times, so the researchers could chart any changes in their outlook. All the while the participants went on seeing their own private doctors, taking whatever medications their doctors prescribed for them. This was a watch-and-see study, and the researchers made no attempt to work with any of the volunteers to teach them particular coping strategies or educate them about arthritis.

As it turned out, the individual helplessness scores stayed pretty much the same throughout. And the volunteers who felt the most helpless fared the worst with their arthritis, from start to finish. They reported more pain and disability than those who did not feel helpless. In fact, the researchers concluded, a high helplessness score could serve as a red flag for physicians, to help them identify, at the outset of treatment, those patients who will likely need extra attention and assistance.

An Antidote for Helplessness

Let's take a close look at an extremely thorough, well-thought-out program for helping people with arthritis take charge of their pain control and defeat the feeling of helplessness. Psychologist Jerry C. Parker, Ph.D., and his colleagues at the University of Missouri School of Medicine devised this particular regimen, and tested it recently on patients at the Harry S Truman Memorial Veterans' Hospital in Columbia, Missouri. Compared to a purely educational program, or routine rheumatology care, this combination-treatment approach to arthritis proved to make a substantial difference in the way people felt, in terms of both pain perception and feeling in control of their lives.

To start with, the twenty-nine volunteers spent a week as inpatients at the hospital, where they were tested and treated to a five-day crash course in the following subjects:

- the nature and treatment of rheumatoid arthritis
- theories and facts about pain, including its emotional aspects
- stress management, including relaxation training
- distraction strategies for taking their minds off arthritis pain

- problem-solving techniques
- marriage and family dynamics
- communication skills

Every one to three months over the next year, whenever the volunteers returned to the hospital for a routine clinic visit, they also attended a meeting of a support group, where they talked about using the techniques they'd learned in their everyday lives. As a result, they made great gains in their ability to control pain. When the researchers contacted them a year after the study ended, they reported that they were still applying the lessons, because the strategies were still helping.

'If you break a leg, you know why you feel pain, and you know why it happened,' Dr. Parker explained when he presented the results of this study to the national meeting of the Arthritis Health Professions Association in Washington, D.C., in 1987. 'With rheumatoid arthritis, we don't understand why one person gets the disease and another doesn't. If a sense of helplessness develops, it often starts a vicious cycle in which pain causes depression, which in turn can increase pain and even the disability. Based on what we've learned in this study, clearly, there are pain relief and quality of life benefits beyond standard medical treatment.'

The Art of Stress Management

Fully 670 of the US survey participants, or 64 percent of the survey group, found that stress aggravated their pain, whether they had osteoarthritis or rheumatoid. 'I have found that stress affects how I feel a great deal,' said a bookkeeper from New York. 'When I let things get to me, my pain increases, which causes more stress, which causes more pain, and so on, round and round.'

A composer from California wrote, 'My arthritis was pretty much restricted to my finger joints, and fairly mild until about three years ago, when I went back to school for advanced studies, living four hundred miles from my wife and kids, and commuting home every two weeks. It was a high-stress program. My arthritis got *much* worse, I think largely due to stress.'

Since controlling stress is tantamount to pain relief for these people, you can bet they take their relaxation seriously. Here are the US survey's top ten favourite stress beaters.

Technique	Number of Participants Who Use it
1. Deep breathing	210
2. Avoiding stressful situations, including crowds	128
3. Attention-diverting, including hobbies and reading	127
4. Exercise or other physical activity	116
5. Relaxation technique, including self-hypnosis	88
6. Reducing anxiety through self-control, self-affirmation	87
7. Rest	80
8. Imagery or visualization	71
9. Meditation, including prayer	61
10. Resolving the problems that are causing stress	54

Most participants who practised stress control combined two or more of these strategies. The bookkeeper mentioned above, for example, used several: 'When I feel things piling up, I do the relaxation techniques I learned. I also try to busy myself with things I enjoy – whether it's reading or watching TV or working on a craft. Anything to take my mind off what's bugging me. At work when I feel uptight I get up and take a little walk. I am lucky in that I am free to move about as I please, and if I need a break I can take it. I also make it a point, when I'm stressed up, to go to a quiet, relaxing place for a nice lunch. It allows me quiet time to unwind.'

Each technique has its own special virtue.

Deep breathing. Your breathing is the most accessible part of the stress reaction, which also includes a speeded-up heartbeat, tensed muscles, and an outpouring of adrenaline. Gently force yourself to breathe deeply and evenly, and the change of pace will slow down the rest of your body. Deep breathing is the beginning of most formal relaxation techniques. Do it by inhaling through your nose for several seconds as you expand your abdomen. (Raising your shoulders doesn't help.) Hold the breath for a moment or two and then exhale through your mouth. Try to make yourself as comfortable as possible. 'I sit in my recliner with my feet up,' said a former teacher from Idaho, 'do deep breathing, listen to music, and sometimes swear a lot.'

Avoiding stressful situations. This works well, insofar as you can manage it. Not all stress is avoidable, but try to identify the people or things you don't have to put up with. 'I was under a lot of stress during my marriage,' an Arizona homemaker recalled. 'Once divorced I got relief and a remission which I have enjoyed for twelve years.' A forty-two-year-old former television producer writes: 'I have changed my home to northern Wisconsin, where the pace of living is laid back. I have removed myself from a high-powered job, loaded with stress and competition. I involve myself with things I enjoy, and not with things I feel I'm supposed to do.'

Attention-diverting activities. These get your mind off stress and pain and can be rewarding in themselves. Many participants said that the hobbies they enjoy, including needlecrafts of all description, also provide good exercise for their affected joints. 'I go to my workshop and build shelves,' reported a retired pharmacist from Illinois with arthritis in his knees and shoulders. 'The hammering and sawing help. I probably have enough shelves to open a store!'

Exercise. This often chases tension away in short order. The participants particularly liked exercises that got them out of the house, too, such as walking, swimming, and bicycling.

Relaxation techniques. Those mentioned in the survey include self-hypnosis, biofeedback (see Chapter 8), and audio-cassette tapes that calmly talk to participants and help them clear their heads and relax every muscle. A retired policewoman from New York explained, 'I lie down and tell myself to think of nothing and to feel no pain from my head, then face, then neck, and so on, down to my toes.' Some learned their technique from a mental-health practitioner, and some from books and tapes. In any case, becoming proficient at therapeutic relaxation takes practice, and any technique works best when practised every day. One form of self-hypnosis that has been used successfully by people with arthritis, called 'glove anaesthesia,' teaches you to picture your hands covered with gloves upon gloves, so that your fingers feel no pain or other sensations, and then to think of touching the places that hurt, allowing the gloves to absorb all the pain.

Reducing anxiety through self-control, self-affirmation. This boils down to getting a grip on yourself, and giving yourself as much support as you can muster. 'I use lots of breathing exercises, in fresh air,'

said a California housewife, 'and remember *I'm somebody important.*'
An Army officer used 'positive thinking – envisioning success,
accentuating positive factors, downplaying the negative.' Many
reminded themselves, 'This, too, shall pass.'

Rest. Get the sleep you're entitled to at night, participants
advised, and slow down or stop during the day if and when you
need to.

Imagery or visualization. Some of the survey respondents used
their imaginative powers to surround themselves with beautiful,
peaceful scenery, even when they were stuck in a stressful situation. 'I visualize some kind of water – oceans, rivers,' wrote a
graduate student from California, 'and dissociate myself from
the present, if it's impossible to leave.' Another approach to visualization is to try to journey inward and see inside your joints or
imagine specific healing processes going on there. 'I talk to my
pain,' said a New York health consultant, 'or to a specific part of
my body to find out why it is hurting. I sometimes get immediate
release from pain this way.'

Meditation. This combines relaxation with an attempt to focus
on a word or phrase that clears your mind of other thoughts.
(For some participants, prayer achieved the same deeply relaxing,
closed-eyed, totally focused state.) Dr. Joan Borysenko of
Harvard Medical School, director of the Mind/Body Clinic at
Boston's Beth Israel Hospital and author of *Minding the Body,
Mending the Mind* (Addison-Wesley, 1987), offers these basic
instructions for meditating.

* Choose a quiet spot, away from all distractions.
* Sit in a comfortable position.
* Close your eyes.
* Relax your muscles sequentially from head to feet.
* Become aware of your breathing without trying to control it.
* Repeat a focus word silently in time to your breathing.
* Don't worry about how you're doing, but take note of where
  and how your mind wanders.
* Practise meditating every day for ten or twenty minutes.

Resolving problems. Sometimes the only way around stress is to
face the situation squarely and deal with the problem causing

the stress. 'I look inside to see what the problem is,' reported a homemaker from Vermont. 'Sometimes I write on a legal pad until I feel better and can see solutions.' Several other participants also used writing as a means of problem-solving. Interestingly, an experiment at Southern Methodist University, which required a group of college students to write for twenty minutes a day about traumatic events in their lives, showed that the students' immune-system activity increased as a result of this exercise.

A Few of Their Favourite Things

The US survey participants were asked what they did to lift their spirits, and the answers were as varied as the participants themselves. Hundreds of them had a favourite hobby that cheered them. They painted with watercolours, played a musical instrument, sewed quilts or clothes, built model ships, trains, and planes, took pictures, made pottery, knitted, crocheted, and collected everything from stamps and baseball cards to china and doll-house furniture. Staying busy, most of them agreed, is therapeutic. And many of them were still busy with their careers, too, getting a great lift from doing their work well.

They loved to get out and go fishing, boating, camping, horseback riding, sunbathing, or bird-watching. Some travelled far, but many settled happily for a walk or a car ride just to enjoy the change of scenery.

The physical exertion of exercise did the most good for some participants, who beat out the blues by bicycle riding, for example, or walking, swimming, or practising judo, karate, or Tai Chi. A few chose sports such as golf or volleyball.

Getting things done around the house was soothing for those who liked to make home improvements, fix cars, get absorbed in gardening, clean, cook, or bake.

Some participants found their greatest enjoyment in helping others, by volunteering their free time to church activities, community groups, political causes, mental institutions, hospices, hospitals, and senior centres. Others were buoyed up by looking after their children, grandchildren, or pets. 'What I have done to lift my spirits,' wrote a former teacher from Massachusetts, 'is to bring home a five-week-old puppy, against my doctor's orders (he was afraid I would trip over her) and against my husband's wishes. My "puppy" was three years old in July, and weighs eleven pounds, fully grown. She has brought so much pleasure to the family, that even my husband now loves her. When you hold her, you forget about yourself, tension goes down, and you're happy all over. Better than any medicine you can buy. She is a joy and a treasure.'

Many participants chose to pamper their bodies with a bath, a massage, or a nap. They might treat themselves to a favourite food or drink, too, and perhaps go shopping just to buy something frivolous but affordable.

There were great rewards for many in the social support of their families and friends, clubs, community activities, and self-help group meetings held by their local chapter of the Arthritis Foundation or Alcoholics Anonymous. Some get-togethers were game times, for playing bridge, backgammon, bingo, chess, or horseshoes.

Entertainments needn't be lavish to be cheering. Many participants were happiest when reading a book, they said, listening to the radio, or watching television. 'It's hard for me to go to the movies,' noted a former cabdriver from Nevada, 'because long sitting periods increase my discomfort. I'd rather rent a movie to watch on my VCR, so I can stop, take a break, and move around from time to time.' Other participants enjoyed attending movies, plays, concerts, baseball games, and car races.

Some went to museums, some went back to school, or took correspondence courses. They lost themselves in murder mysteries, Westerns, romances, and fantasies, but they also liked to read newspapers, magazines, and the Bible. They might meditate to improve their outlook, or daydream, or pray, or bend their minds to some conundrum to keep themselves preoccupied. 'I do difficult crossword puzzles,' wrote a veterinarian from New Hampshire, 'or try to work out chess moves, or try to think through complex economic theories.'

Sometimes they lifted their spirits by giving their emotions free expression. 'When I'm really down,' confessed a former copy editor from Iowa, 'I write limericks and insulting greeting cards.' 'I really need to cry and yell sometimes,' said a homemaker from Virginia, 'and if I'm not alone, then I do it in the bathroom with the water running.' 'I have learned to laugh,' countered a nurse from Michigan. 'Surprisingly, laughter often reduces pain.'

Summary of How and Why to Build a Positive Mental Outlook

Though not caused by emotional factors, arthritis can generate anger, denial, anxiety, depression, and feelings of helplessness.

Addressing the emotional problems associated with arthritis is important because:

- Denial can make you ignore proper precautions.
- Depression may keep you from following your treatment plan.
- Anxiety and depression tend to lower your pain threshold.
- Helplessness may lead to depression, and aggravate your pain and disability.

Treatments for relieving or avoiding emotional problems include:

- Psychotherapy (one on one, or in a group)
- Medications, such as antidepressants
- Programs to teach relaxation techniques, 'coping statements,' family dynamics, communication skills, and the like

Stress frequently exacerbates arthritis pain. Stress-management techniques that may relieve pain include:

- Deep breathing
- Avoiding stressful situations
- Attention-diverting activities, including hobbies and reading
- Exercise or other physical activity
- Relaxation techniques, including self-hypnosis
- Reducing anxiety through self-control and self-affirmation
- Rest
- Imagery or visualization
- Meditation or prayer
- Resolving the problems that are causing stress

Chapter 16
The Twenty-Five Top-Rated Techniques for Fast Pain Relief:

At-Home Treatments You Can Use to Enhance Your Overall Care

• *Rest* • *Heat* • *Ice* • *Baths and showers* • *Exercise* • *Massage*
• *Over-the-counter products* • *Joint protection* • *Biofeedback and more*

Many participants in the Arthritis Survey no longer saw a doctor, a physiotherapist, or any other kind of practitioner for arthritis treatment. They cared for themselves, at home, using the techniques covered in this chapter. The others, whether they took monthly gold shots, weekly physiotherapy treatments, or daily doses of a prescription drug, also used these techniques to boost the effectiveness of their professional care. These are simple but powerful tools that our participants use for *immediate* pain relief.*

The twenty-five pain-relief strategies in this chapter are arranged according to their popularity among the UK participants, beginning with the ones used by the greatest number of people. Although not all of these techniques are appropriate for

---

* Participants also practised a variety of techniques at home for long-term improvement, which are discussed in other chapters, such as modifying their diet to lose weight and improve nutrition (Chapters 12 and 13), following an exercise routine (Chapter 17), building a positive mental outlook (Chapter 15), making their surroundings more comfortable (Chapter 18), and learning how to perform everyday activities with minimum pain (Chapter 19).

Pain Relief Strategy	No of UK participants	Percentage
Comfortable positions	233	(53%)
Exercise	218	(49%)
Heat from a heating pad	193	(44%)
Dressing for warmth	178	(42%)
Rest	184	(40%)
Walking for relief and relaxation	173	(38%)
Massage of painful areas	170	(38%)
Keeping busy with pleasant activities	165	(37%)
Aspirin	154	(36%)
Warm or hot baths	132	(29%)
Shower	99	(23%)
Heat	94	(22%)
Relaxation	86	(20%)
Time outdoors	92	(20%)
Joint coverings	87	(20%)
Herb teas and other warm drinks	82	(19%)
Hot tub	82	(19%)
Ice	76	(18%)
Liniments	58	(14%)
Sauna	54	(12%)
TENS	45	(10%)
Local rest	44	(10%)
Meditation, self-hypnosis	39	(9%)
Comforting food	33	(7%)
Cool soaks	20	(4%)
Wax dips	16	(3%)

all people with arthritis, we'll wager that you'll find at least half a dozen suggestions on the list that will work for you. The UK results were somewhat different to the US results. Comfortable positions was the most favoured strategy, followed by exercise, heat from a heating pad, dressing for warmth and then rest. The full results are shown above.

The top US strategies were rest, warm baths, heat, showers and ice.

Comfortable Positions

Many people have a favourite position that can instantly improve the way they feel. 'I have no pain when my legs are stretched out, as when I'm lying on my back,' found a retired salesman from Ohio. A teacher from Indiana liked to be sitting down with her knees bent at a 90-degree angle. And a retired railroad carman from Missouri said he needs to get out of bed every night for a while and sit in a chair for pain relief.

Exercise

Given that a regular exercise program, faithfully followed, can go far toward controlling pain and improving general well-being, there are also specific exercise movements that can be used for on-the-spot relief of pain or stiffness. If housework or office work builds up pain in your neck and back, for example, try doing a few simple *head rolls* from a standing or sitting position. You can even do them lying down. (If you have advanced rheumatoid arthritis check with your doctor before attempting this one, since there's a chance the movement could injure you.) Follow these steps in one very slow continuous motion, breathing deeply throughout:

- Tilt your head all the way right as though you were trying to touch your right ear to your shoulder (but don't lift your shoulder to your ear).
- Let your head fall slowly forward to drop your chin almost on your chest.
- Rotate to the left, stretching to get your left ear near to your left shoulder.
- Lean your head all the way back and look at the ceiling; repeat in the same direction, and then go the other way twice.

For low back pain, lean your back against a wall with your feet about ten inches away from the wall; tighten your buttocks and your abdominal muscles until you feel the small of your back touch the wall; release; repeat. Shoulder shrugs, rolls, and stretches, finger curls and spreads, and foot circles are just a few of the many other movements you can do during the day, no matter where you are, whenever you feel the need. (See Chapter 19.)

Heat

Whether it comes from a heating pad, an electric blanket, a hot-water bottle, a hydrocollator, a heat lamp, or a hot pack made from a washcloth or towel, heat works to drive out pain and stiffness. 'I swear by my heating pad,' and 'I'd be lost without my heating pad,' are typical comments from survey participants. In fact, an electric heating pad is the item most likely to be purchased for arthritis pain relief. It's a good investment, to be sure, but here are some homemade alternatives from participants who use them.

- Iron over a wet towel until it is packed with steam. Place a thin towel on your skin, put the steam towel over that, and cover both with another dry towel.
- Run hot water on towels or washcloths, wring out excess, and wrap them around affected areas. When they lose their heat in a few minutes, repeat the process.

An entrepreneur from British Columbia found great relief for his hands under the wall-mounted electric dryers that replace paper towels in some public rest rooms. In fact, they helped him so much that he was thinking about buying one for home use. Most participants who used heat therapy found the dry heat from hand dryers and heat lamps to be not quite as soothing as the moist heat provided by hot towels and many types of electric heating pads, but this is a matter of personal preference.

WARNING: Do not apply heat to a hot, swollen joint.

Dressing Right

Many participants felt a pain when they felt a chill, whether it came from a wintry blast, an air conditioner on a hot summer day, or a problem with blood circulation. 'Above all keep those joints *warm*,' said an antiques dealer from Texas, who sometimes wore three pairs of slacks in the winter to keep her knees free of pain. A nurse from another part of the state put her hands in special moist-heat mittens when they ache. 'I'm obsessed with being cold,' admitted a public relations consultant from Ohio. 'At home, I always wear knee socks and a flannel and wool dressing gown.' Many people said they slept with cotton gloves on, or socks, or both, to ease pain and morning stiffness. And they stressed the importance of choosing shoes and clothing they could put on and take off easily.

Rest

Two-thirds of the US participants and 40 percent of UK participants stressed the importance of rest for pain relief and prevention. Many of them led extremely active lives but used rest when and as they needed to. 'Rest' may simply mean a few minutes of sitting in a comfortable chair or taking a break from an activity that causes pain. 'Even though I have to work ten to twelve hours every day,' wrote a forty-nine-year-old dairy farmer from Missouri, 'I lie down and rest my back in midday or the pain becomes intolerable.' Rest can also mean ample sleep at night and naps in the afternoon to both relieve and ward off pain. A thirty-eight-year-old mother of three from Connecticut observed, 'Rest is *extremely* important, no matter how foolish you feel taking a nap or going to bed early. If you're tired, you hurt!'

Walking

Even before walking became a hot new trend, complete with fancy required equipment and magazines and videotapes for its devotees, survey participants knew the therapeutic benefits of walking. A daily walk was part of most of the regular exercise programs described by our participants. And many of them headed out for a walk precisely when they felt their worst, for relief of both pain and stiffness. 'Whenever I get painful joints,' wrote a New York housewife, 'I walk until I feel better. Even if I don't go outside, but just walk around the house, it helps me.' A Texas homemaker said that if she is troubled by pain or stiffness during the night, she gets out of bed to walk it off. Walking outdoors, provided you are up and ready for it, has the added advantages of fresh air, a break from other activity, and the mental stimulation of the people and things you encounter on your way.

Massage

It's practically a reflex to put your hands on a painful area and rub it gently to bring relief. The warmth and increased circulation do help chase the pain – a fact that has kept massage in vogue for many centuries. Self-massage is quite effective, provided you can reach the parts that hurt. And if you're lucky enough to have someone else give you a good massage, you can let yourself drift into a state of relaxation that may bring you an even greater sense of well-being.

'Deep muscle massage done on a regular and sustained basis has proven to be the most beneficial treatment,' wrote a fifty-nine year old man from Vancouver, 'followed by stretching and strengthening exercises.'

'Massage helps a lot,' said a university student from California, 'because when my body is relaxed, it makes a world of difference in the pain level, especially for shoulder, neck, or back pain. I also find that a good foot and leg massage after walking or working relieves the stress and pressure I feel in those joints.'

Some participants liked to electrify their massage by using a hand-held massager, or a vibrator unit that slips over the hand doing the massaging, or by leaning against a massage/vibrator pillow.

Keeping Busy

Family life, jobs, education, volunteer work, sports, group activities, and hobbies distracted survey participants' minds from pain, and then some. 'I try to ignore the pain as much as possible,' said a machinist from Texas, 'and get on with my life. I enjoy everything I do, and do it as much as I can. I was told I had only seven or eight years to walk and then I would need a wheelchair. That was nine years ago.'

'I have pets and plants to care for, to need me,' wrote a forty-two-year-old widow from Montana. 'I keep active, and if I can't do the thing I want to do at the moment, I do something else until I feel I can. I don't do things just to show off, only to suffer later for it. I use common sense, but I don't fall into the "I can't" syndrome.'

Aspirin and Other Over-the-Counter Pills

Just as arthritis isn't 'minor aches and pains,' plain old aspirin isn't ordinary medicine. It's a heavy-duty drug that plays a pivotal role in arthritis treatment. (See Chapter 6.) However, aspirin and aspirin substitutes have another use – as staples in the home medicine chest. And that is where survey participants who usually get by without drugs sometimes look for pain relief.

If you take aspirin once in a while, try taking it with some food or milk, or even an antacid, so that it doesn't upset your stomach. You can choose plain, buffered, coated, or liquid aspirin, but the brand you use is irrelevant as far as anyone can tell.

The best-known aspirin substitute is Tylenol, which is made of acetaminophen. Some other brand names for acetaminophen are Datril, Panadol, and Anacin-3. Tylenol was quite popular among US participants and was mentioned at least three times more often than any other brand-name, over-the-counter pill. It relieves pain extremely well for many people, but it does not affect inflammation.

Another non-aspirin formula is ibuprofen – the key ingredient in the popular prescription drug Motrin. Ibuprofen is sold over the counter, too, in non-prescription strength, as Advil, Nuprin, and Medipren, to name a few brands. Like aspirin, ibuprofen works against both pain and inflammation.

WARNING: Aspirin and ibuprofen are related to each other and to all of the prescription non-steroidal anti-inflammatory drugs. Do not take aspirin or ibuprofen if you are regularly using one of these drugs, such as Motrin, Indocin, Naprosyn, or Feldene, to name some of the most popular ones. If you do, you may increase the risk of side effects from them. Acetaminophen, however, can usually be used with these drugs because it is not an anti-inflammatory. When in doubt, check with your doctor.

Warm or Hot Baths

'I love hot baths,' said a South Carolina secretary, and so do many, many others. 'I have only been diagnosed with rheumatoid arthritis for little over a year and so far I have found that long hot baths, splinting and not thinking about it work best for me,' wrote one woman from Greatham. Some like it hot, and some prefer it warm, but the bathtub was where half the US participants and 29 percent of UK participants sought pain relief. 'Sitting in a tub of warm water, not hot, for a good long time – half an hour, say – twice a day, helps about the best of anything,' swore a Wisconsin businessman, comparing his tub to prescription drugs, including steroids. An Iowa housewife rates the tub

right up there with one of the most popular forms of professional treatment: 'Physiotherapy helped my back, but I'm better
off with hot baths.'

A bath is also an effective antidote for stiffness. 'I sometimes
have to take a bath the moment I get up in the morning,' said a
Michigan homemaker, 'just to get my body moving.' Because of
the easier movement the water allows, several of our participants
liked to do their range-of-motion exercises in the tub. 'During
my hot soak every morning,' wrote a cafeteria server from
Colorado, 'I try to manipulate, rotate, and bend the fingers and
toes that are affected, as well as move my ankles, shoulders, and
elbows.'

A tubful of plain water was soothing enough for most people,
but a few liked to bathe with salts, oils, or bubbles.

The only thing wrong with a hot bath, according to a
California shipping clerk, is that you have to get out sometime.
After twenty to thirty minutes, a hot bath stops being therapeutic
and starts to tire the muscles.

Showers

'During serious flare-ups,' wrote a seamstress from Illinois,
'I take about three showers daily. It helps.' Most people would
rather soak in a tub for pain relief than stand in a shower (or sit
on a shower seat), but showers do offer a few unique advantages
participants enjoyed: (1) The temperature of the water can be
changed instantly to give alternating hot and cold treatments; (2)
the force of the water can be focused directly on the painful
areas, especially if you have a hand-held shower-massage attachment; and (3) it's easier to get in and out of a shower than a
bathtub.

Relaxation and Stress Reduction

With the majority of the US participants noting that stress aggravates their pain, it follows naturally that a number of them got
relief by reducing stress – or removing themselves from
extremely stressful situations when they could. Since that's not
always possible, and since no life is free of stress, they also relied
on stress-reduction techniques to calm themselves and their
pain. Meditation and visualization, mentioned earlier, can be

used for stress reduction. (These and several other stress-beating techniques are described in Chapter 15.) Here are some steps participants liked to take for a quick fix.

- Concentrate on your breathing. Take very deep breaths by expanding your chest without lifting your shoulders. Inhale slowly through your nose for five seconds, hold the breath for another five, and then slowly exhale through your mouth. Repeat until your heart stops racing.
- Let out your feelings. Cry, curse, laugh, pray, or whatever the situation calls for.
- Dive into a good book.
- Repeat some encouraging words to yourself – your own ('I can manage this'/'I know this will turn out fine') or someone else's (a line of poetry, a psalm, a song).

Although we usually think of stress as being mental or emotional or both, some survey participants cited *physical* stress as their worst enemy. A Wisconsin postal clerk's definition of stress reduction, for example, was to avoid any unusual strain on his body, such as heavy lifting and high reaching. When your body is overloaded, the arthritis pain inevitably increases, so it makes sense to try to control both kinds of stress.

Time Outdoors

Spending part of every day outdoors was a ritual with many of the participants, who got a general feeling of well-being from fresh air – and a few specific benefits, too. Some found special comfort at the beach, for example, where they could bury their hands and feet in the hot sand. And even though sunbathing to get a tan is no longer considered a healthy pastime, sitting in the sun with sunblock or clothes on just to revel in its warmth still feels good.

A writer from Illinois found a surprising source of pain relief when she went camping in Minnesota. At first, she could barely enjoy anything about the trip because her hands hurt so badly, but when she agreed to go fishing with her husband – and repeatedly washed the bait off her hands by dipping them in the icy water of the lake – her condition soon improved.

Joint Coverings

Many a wrist and knee has gone into an elastic bandage for a while to find relief. The wrapping could be an Ace bandage, an athletic ankle support, a Futuro Knee Thermo Comforter, a Barlow Knee Support, or any product that allows you to put gentle pressure on the affected joint. Even Band-Aid strips will do, according to an insurance underwriter from Nebraska who found them just the right size for the small joints of her fingers and toes. Ace and other elastic bandages are reusable, up to a point. 'I keep a supply of several elastic bandages in good condition, with lots of stretch,' wrote a housewife from California, 'and wash them by hand as needed.' Some of the participants said they get an added measure of relief by applying a liniment before wrapping the joint.

Under their feet, several participants liked the feel of an arch support or cushion insert in their shoes. Some of them used orthotics specially made for them by podiatrists or orthotists. Others shop for inserts at drug, shoe, or department stores, or shoe-repair shops. 'I am on my feet an average of twelve hours a day,' wrote a surgical nurse from South Dakota. 'The arch supports I bought at a shoe-repair shop for twelve dollars really help.'

Herbal Teas and Other Drinks

Hot caffeine-free drinks, especially herbal teas, are not only good-tasting and relaxing, participants said, but also help alleviate pain. 'I like chamomile or peppermint/chamomile mix or comfrey for soothing and relaxing me in general,' said a twenty-two-year-old California student who's had arthritis since she was seven. 'Maybe it's more mental than physical, but these help, especially on rainy days.' A retired office manager from Oregon who can no longer take anti-inflammatory drugs is now preparing her own teas with dried herbs she buys at health-food stores. 'In the past, I've taken Nalfon, Clinoril, and Feldene,' she wrote, 'but I can't any more because of a problem with my blood platelets. The only drug I use now is Tylenol, and I'm drinking herbal teas. Alfalfa with nettle seems to help the overall condition for me, and I'm still experimenting with other combinations.' Even when the herbs have no noticeable effect on their pain level, some participants enjoyed sipping hot herb or spice tea, or hot chocolate, just for the warmth it brings from within.

WARNING: Although herbal teas seem 'natural' and harmless, excessive quantities of herbs used medicinally can cause a variety of toxic effects.

A number of survey participants said they sometimes used a glass of wine, or a cocktail, or a 'good stiff drink' as a pain reliever. 'I like a glass of wine while I cook supper or after a rotten day at the office,' said a Kansas computer programmer, 'but too much creates problems of fluid retention and - self-recrimination.'

WARNING: Alcohol creates many other problems, as well, which are all too well known. Speaking strictly about arthritis, however, we noted that more than thirty of the US participants had a sensitivity to alcohol and suffered increased joint pain after they drank even a small amount of any alcoholic beverage. (See Chapter 12.) 'Don't turn to booze for relief,' warned a Virginia nursery and greenhouse worker. 'Although it gives some quick relief, I drank myself into being an alcoholic while trying to kill that last bit of pain.'

Hot Tub or Whirlpool

Most participants raved about plain baths, because most people have plain bathtubs, but those who owned whirlpools and hot tubs had the most to rave about. These minispas can combine the soothing comfort of soaking in a wide deep bathtub with the water-jet action of a shower massager. A few technical differences separate the whirlpool from the hot tub: A whirlpool is a tub of any size with a swirling current of water. A hot tub is also a bathtub with churning water, but it is usually made of wood, usually big enough for two or more, and has a heating element in it. A Jacuzzi could be either of these; it's really the name of the company that manufactures some of the most popular models. A California car dealer gave his Jacuzzi a plus-3 rating – higher than he gave to any of the practitioners who treated him. He spent twenty minutes a day in it at 98 degrees, and found it the best help of all. Our participants also used portable or 'home spa' units that work in any standard tub. 'I bought a two-hundred-dollar home whirlpool,' wrote an executive secretary from Texas, 'and it was the best two hundred dollars I ever spent. The whirlpool helps loosen tight muscles and relieves the pain. I use it every day.'

We're talking about 'at-home' treatments in this chapter, but you don't have to have a hot tub or whirlpool at home to enjoy its benefits. Several participants gladly make the trip to a health club or spa to use one. 'No matter how swollen I am or how much pain I'm in,' wrote a legal secretary from Ontario, 'five to ten minutes in a whirlpool gives me almost total relief.' And an office manager from California said she has kept a trailer at a county park for the past three years, just so she can use the Jacuzzi there.

Ice

Some participants favoured ice over heat for general pain relief, and some used it only on swollen, inflamed joints. 'The joint, if inflamed, is hot enough,' reasoned a retired nurse from New Jersey, 'so I apply ice instead of heat.' Gel-type ice packs that can be left in the freezer and then moulded to fit the painful part were quite popular, but many people got just as much relief from a well-placed bag of frozen peas or a plastic bag filled with water and ice. 'I fill a paper cup with water and leave it in the freezer,' said a Washington homemaker. 'Then I always have a quick pain reliever ready to rub over the joints.'

'What treatment works on one occasion may not work on another. Overall, the best treatments are a combination of ice, heat, exercise and massage with essential oils,' wrote a woman from Canvey Island.

WARNING: Remember that ice carries the danger of frostbite. If you use an ice pack, put a thin dish towel or cloth nappy on your skin for protection, and don't leave the pack in place for more than twenty minutes at a time. The ice-cup massage is safe for a minute or two on any one area – so long as you keep the cup moving.

Liniments

Ointments, creams, and liquids that survey participants rubbed on their joints gave many of them relief from pain, stiffness, and muscle soreness and helped them get through the day or sleep through the night. 'Aspercreme works well at night for a good night's sleep,' wrote an electronics technician from Minnesota.

Most liniments bring a feeling of heat to the area where they're applied, and this effect was enough for some people. 'BenGay is my best friend,' said a dressmaker from Illinois. 'I use it for warming up my joints.' Liniments may irritate your skin if it is sensitive, however, and you may or may not like their strong smell. A New Jersey homemaker jokingly reported that while BenGay was temporarily relieving her joint pain, it completely cleared her husband's nostrils.

The top-rated US favourites were Ben/EGay, Aspercreme, Icy Hot, Heet, Mentholatum, Absorbine Jr., Mineral Ice, and Myoflex, followed by Tiger Balm, Banalg, Sportscreme, and rubbing alcohol. Here are a few of the 'also-rans' (arranged alphabetically) that got five mentions or fewer: Aloe Vera Rub, Blue Star Horse Liniment, Deep-Down, InfraRUB, Mobisyl, Musterole, Myodyne, Oil of Wintergreen, Omega Oil, Pronto Gel, Rumal, Sloan's Liniment, Soltice, and Triple Liniment.

For cost or other reasons, a few participants prefered their own homemade rubs to any available in stores. A North Carolina church organist, for example, occasionally used her aunt's recipe – a mixture of one pint of rubbing alcohol and one ounce of Oil of Wintergreen, with one hundred aspirin tablets dissolved in it. An Illinois housewife relied on the same basic concoction, made with thirty-six aspirin instead of one hundred, which she rubbed on her knees before going out to walk.

WARNING: If you are allergic to aspirin by mouth, don't use Aspercreme or its equivalent on your skin. If you are unsure about a particular product, show it to your doctor. (Also see Chapter 6 for more information about liniments.)

Saunas and Steam rooms

The major difference between these two kinds of very hot rooms is their humidity. The sauna, heated with hot rocks, is drier than desert air, while the steam room, as its name suggests, is extremely moist. (The relative humidity in a sauna ranges from 5 to 25 percent, compared to about 95 percent in a steam room.) Participants recommended both for the soothing warmth they provide, but the steam room has the greater capacity to deep-heat your joints, partly because the steam makes it hard for your own sweat to evaporate.

TENS, Biofeedback, and Other Gadgets

Many types of professional pain-treating equipment seen in hospitals and practitioners' offices are also available for home use. On the advice of their physicians and therapists, participants bought or borrowed devices that stimulated their nerves electrically (TENS units, for *t*ranscutaneous *e*lectrical *n*erve *s*timulation); made them aware of some internal bodily rhythm (biofeedback); stretched them out (traction); or turned them upside down (gravity inversion). (See Chapter 8 for a more detailed explanation of the way practitioners apply these techniques.)

Sometimes called 'electric aspirin,' TENS units are small but complex machines that can give a gentle analgesic jolt. The unit itself, about the size of a transistor radio, generates electrical impulses. It attaches to your body via wires and electrodes taped to your skin at certain points, depending on where you hurt. No one knows exactly how or why it works, and the effects vary from one person to the next. 'I frequently rely on my personal TENS unit,' wrote a dental hygienist from Delaware, 'since I no longer want to take medication. After almost three years of popping pills – Dolobid, Feldene, Naprosyn, Parafon Forte, prednisone, and some others I can't remember – I was tired of them, and tired of the nausea and dizziness. So now I just tolerate the pain with the help of TENS.'

The equipment used for biofeedback can be as elaborate as a computer, as simple as a thermometer. More than forty US participants tried one type or another to learn how to gain conscious control over some ordinarily self-regulating bodily phenomenon, such as their pulse rate or the skin temperature of their feet. In operation, the machinery gives you *feedback*, in the form of light or sound, for example, that tells you how well you are controlling your internal *bio*logy. With practice, an Ohio housewife learned how to decrease her pain by raising her body temperature, and a Mississippi real estate agent found that he could avoid pain and stiffness by using biofeedback to relieve tension. If you want to learn biofeedback, look for a reliable teacher, perhaps a psychologist who is familiar with the technique.

Back or neck traction has helped some of our participants, and a few continue the treatments at home, including this bridge builder with the Santa Fe Railroad: 'I have a traction device that hooks over an open door. It has two pulleys and a clothesline rope, with a head-jaw harness on one end and a ten-pound bag of sand on the other. I sit under this occasionally, half an hour at a time, and try to work my crossword puzzle while it pulls apart the vertebrae in my neck.'

Only one of the participants, a California nurse, owns and uses the gravity-inversion equipment that was fairly popular a few years ago. It allows her to lie down and then turn herself upside down for ten minutes a day, which relieves the pain in her spine.

WARNING: Don't attempt traction (or inversion traction) on yourself without the direction of a physician or a physical therapist.

Meditation, Self-Hypnosis, and Other Mind-Control Techniques

Believing in the power of the mind over the body, many participants used some formal technique for guiding their thoughts away from pain. 'The basic philosophy here is "Heal thyself," and "I can overcome,"' explained a clinical psychologist from Tennessee with arthritis in his back and shoulders. 'Self-hypnosis has worked for me,' he added, 'and not just as a mask for pain.' Some found that the deep concentration required for these techniques serves to distract their minds from the pain in their joints. Others felt so relaxed after practising meditation or self-hypnosis that they were less troubled by pain, and a few actually managed to think their pain away. This is *not* to say that their pain was imaginary, or so minor that it could be easily quelled. Rather, it seems to reinforce what many medical researchers have shown about the mind/brain's ability to generate its own internal pain-relieving drugs, called endorphins. 'I could not function while on painkillers, and I was afraid to start using cortisone at the age of twenty-six,' wrote a production coordinator from Minnesota. 'I found I could control my pain with self-hypnosis, heat, and aspirin.'

Participants endorsed a wide range of mental techniques, from training in Transcendental Meditation, to seeing a psychologist for instruction in self-hypnosis, to simple visualization exercises that originate in their own fantasies. 'I sit or lie comfortably,' said a Colorado college professor, 'relax completely, close my eyes, and think of favourite scenes, such as my childhood home, sunsets, lighthouses against surf, and trout streams.' A New York tennis instructor said, 'I focus on my goal to be healthy and visualize in my mind all that good health means to me.'

If you would like to try your own form of meditation, give yourself the benefit of solitude and privacy for at least ten or twenty minutes a day. Take the phone off the hook, too. Pick your most comfortable position, so that you'll be able to relax your body. In fact, some people's entire 'meditation' consists of consciously trying to relax each body part in order, from the forehead to the toes, or vice versa. Closing your eyes and breathing deeply and evenly are also important. Deep breathing, like relaxing, is such potent medicine for some people that they can feel relief just by focusing their minds on inhaling and exhaling, perhaps repeating a sound or word with every breath. The more you practice meditation, proponents say, the better you get at it, and the better it can make you feel. For some participants, prayer confers the same benefits.

Food

Whatever they generally ate or avoided eating because of arthritis, several participants had a favourite food that figured in their pain-relief programs. Here are a few examples.

An Oklahoma bank teller: 'When I hurt, I baby myself. I get extra rest, I take warm/hot baths and soak for twenty minutes. I take extra aspirin, I dress warm from the neck down, including my feet, I drink hot tea, read, and eat oatmeal.'

A thirty-five-year-old artist from Ohio who's had both knees and hips replaced: 'I feel better once I've eaten a nice salad, fruit, or vegetables.'

An Idaho homemaker: 'I notice a lot of what I eat depends on how I feel on certain days. The fresh fruits are so refreshing when you don't feel too perky.'

Sometimes the absence of food is the therapy. 'I find that occasional fasting helps the way I feel,' said a newspaper reporter from Tennessee. Several clinical studies by medical researchers have shown that some people with arthritis definitely feel less pain after a fast, possibly because the fasting eliminates whatever food(s) may aggravate their symptoms. (See Chapter 11.) However, not enough of the participants used this technique for us to be able to evaluate it. On the contrary, we can see several good reasons for *not* fasting: (1) If you need to take pills regularly to control pain and need to take them with meals to minimize the drug side effects, fasting would disrupt your medication regimen. (2) If your appetite is poor and you have trouble eating, fasting might weaken you further. (3) If you are overweight or have an eating disorder, fasting one day may induce you to binge the next. (4) If you have any other medical conditions, such as diabetes, fasting poses even more serious dangers.

Combining Heat and Cold

Thermotherapy and cryotherapy, otherwise known as heat and cold, can make a great team when used one right after the other for combination therapy. Whatever the heat fails to soothe, the ice anaesthetizes. The owner of a small business in Utah wrote, 'I use a heating pad and ice when I have the worst pain. The alternating hot and cold really helps.' Participants mixed virtually every form of heat and cold for this technique, such as taking a hot shower and then turning it into a cold shower, using a hot-water bottle or a heating pad followed by an ice pack, and setting up two dishpans full of water for contrast baths. A bookkeeper from California treated her hands and feet this way, immersing them in warm and then cold water, back and forth every few minutes for a total of thirty minutes.

Cool Soaks and Mineral Springs

Not as well known as warm baths or hot showers, and not as popular as whirlpools or hot tubs, cold baths held a place in the hearts of some participants. A machine operator from Washington said they helped him more than anything, and several others talked about the virtues of soaking their swollen, painful hands or feet in cool water.

Only four of the US participants had visited natural springs reputed to have healing powers. They all enjoyed the experience, especially since they happened to have the natural wonders practically in their backyards in Nevada, Oregon, and Hot Springs, Arkansas. A photographer from Massachusetts, who was able to try the hot sulphur baths at the Dead Sea Spa while on assignment in Israel, pronounced them 'wonderful.'

Wax

Few things warm and soothe aching hands as thoroughly as a dip in hot wax. Paraffin treatments are a popular offering from physiotherapists, but several participants treated themselves at home. 'It was costing me fifty dollars a visit to see the physiotherapist,' recalled a retired telephone repairman from New Jersey, 'and Medicare only picked up twelve dollars of that. The wax felt so good that I wanted to go three times a week, but couldn't possibly afford to, so the therapist helped me buy my own paraffin bath for about $150. Now I use it twice every day.' You don't really need a special machine to try this treatment. Here are directions that a Massachusetts yarn-shop owner learned from her physiotherapist.

- *Materials:* 3 packages paraffin wax, available in grocery stores. Tall pot, pint of mineral oil, plastic bags big enough to fit over your hand, towel (warmed, preferably).
- Melt enough paraffin in the pot to fill it about halfway.
- Add mineral oil until the pot is three-quarters full. Stir well.
- Remove pot from heat and let cool until a light skin forms over the paraffin. Test the temperature.
- Keeping your fingers slightly apart, dip one hand and wrist in quickly and out again. Letting the paraffin dry slightly between dips, repeat this step ten times.
- Cover your hand with the plastic bag and wrap the warm towel over that, leaving them on for twenty minutes. Keep your hand still, or do your hand exercises in the soothing heat.
- Peel off the paraffin and save it to use again another time.
- Repeat the process on the other hand. When you're finished, massage your hands and fingers with the mineral oil that remains on your skin.

You may want to try the wax dip on your feet, too.

WARNING: The hot wax carries two dangers. (1) If you spill the paraffin or the mineral oil during heating, you could start a fire, so be extremely careful, or get a crockpot to use just for this purpose. (2) To avoid burning your skin, be sure to let the wax cool sufficiently before immersing your hand. You can also burn your hand or arm on the hot pot, so dip carefully. Burn safety is what makes paraffin bath units cost about one hundred dollars. They are temperature-controlled to keep the wax between 126 and 130 degrees, and made of heat-resistant plastic.

Summary of Top-Rated Self-Help Measures for Immediate Pain Relief

1. Comfortable positions
2. Exercise
3. Heat from a heating pad
4. Dressing for warmth
5. Rest
6. Walking for relief and relaxation
7. Massage of painful areas
8. Keeping busy with pleasant activities
9. Aspirin
10. Warm or hot baths
11. Shower
12. Heat
13. Relaxation
14. Time outdoors
15. Joint coverings
16. Herb teas and other warm drinks
17. Hot tub
18. Ice
19. Liniments
20. Sauna
21. TENS
23. Meditation, self-hypnosis
24. Comforting food
25. Cool soaks
26. Wax dips

Chapter 17
The Best Fitness Exercises for People with Arthritis

• *Walking* • *Swimming* • *Bicycling* • *Gardening and other physically demanding work*

Believing as they do that 'using it' keeps them from 'losing it,' the great majority of Arthritis Survey participants exercised regularly. Most of their workouts were a combination of stretching or strengthening exercises for their affected joints, together with some general fitness activity – such as walking or bicycling – that they enjoyed over and above its therapeutic value.

Some health experts have looked askance at vigorous exercise for people with arthritis, fearing that it would injure rather than improve their joints, but the latest studies show that physical exertion can actually reduce the symptoms of arthritis, provided it's done carefully, with medical approval, and *not* pursued during an arthritis flare-up. Exercise relieves pain for many of the survey participants. It also increases their joint flexibility and range of motion, offers them some protection from deformity and disability, and improves their muscle tone, which in turn builds strength and guards against contractures and spasms. Some of them find exercise an aid to weight loss. There are other health rewards, too, that you can reap from regular exercise, although they are unrelated to arthritis, such as lower blood pressure, reduced anxiety, a decreased risk of heart attack, greater mental alertness, and even a longer life expectancy.*

This chapter takes a look at the participants' favourite fitness exercises, and sees what exercise physiologists say about

---

* A continuing study of thousands of Harvard University alumni, reported in 1986 in the *New England Journal of Medicine*, shows that physically active men live longer than those who get no exercise.

the relative merits of each. But the most important goal here is to encourage *you* to talk to your doctor about taking up one of these physical outlets if you don't already take time to exercise.

Nothing to Fear, Much to Gain

The fitness boom that filled the streets with joggers may have left you feeling left out. All that running and pounding couldn't be good, could it? And if injuries ground so many people who start out with no musculoskeletal problems, what would happen to someone with arthritis who attempted jogging or aerobics?

The fact is that many people with arthritis can jog – in waist-deep water. And researchers at the University of Missouri Multipurpose Arthritis Centre, who enrol many of their patients in twelve-week exercise programs, say that a modified regimen of aerobics can improve the physical function of arthritic joints quite a bit. Even a short walk, if you take one every day, can work a substantial increase in your well-being within three or four months' time.

A fifty-three year old woman from Gloucester wrote, 'Prior to daily exercise I would experience stiffness and tenderness that led me to restrict movement, which made things much worse. When I exercise I warm the muscles around the inflamed joints. This is what seems to restore mobility and strength.'

'Exercise takes your mind off arthritis,' said a writing teacher in the survey, 'and fortifies your body to resist its effects.' Indeed, a fitness exercise such as walking can help prevent osteoporosis, because it strengthens the bones. Doctors at Washington University and the Jewish Hospital in St. Louis have found that exercise and calcium supplements can even help prevent osteo-porosis among women who are already past menopause.

'I walk and swim, play Ping-Pong, and do mild aerobics,' wrote a seventy-two-year-old retired pharmacist from New York. 'I've had to forgo baseball, badminton, tennis, and golf, though. After one good slam in a tennis match, my shoulder is useless, and a golf swing that really twists my knee sends me right to the club-house. But I try to exercise in some fashion for an hour or so a day, even if it's just gardening or washing my car. Sweating seems to help, and the activity *seems* to 'lubricate' my affected areas.'

This may be precisely what does happen. The heat you generate by exercising will warm your joints as well as any heating pad. And the motion of the joint is self-nourishing. As Dr. James F. Fries, director of the Stanford Arthritis Clinic, explains in his book *Arthritis. A Comprehensive Guide* (Addison-Wesley 1985), 'The cartilage of the joint . . . does not have a blood supply. It gets oxygen and nourishment and gets rid of waste products by compression – fluid is squeezed into the joint space, then removed and replenished. The health of the cartilage depends on motion, because without motion there is no nourishment of the cartilage.'

What kind of fitness exercise should you do? Here's a rundown of the ones the US participants like.

Exercise	Number of US Participants Who Do It
Walk	572
Swim or other water exercise	228
Bicycle or exercycle	116
Physical work, such as gardening	77
Rowing machine, Nautilus, etc.	21
Yoga	19
Dance (ballet, jazz, or 'slowly')	11
Aerobics (low-impact or dance)	10
Run or jog	10
Tennis or racquetball	10
Climb stairs	9
Bowl	7
Callisthenics	7
Golf	6
Handball, basketball, or volleyball	4
Exercise class at gym	4
Jump (rope or trampoline)	3
Karate or Tai Chi Chuan	3
Fish	1
Play indoor horseshoes	1
Roller-skate	1
Softball	1

And here is the list of favourite UK forms of exercise together with the ratings for improvement in mobility and pain relief: as you can see swimming comes out tops for both maintaining and improving mobility and pain relief.

Type of exercise	Number of UK participants taking it for mobility	Number taking for pain relief	Percentage who found the exercise maintained or greatly improved mobility	Percentage who found the exercise somewhat or greatly reduced arthritic pain
Walking	235	200	89%	56%
Swimming	155	144	93%	72%
Floor exercises	130	113	61%	54%
Gym	102	94	88%	56%
Yoga	39	32	86%	60%
Pilates	33	28	87%	46%

Almost any activity beats being sedentary, but some activities are better than others. Let's consider the favourites, in order of their popularity.

Walking

The oldest and best of the weight-bearing exercises.

'We no longer dispense eye of newt,' Dr. Gene H. Stollerman quipped in his regular column for *Hospital Practice*, 'but we certainly should be prescribing shanks' mare.' Dr. Stollerman called this exercise 'walking therapy,' and the 572 US survey participants and 235 UK participants who walk for fitness would probably agree with his terminology.

'I walk for at least an hour a day at a brisk pace,' reported a fifty-three-year-old Mississippi real estate agent, 'and the exercise seems to relieve the tension that can cause pain and stiffness.'

'I walk anywhere from one to six miles a day, depending on the season,' said a communications consultant from North Carolina, age fifty-six, who treats herself to high-quality hiking boots. 'In the winter I take a daily short walk, but in the summer

I build up gradually until I'm ready for my outdoor vacation, when I hike long distances in the wilderness. Activity is an important part of my pain management. If I hike too far, my ankles swell and hurt, so moderation is essential. But the improved muscle tone I have from walking helps me prevent falls or other injuries, and adds something positive to my self-image and my outward appearance.'

The ideal distance or speed you should walk depends on your overall fitness and the degree of joint damage you already have. This is why experts are always telling you to consult your doctor before you begin walking for exercise, even though you've been walking since age one. The general rule is to start out slowly and build up gradually, always listening to your body and your own common sense. One participant began by walking fifty feet a day, confident that if she could do that much initially, after being sedentary for years, she would eventually be able to walk more.

Physicians who study the physiology of walking, including Dr. James M. Rippe of the University of Massachusetts Exercise Physiology Laboratory, point out that anyone can start a walking program, indoors or out, that is easy on the joints and doesn't call for a big investment in fancy paraphernalia. Susanna Levin, an editor at *The Walking Magazine*, ticks off some of the other advantages.

- Walking, especially brisk walking, is definitely a good workout that will benefit your heart as much as your joints.
- Since most people can walk for a longer time than they could run, for example, or play tennis, walking tends to build muscular endurance and burn calories.
- Walking is so accessible and do-able that you're far less likely to quit this exercise regimen than any other you might try.

'Do something!' urged a forty-four-year-old factory worker from Wisconsin. 'Don't sit around feeling sorry for yourself. Even if it's only a short walk, you'll begin to feel better. I now walk at least three times a week. I go for about an hour, walking briskly for about two and a half miles. It's true that exercise gives you a sense of "well-being." And it *doesn't* increase your appetite. For me, it takes *away* the "munchies" feeling!'

For the UK participants walking maintained mobility for 41 percent, improved mobility for 24 percent and greatly improved mobility for 24 percent. In terms of pain relief 37 percent found walking somewhat reduced their pain while 19 percent found it greatly reduced their pain.

Swimming

Get the most out of exercise with the water's support.

Most of the 228 US participants who took to the water did so because of the buoyancy of the element, and the way it cushioned their joints from shock. 'Swimming is the best exercise,' said a Michigan homemaker, 'since you don't stress the joints. If you can't swim, just kick your legs and do range-of-motion exercises in the water.'

'My rheumatologist at the Mayo Clinic told me to swim every day for the rest of my life,' reported a forty-year-old social worker from North Dakota. 'I try to, and I've also taken the "Rusty Hinges" water exercise program at the YMCA. The water exercise is good, since you can move without much stress on your joints.'

The stress-free environment that the water provides had pretty much convinced exercise physiologists that swimming couldn't have the same bone-building advantages as weight-bearing exercises such as walking and running. However, researchers at the Veterans Administration Medical Centre in Portland, Oregon, say that the exertion of swimming *does* put enough force on the bones to strengthen them. They examined men whose only exercise was swimming, and then they compared the thickness of their bones to those of men who took no exercise. They found that the swimmers had a clear edge over the other men.

'I swim for half an hour, six days a week,' said a thirty-seven-year-old home health aide from Florida, 'and the only reason I don't swim on Sundays is that the pool is closed. I find that regular swimming eliminates pain. I swear by swimming.'

'I do aquafit three to four times per week. It has made a big difference and I now have strong muscles to support my joints. I also try to have a positive mental attitude, looking at what I can do rather than what I can't,' wrote a woman from Montreal.

As much as they raved about the sport, our participants railed about the water temperature of some of the pools they have used. 'I used to swim a mile to a mile and a half every day,' wrote a retired office manager from California, 'but now I cannot tolerate the cold water the pool has. I've found a private pool that should be available soon with 80-plus-degree water. Swimming really helped me, but the cold water only made the pain and stiffness worse.'

Swimming and other forms of water exercise are touted as being virtually injury-free, but one of the participants, a retired librarian from Missouri, did run into trouble in the water: 'I took a swimming course which was to help arthritics through exercise. This proved harmful because the up-and-down movements we were to make with our wrists only made mine sore, and they swelled more. I stopped going to the class. Swimming on my own, though, was very helpful. I am not an expert swimmer by any means. I learned to swim when I was forty years old, when my doctor told me just to go in the water, even if I couldn't swim. Eventually I learned, and my knee improved markedly.'

For UK participants swimming gave excellent results. For 30 percent swimming improved their mobility while for a whopping 33 percent swimming greatly improved their mobility. For another 30 percent swimming at least maintained their mobility. The results for pain reduction were also excellent – for 46 percent swimming somewhat reduced their pain, while for 26 percent it greatly reduced their pain.

Cycling

Bicycles and exercycles for indoor or outdoor exercise.

'A little over a year ago, I started riding a stationary bike daily,' said a secretary from Georgia. 'I very much feel this has helped keep me limber.' She wheeled through two and a half miles by the cycle's odometer before leaving for work in the mornings, and found, 'I loosen up, I feel better, and I now miss my exercising if I am unable to do it for any reason, because the stiffness returns.'

There is some controversy in cycling for arthritis, however. Dr. Willibald Nagler, physiatrist-in-chief at The New York Hospital-Cornell Medical Centre and author of *Dr. Nagler's Body*

Maintenance and Repair Book (Fireside 1988), says that pedalling puts too much stress on the knees and can cause inflammation. If your knees are affected, check with your doctor before making cycling part of your exercise routine. 'I tried to continue riding five miles daily on an exercise bike,' reported a housewife from Minnesota, 'and ended up with swollen knees.'

Exercycles are more flexible than bicycles, since you can reduce their wheel tension to zero, and with it the force your legs must fight. On the other hand, bicycling gets you out and about, and is therefore more appealing as a pastime, giving you a better chance of sticking with your exercise program.

'Exercising is much more enjoyable when done with others,' noted a retired family counsellor from California who rode her bicycle for thirty minutes a day. 'Establishing a regularly scheduled time and place also helps the maintenance of a good exercise program.'

Many participants built variety into their workouts by combining more than one type of fitness exercise, including this retired school superintendent from Massachusetts: 'I walk at least two miles a day, or in summer swim a half a mile a day. During the winter months I ride an exercise bicycle and work out on Nautilus machines three days a week for an hour at a time.'

Physical Work

You don't have to be a 'jock' to get your exercise.

The fact that 'activity' is now considered the equal of exercise by many doctors is proof that fitness has come home. Not everyone can be a marathon runner, but anyone can make some slight increase in everyday activities that could lead to better fitness.

'I work in my garden for exercise,' wrote a homemaker from Illinois, 'hoeing, weeding, and so on, all of which really helps, for as long as two to three hours a day in summer.'

The idea that physical exertion 'counts' as exercise is a new one, however, and for every participant who named gardening or housework as an exercise, there were others who explained that they couldn't follow an exercise program because they were too busy doing physical work. 'I am a waitress,' wrote a fifty-two-year-old survey participant from California. 'I am on my feet a minimum of eight hours, five days a week. I move. When I stop and relax, the pain starts. I use my hands and my shoulders carrying and serving an average of a hundred customers a day. I have a degree in library science, but I cannot do a job that is not physical. When I am sedentary, I stiffen up and can't move at all. I feel that my job as a waitress keeps me alive and moving.'

Here's another person who answered *no* to the question, Do you exercise for arthritis? 'I do not exercise in a set pattern,' said this retired advertising director from Illinois. 'However, I keep a two-storey house, paint it inside and out, refinish antique furniture, and do garden and lawn work.'

'I try to swim laps two to three times a week, and walk constantly,' said a thirty-six-year-old freelance writer from New York who has had two joint-replacement operations. 'I also do house, garden, and yard maintenance. Sometimes it's exercise enough trying to live a normal, active life.'

Summary of Fitness Exercises for Arthritis
Walking is an excellent form of exercise for most people with arthritis because:

- It is weight-bearing (and therefore bone-building).
- It offers an easy start and great room for advancement in terms of distance covered and pace achieved.
- It is low-risk, compared to jogging or other fitness activities.
- It can be done indoors or out, with no special equipment.

Swimming and other water exercises are also excellent because:

- The buoyancy of the water protects your joints from shock.
- The water makes possible many kinds of movements that would be difficult or dangerous on dry land.
- The exercise may be bone-building even though it's not weight-bearing.

Cycling is often an ideal path to fitness because:

- Exercycles and multispeed bicycles offer a wide range of tension settings (or speeds) to accommodate different levels of strength and ability.

- The exercise challenges and builds up the leg bones and muscles, although it may aggravate arthritis of the knee.

Physical Activity, such as gardening, is thought to be good exercise because:

- It confers some of the same bone and muscle benefits as other forms of mild exercise.
- It offers the chance for people who are not athletic to become more active, and consequently more fit.

Chapter 18
How to Make Your Environment More Comfortable

• The best mattress • Kitchen conveniences • Chairs and stairs • Bathrooms as home hydrotherapy centres • Workplace changes • Car comfort

Every room in your house, every workplace, every mode of transportation, and every spot you visit contains something that can become a problem because you have arthritis: the couch is too soft to sit on comfortably; the toilet seat is too low; cooking and eating utensils are too hard to hold. But every one of these problems has a solution, as the US participants in the Arthritis Survey have found.

Nearly half the 1,051 US survey group members said they got along splendidly *without* any special aids or adjustments, either because their successful treatment plans allowed them full function or because their arthritis had not yet restricted them. Some participants were planning to make certain changes in their surroundings, and a few asked for advice on what to do and how to do it. The other half of the participants, on whose experience we base this chapter, have met and mastered countless challenges by modifying their environment – at home, at work, or on the go. These changes run the gamut from the simple purchase of a single item, such as a jar opener or a back-support cushion, to major overhauls, such as finding a different job or moving to a one-storey home. They can be as cheap as a strip of foam rubber to wrap around a pencil or as expensive as an indoor heated swimming pool. Here are all the alternatives learned about in the survey – both the general suggestions and the many specific items, whether handmade or store-bought. Most of the items can be found at drug or discount stores, in medical supply outlets, or ordered through the mail from the companies the survey participants recommended.

At Home

When a powerhouse electrician and his wife from Pickwick Dam, Tennessee, built their new house three years ago, they used the fact that they both had arthritis as a basic element of the design. Their home is a model of what good planning can do in the interest of comfort. 'We installed a heat pump instead of a fireplace or wood stove. We placed all of the electrical outlets high on the walls where they can be reached without stooping. The bathroom is only ten steps from our bed, and the commode is on a six-inch raised platform for easy on and off. We also installed a large bathtub with a whirlpool. Our bed can be elevated at the head and foot, and has a built-in vibrator. The kitchen is small, with all the storage space placed at a height that requires a minimum amount of stooping and lifting.'

About fifty participants left a large two- or three-storey house for a one-level home, an apartment in an elevator-service building, or a new start in a warmer climate. Others, who stayed within the confines of their existing homes or limited budgets, were quite successful in their efforts to revamp their surroundings, as you'll see. Before we trail them around from room to room for special tips about beds, bathtub railings, and the like, here are a few ideas that could work anywhere.

- Rearrange your cupboards, closets, or other storage areas to make sure you put your most frequently used items within easy reach.
- Arrange your furniture for safe and easy passage through the room. Eliminate unnecessary items as you do this, and you'll also simplify your housecleaning. Where possible, position a super-sturdy table or bookcase near the places you like to sit, in case you need some help getting up.
- Find out where the draughts are coming from and eliminate them.
- When buying items that you must carry or push – dishes, iron, vacuum cleaner, etc. – choose the lightest ones you can find.

- Make doors easier to open with lever handles that fit over standard knobs.
- Carpet the floors if you can. At least put a rug or a rubber mat wherever you stand for any length of time – in front of the kitchen sink, for example – but get rid of other scatter rugs before you trip on them, especially if you walk with a crutch or a cane.
- Build up the handles of hard-to-hold utensils or tools with pipe insulation, bubble wrap, or even the foam from a plastic hair curler.
- Equip your home with step stools and long-handled utensils (from shoehorns to feather dusters) that save you the discomfort of reaching up and bending down.
- Replace hard-snapping light switches with soft-touch wall switchplates and touch-on attachments for lamps.

An Ohio artist asked a student from the local vocational school to advise her in rearranging her kitchen to save steps, ease traffic flow, and prevent falls and bumps. ('Knee against table legs – ugh!') Then she used the traffic-flow idea throughout her house, keeping furniture in small groupings, and she is well pleased with the results. 'I also love my bedroom more,' she writes, 'since I added pillows, a well-lighted vanity, and soul-feeding things like my own corner and my own art creations.'

Bedroom

A good mattress is the cornerstone of comfortable living, although the definition of 'good' may vary from extra firm, which is the survey favourite, to relatively soft. Most participants who stressed the importance of a good mattress slept on a combination of layers – and recommended it highly. They begin with a bedboard or platform bed to give a solid base, put a firm mattress on that, and top off the whole with a layer of egg-crate foam. (You'll know egg-crate foam when you see it, with its flat bottom and convoluted top layer that looks as though it could hold a few dozen eggs.) This arrangement combines the firmness needed for good back support with the right amount of soft padding to cushion painful hips or shoulders. The nice thing about egg crate, participants reported, is that it handles your body gently – as though it were as fragile as an eggshell. Manufacturers claim that it cushions and buffers the body by virtue of its many small pockets of air, keeping pressure off the sore spots. Other kinds of mattress pads, made of dimpled foam, achieve the same results for other satisfied participants.

Some people preferred a mattress made entirely of foam, instead of a standard mattress with a foam pad on top. 'I have been sleeping on polyurethane – that's the technical name for foam rubber – for over eight years,' wrote a retired court stenographer from Massachusetts. 'This helps to relieve the pressure on my hips, spine, or legs. Regular mattresses caused me much pain. There is nothing that can compare with foam rubber!'

A luxurious covering for any kind of mattress is a woollen bed pad (sheepskin) or electric mattress pad/bed warmer. The luxury comfort of these items frequently comes with a luxury-level price tag as well, but some participants consider them necessities. Flannel or thermal sheets (preferably flat for easy handling, not tightly fitted) are another, less expensive, way to warm up a cold bed. And over the sleeper, the top choices are electric blankets, followed closely by sleeping bags, down comforters, or other warm but lightweight covers. 'My electric blanket is a lifesaver,' saaid a New York saleswoman. 'It allows me to get out of bed each morning.'

A bed board is typically a ¾-inch piece of plywood cut to fit your bed and placed between the mattress and the box spring. Once you get used to the support it provides (for sleeping and for helping you get out of bed), you may wish you could carry one along on trips – and several of our travelling participants said they use a lightweight version that folds to become portable.

A few additional words about the bed board: it doesn't work for everyone. 'My backbone and yours are *not* a straight line like the bed boards so many swear by,' said a mechanical engineer from California. 'I don't get their geometry.' A glassmaker from West Virginia, who's had both hips replaced, agreed: 'Yes, I tried a bed board once, for about two weeks. It caused me more pain, so I quit using it. I do need to change mattresses every so often, though, because even a firm mattress finally wears out.'

What *does* seem to work in bed for everyone is an extra pillow, or several extra pillows in a variety of shapes and sizes to raise the knees just so, for example, to give the neck a special cradle, to support the hips during sex, or to keep the blankets off feet that hurt. Participants named a variety of specialized items, including neck rolls, butterfly pillows, cervical pillows, orthopaedic pillows, arthritic pillows, leg rests, and bed wedges, but an ordinary bed pillow or a piece of foam cut to your exact specifications can work just as well. 'I need at least two bed pillows to prop up my legs,' noted a Mississippi homemaker. 'I don't just put my feet on them, but push them up under my legs for support while resting.'

Thirty-two of the participants mentioned that they sleep on a water bed, and most of them raved about its comfort. 'Without my 'Flotation System' water bed I could not sleep for more than three or four hours,' wrote an assembly-line worker from Wisconsin, 'and the good night's sleep I get now works wonders for me!' Only one other water bed was mentioned by brand name, the Semi-wave water bed from National Bedrooms, and the rest were just called 'wonderful.' Why? 'The water bed helps a lot because it gives me firmness and heat,' explained a Pennsylvania housewife, 'with nothing pressing on the bone spurs in my spine.' A few men and women said the water bed was the best boon to lovemaking they had found, and an artist swore that if it didn't wiggle so much, she would stay in it all day in wintertime to do her painting. In fact, the only two complaints we heard about water beds came from women who really had no problem sleeping in them but had considerable trouble struggling out of them in the morning. (A water bed must be kept properly filled to give firm support.)

Any bed, truth to tell, can taunt you getting in and trap you once you're there. Many participants licked this problem by raising their beds to a more manageable height – approximately six inches above the norm, or whatever feels comfortable. Beds can be elevated on wood or cement blocks, or, as one disabled civil servant did, by piling on an extra mattress. Several people purchased or built high platform beds, and then found to their delight that the platform offered even better support than their old box spring and mattress. A platform is the ultimate bed board. Hospital beds are also higher than standard bed frames and have the added advantage of motorized movement to elevate your head or legs as you desire.

Two women in the survey said they've had to stop sleeping in a double bed with their husbands and switch to twin beds. Six participants liked to put their mattress or a couple of egg-crate pads right on the floor for firm (and inexpensive) support, and another five preferred, at least some of the time, to sleep in their reclining chairs.

Aside from the ideal sleeping arrangement, several participants made their bedrooms more comfortable with a good chair to sit in while reading, a bedside lamp that turns on with the gentlest touch of a button, and a television set. (Remote control is ideal, if you have it, but at least position the TV so you can turn it on without stooping and watch it without straining your neck or back.) A former insurance secretary from California with very limited use of her hands has replaced the door of her bedroom closet with a curtain, and she uses open shelves hanging from the closet pole, instead of the formal bureau with its stubborn drawers.

'I keep a footstool in the bedroom to help me get dressed,' wrote a retired salesman from New York. 'I'm slightly over six feet tall, and it's a long way down to the shoes these days.'

Kitchen

With so much time spent here and so many different kinds of tasks to be done, the kitchen becomes a home's haven for gadgets. The most popular of these, by far, among the survey participants were the ones that let everything but genies out of bottles, cans, and jars. There are electric can openers, of course, plug-in and portable models, stationary jar openers that attach to the wall or under a cabinet, rubber grippers that fit over screw tops and make them easier to open, plastic moulds that hold on to the bottoms of bottles while you turn the tops, hand-held gizmos that adjust to fit every size top or cap and remove them with lever action, 'tab grabbers' for aluminium drink cans, and the old standbys – pliers and nutcrackers. It seems as though no one can get along without one of these devices.

The most frequently mentioned aid for meal preparation was not a cooking utensil per se, but a high stool that lets one sit comfortably at the kitchen counter or the sink. A few participants had gone a step beyond the stool and actually changed the height of their counters, either raising them to eliminate a lot of leaning over or lowering them to accommodate a cook in a wheelchair. Appliances, too, can sometimes be height-adjusted. 'The stove in my kitchen was too low,' said a forty-three-year-old secretary from Idaho. 'Raising it just four inches lessened the pressure and pain in my knees.' Consider yourself lucky if you have a waist-height wall oven.

Under and over the counters, the cupboards themselves can be made more user-friendly by replacing small knobs or handles with ones that are easier to hold, by raising or lowering the handles, by removing snap locks, or by taking off the doors altogether. Inside, you can arrange your foods and utensils so that the heaviest and most-used items are closest at hand. Revolving shelves, or lazy Susans on the existing shelves, can save a lot of reaching, too.

Cadillac appliances for simplifying cooking are the food processor and the microwave oven. The processor makes short work of dicing and chopping, it's true, but not everyone can afford one. A retired educator from Georgia and an Ohio farm wife had both hit on the same strategy to simplify slicing vegetables by hand. They drove a long nail through a cutting board to keep onions or what-have-you in their place. Some participants said that just *using* a chopping board, rather than cutting foods in their hands as they had always done, makes the work easier. A North Carolina homemaker solved the peeling problem by cooking her potatoes with the skins on, and she reasoned that she not only saved herself the aggravation of peeling but added a few extra nutrients to her family's meals. Participants who insisted on peeling, though, preferred bona fide vegetable peelers to paring knives. Some found that a peeler with a U-shaped handle is easier to use than the straight-handled peeling/coring type.

As for the microwave, it is the first choice of those who like to cook early in the day for reheating at dinnertime, those who cook huge quantities of food on good days to freeze for bad times, and those who rely heavily on packaged frozen foods such as potpies and TV dinners. Any oven can heat up frozen foods, of course, but the microwave does it faster *and* – even more important to some participants – doesn't require the use of pots or pans. If you're sticking with your conventional oven, you may want to trade in your heavy cookware and dishes for lightweight ones.

The other appliances cited in the survey for comfort and convenience were the large electric mixer with dough hook for those who make their own bread, the dishwasher, and the electric pot scrubber. However, many participants didn't use the dishwasher even though they have one, on the grounds that a sinkful of warm water and dirty dishes was good therapy for the hands. Several of them said they intentionally left dishes in the sink overnight, so the chore of washing them first thing the next day could help banish the morning stiffness in their fingers.

As mentioned earlier in this chapter, almost any utensil with a handle can be made into a custom-fitted tool by wrapping and fattening the handle until it's easier to hold. Here are the materials survey participants used for this purpose.

- sponges fastened with tape
- foam or rubber tubing, which can be cut to any length, with centre holes of various diameters
- foam-type hair curlers
- dish towels or washcloths
- plastic bubble wrap used to protect fragile items for shipping

If none of these works on your kitchen sink, consider trying one of the commercially available tap turners that come in a variety of designs and shapes to fit over any type of faucet. A few of the participants replaced the existing taps on their sinks with flat blade-shaped handles – or a single lever-type faucet that controls both the volume and the temperature of the water.

There are also many specialty utensils manufactured with extra thick, extra light, or angled handles, all available by mail order, as well as lightweight mugs with easy-grip handles, and some with *two* easy-grip handles.

Bathroom

The bathroom is typically the home hydrotherapy centre for arthritis self-care. Well over half the participants turned to it at least once a day for the soothing powers of a hot shower or a warm bath. A good number of them said they also exercise while bathing, because the warmth and buoyancy of the water make movement more manageable. Home hot-water therapy was so important to one Illinois lawyer that he installed a special large-capacity hot-water heater in his home to assure himself an abundant supply.

You may find it easier to turn the water taps if you exchange your round or four-pronged faucet handles for lever shaped ones, or use a cushiony rubber jar grip from the kitchen for this purpose.

For safety, participants favoured some kind of handrail on the tub side, which also eases entry and exit. In the stall shower, too, they said, a rail or 'grab bar' makes a good investment. Your tub should of course be equipped with a no-slip bathmat, and for comfort, you might like to try a bathtub mattress or a cushion made of inflatable plastic. The ultimate luxury though, is a home spa unit that churns the bathwater with whirlpool action.

'I found that I was in a hot tub of water so much,' wrote a hairstylist from Virginia, 'that for Christmas I asked for a portable whirlpool. I love it. I use it a couple of times per week, and to me it's worth its weight in gold. The one I have is by Pollinex, and it allows me to adjust the speed and direction of the water flow, so I can let the water pulsate just where I need it – and at different times, I need it at different places. For about $150, I have found my salvation. It was my idea, too, not the doctor's, and it's better than any medicine he has prescribed to date!'

The shower version of the whirlpool bath is the pulsating or massage-type attachment, such as the ones manufactured by Pollinex and Water Pik. Some of these replace the existing shower head, changing the force and flow pattern of the water. Other types attach to the tub faucet, serving as hand-held showers that allow for extra attention directly on painful places.

Some participants also liked to shower sitting down, on a homemade or store-bought shower seat. Even those who could stand comfortably chose to use the seat because it helped prevent falls, facilitated washing, and made it easier to take full advantage of the water. 'I use a piece of plywood to straddle the bathtub edges when I shower,' said a Pennsylvania masonry contractor, 'so I can sit down and give my knees a shower-massage treatment.'

A few of the participants, however, found the height of the tub side to be an insurmountable obstacle. A Michigan housewife reported, 'We removed our old bathtub, because it was difficult to step high to get into the tub. We now have a walk-in shower with a seat and a pulsating shower head. This is a tremendous help to me.' One retired plumber from Wisconsin who had an old-fashioned high bathtub with feet built an elevated platform to help him get in and out of it.

Once you have gone to any trouble or expense to avoid extra stooping and reaching while you bathe, you don't want to be foiled by something as simple as a slippery bar of soap. A resourceful Arizona craftswoman said she crocheted a small mesh bag to hold her soap, and she keeps it tied to the shower head on a long string. Avon and several other cosmetics manufacturers achieve the same end with a 'soap on a rope' that hangs conveniently from the faucet or around the bather's neck. A long-handled back brush is another nicety – or even a yardstick with a sponge on the end of it, as suggested by a North Carolina maintenance man.

An extremely popular way to raise the comfort level in the bathroom is to raise the height of the toilet seat. There are several models of raised seats, from specially shaped foam pads about two inches thick to steel-and-plastic additions that elevate the seat level as much as eight inches. Any of them can be installed or removed quite readily, so it needn't be considered a permanent change. In fact, several participants said that they have used a raised toilet seat as a temporary measure while recovering from surgery, for example, or during a painful flare-up.

Handrails are also a useful addition to the toilet, whether or not the seat is raised. Some handrail styles automatically raise the seat level an inch or so when installed, and the installation is usually a simple matter of slipping some aluminium rails together and into position.

Several participants liked to use an electric toothbrush, not just because of its brushing action but because of its thick easy-to-hold handle. 'For myself and for my arthritic patients,' said a dental hygienist from Delaware, 'I make a special toothbrush by wrapping bubble wrap (bubbles out) around the handle a few times and securing it with strapping tape.' Two products mentioned by a Missouri National Guardsman, 'Floss Fingers I' by Preventive Dentistry Products and 'Floss Mate' by Butler, will let you floss your teeth with one hand, and without the dexterity usually required to floss the back teeth. Pump-type dispensers for toothpaste, soap, and hand lotion may also simplify your bathroom visits.

Living Room

If you do most of your sitting in the living room, you have many options for making that pastime as comfortable as possible. The simplest is to start with what you have and modify it if you have to. A straight-back chair is many people's favourite, because it combines decent back support with a relatively high seat that is easy to reach and to leave. If the chair has arms to aid you, so much the better. If it feels too hard on your hips or doesn't give enough support for your lower back, you can pad the appropriate places. 'I have straight-back chairs in the kitchen and the living room,' said a retired kindergarten teacher from Rhode Island, 'and I use cushions with them.' Low chairs caused her so much trouble that she never uses them, preferring to stand at friends' houses if no suitable chair is available.

Cushions on chairs also serve to raise them a little higher, which is all to the good. Many styles are portable, and many of our participants carried a favourite chair cushion wherever they go, whether it's an inexpensive piece of flat foam or a costly automatic lifter seat with spring-action that actually helps them to their feet. It is also possible to raise a chair or a couch from the bottom up – by standing it on a platform about four inches high, on risers or wood blocks, or by replacing the existing legs with taller ones. Some of the mail-order catalogues offer 'chair raisers' that attach to furniture legs and raise them three to five inches.

Only a few of the participants felt the need to go out and buy a new chair, but those who did were awfully pleased with the result. The favourite investments were recliners or lounge chairs with footstools, because of the reduced pressure on knees and hips while sitting. Others preferred rocking chairs or posture-control chairs. Some of the armchairs purchased came complete with built-in heating elements for the back, or vibrator/massage units, or both. 'My easy chair is the most useful item I've found,' wrote a retired science teacher from Texas, 'and I found it in a department store. Shopping for it was a time-consuming job, as I had to visit many stores in order to get a properly fitting chair.

A chair that does not fit properly means only one thing: lots of pain.' *Amen*.

Stairways and entryways

'Stairs are my worst enemy,' admitted a retired nurse from Pennsylvania. In her own home, she avoided them with an electrical lift that carries her up or down the stairs along a steel beam. Other participants, who shared her sentiments but couldn't afford this several-thousand-dollar convenience, either moved or resigned themselves to living on one floor of their homes: 'I haven't been upstairs in ten years,' said a seventy-five-year-old Kentucky housewife with arthritis in her knees. 'The last time was when I went to get Christmas decor no one else could find. I was home alone, without a phone up there. I found what I wanted, all right, but I couldn't walk back down. I finally had to throw a leg over the banister and slide down. 'Twas fun.'

Others, who find stairs difficult but not impossible, said they got by with a good sturdy handrail. They said that handrails are essential on *all* stairways, even the two or three steps that lead up to the front or back door.

A few participants have rebuilt their outdoor stairways so that the individual steps are smaller and easier to climb. Others have replaced the steps with wheelchair ramps, and widened the doorways, too, where necessary. Although a wider entry may sound like a major job for a carpenter, it is possible to expand many doorways by about one and a half inches with offset hinges that swing the door free of the door jamb.

At Work

More than 90 percent of the US survey participants continued to work for a living – or did work until they reached retirement age. They did everything from writing sermons to waiting tables; they managed corporations, assembled automobiles, provided health care, created stained-glass windows, and marketed cosmetics door-to-door. Most needed no special allowances made for them at work, but a few really had to modify their activities or change their job descriptions. A North Carolina registered nurse, for example, stopped working in a hospital because it involved too much walking. Now she does private duty nursing, which requires a lot of sitting. 'I sit,' she added, 'in a straight-back chair.'

Changing jobs because of arthritis can be an opportunity for positive growth, as a forty-one-year-old Minnesota woman found when she quit working as a librarian to open her own clothing store and sewing business. 'Lifting books and standing on cement floors was stressful to my wrists, hands, and feet,' she recalled. 'Now I have a carpet in my place of business.'

For most of the participants, though, making the work environment more comfortable was a simple matter of adding the right equipment to get the job done.

If you sit at a desk, whether to type letters or design buildings, the key point is to make sure that the chair is a comfortable one. Although it is not always possible to request and receive a new or different chair, you can at least take your own foam seat pad or back-support cushion to work, to make yourself feel at home. Several participants said they were happiest in a secretary-type chair with wheels, because the seat height and back support can be adjusted to suit them. 'I put my secretary chair to full use,' said an Indiana receptionist, 'because I scoot around in it, too.' Sitters also liked a footstool under the desk, which kept their knees higher than their hips and thus helped them avoid back pain, a major occupational hazard of sitting at a desk. If you use a typewriter or computer that is positioned at right angles to your desk, you may be able to rig a footstool by opening the bottom desk drawer and resting your feet on it.

Desks and drawing boards can sometimes be height-adjusted, too. A desk with easy-to-pull drawers makes a good co-worker. A few forgo the desk altogether in favour of a podium where they can stand to read and write.

On the desk, our participants selected oversize or specially curved pens, preferably with a felt tip because its ready ink flow requires a minimum of pressure to leave bold marks. Those who used a pencil selected the softer leads for the same reason – and electric pencil sharpeners. If the pen or pencil wasn't specially designed, they customized it with a plastic triangle or ring, sold in stationery stores, that widens the implement and softens the grip. (Or use the foam curler trick, described earlier.) They used easy-grip, large-handled or loop-handled scissors, or they cut with a newspaper-clipping gadget that they slide along like a razor, without needing to open and close their hands. A smaller stapler, some said, doesn't have to be slammed with a sledgehammer fist. Another convenience is a speaker phone that leaves your hands free, or a lightweight headset that plugs into any modular phone.

Outside the office setting, many participants worked with their hands for a living or for a hobby. Several have raised or lowered their workbenches for maximum comfort and the safe use of power tools. They also chose lighter-weight machinery, where possible, and got power assistance from gadgets such as the self-charging portable electrical screwdriver, sold at hardware stores. 'I like to work in the garage,' said a foreman and machinist from Pennsylvania. 'A stool with wheels sold by Pep Boys, a national auto supplier, is a big help when working on a car.'

On the Go

Cars – with their thumb-action door handles, their crank-up windows, their strangely positioned controls, their oddly angled seats, and the demands they place on the driver's hands, feet, shoulders, neck, back, and hips – were a necessity for most participants, who have, by necessity, found ways to make them more comfortable.

You can get past the door-handle problem with a plastic door opener that hooks around the handle and presses that annoying button for you. You can turn the ignition more easily with a wooden or plastic key turner or a small crescent wrench. But once inside you've still got to sit in the driver's seat for some period of time. Make it as comfortable as your other chairs by adding a back support or a folding car seat that offers support for your back and your bottom. Some participants also mentioned gel-filled cushions, inflatable cushions, egg-crate car seats, sacroiliac pillows, massage seats that plug into the cigarette lighter, cervical pillows, and the Posture Curve back support from Body Care, Inc., of New York City. Even if you're driving in the backseat, you'll find that taking some kind of pillow along to wedge behind your back or under any painful area can make the trip more pleasant. A few people preferred to lie down on the backseat, and a former photographer from Illinois purchased a van so that she could travel lying on a comfortable mattress in the rear.

Several participants said they traded in their stick shifts and clutch pedals for cars with automatic transmission. Buyers beware, however, that the gear-shift lever on many automatics has a thumb button that may be quite difficult to operate.

Most new cars have a host of electronic conveniences and labour-saving designs that could have been custom-made for people with arthritis, from power steering and power brakes to easy-touch buttons that open and close the windows, seats that change position electrically, and more easy-touch buttons that lock or unlock all the doors simultaneously. Cruise control, which can put your car on automatic pilot for long stretches of highway driving, lets you relax your legs and feet at 55 m.p.h., but it's no substitute for stopping the car every hour or so and getting out to stretch.

Large cars were favoured for their greater legroom and smooth ride, especially four-door models for ease of getting in or out. 'I avoid all cars with bucket seats,' said a psychotherapist from New York, 'which seem to press on the hip bones and lead to pain.'

Once you get where you're going, do you have trouble finding a place to park? Several participants mentioned the value of handicapped license plates or permits enabling them to park right in front of many stores and public buildings.

'Don't use the "Handicapped" parking space if another is nearby,' advised a retired engineer from Florida who follows his own advice. 'Someone worse off may need it.'

Summary of Practices and Products to Increase Your Comfort and Safety

Throughout Your House

Organize cupboards to keep frequently used products within easy reach.

Arrange furniture for safe passage, minimal clutter, and support when rising from a couch or chair.

Eliminate draughts.

Choose lightweight appliances.

Modify door knobs and handles with easy-open levers.

Use soft warm floor coverings that won't make you slip or trip.
Build up handles for easy gripping.
Let step stools and long-handled utensils extend your reach.
Install easy-touch controls for lamps and ceiling lights.

Bedroom Comforts

Good mattress
Foam mattress pad
Woollen or electric bed pad
Flannel or thermal sheets
Sleeping bag

Bed board
Special pillows
Water bed
Raised bed
Hospital bed

Kitchen Helpers

Can, bottle, and jar openers
High stool
Revolving shelves or lazy Susans
Food processor
Microwave oven
Lightweight dishes, pots, pans

Electric mixer
Fat-handled utensils
Tap turners on water faucets
Chopping board (with nail)

Bathroom Aids

Easy-to-use faucet handles
Tub rail
Shower grab bar
No-slip bathmat
Whirlpool unit
Raised toilet seat
Handrails for toilet

Shower massage
Tub or shower seat
Soap on rope
Bath brush
Electric toothbrush
Dental floss tool
Pump dispensers

Living Room

Straight-back chair
Back-support cushions
Chair pads
Footstool

Lifter seat
Chair raisers
Recliner

Stairways and Entryways

Electrical stair lift
Sturdy handrails

Modified entry steps
Widened doorways

Office and workshop

Secretary chair
Footstool (or open desk drawer)
Soft lead pencils
Electric pencil sharpener
Raised (or lowered) work-bench
Power tools
Lightweight machinery

Electric typewriter
Word processor
Fat felt-tip pens
Stool with wheels
Easy-grip scissors or clipper
Speaker phone or head-set
Small stapler

Car

Car-door opener
Key turner
Car-seat cushion
Automatic transmission
Power steering and brakes
Electronic windows and locks

Automatically adjustable seat
Cruise control
Handicapped plates or permit

Chapter 19
How to Go About Your Everyday Activities with Minimum Pain and Maximum Ease

• Smart tips for joint protection • Gadgets that get things done • Scheduling activities and rest to help you accomplish more • New ways to keep doing what you need to do, what you love to do

Among them, the 1,051 US Arthritis Survey participants have racked up some fifteen thousand man- or woman-years of living with arthritis. That's many lifetimes' worth of persevering in the face of pain or disability or both. Through trial and error, these individuals have learned how to go on doing the things they want to do and the things they have to do. Their cumulative experience is an excellent teacher.

No doubt you have devised some of your own methods for handling various chores. Here's your chance to pool your ideas with those of a thousand other people.

The advice participants offered ranges from general principles, such as 'Take it easy,' to ingenious specifics, such as, 'Tie loops of yarn around the handles of the oven, refrigerator, and kitchen cupboards so they can be opened with the forearm instead of the fingers.' It covers everything from keeping house to making love. It includes timesaving tips, work-saving devices, safety precautions, household modifications, and gadgets you can make yourself to make life easier. We have condensed and organized participants' comments into twenty-five strategies for performing everyday activities in spite of — and without worsening — arthritis pain. We begin with the most frequently mentioned suggestions.

Pace Yourself

Keeping active is extremely important for mental and physical well-being, but finding the right activity level can spell the difference between happy involvement and painful overexertion. Participants stressed the importance of pacing themselves to go whatever distance they must cover in a day. 'I've slowed down,' reported a graphic designer from Oregon, 'and in doing so I've found that I have less pain than when I'm in a hurry.'

Pacing yourself is as much a mental as a physical activity. It means knowing your own limitations, so you can work within them instead of against yourself. It means exerting a steady flow of energy, instead of erratic bursts. It means, in the words of one retired engineer, 'One thing at a time. One day at a time. One life at a time.'

Break One Big Job into Several Small Chores

You can do as much as you ever did, in many respects, by taking a different approach to big jobs. Almost any task can be broken into component parts, so you can accomplish each one separately, allowing yourself many small breaks before you reach the final goal. A supervisor in a New York credit bureau planned her housework and laundry so that she did about two hours' worth every night, in lieu of eight hours on Saturday – and she skipped the night or nights when her arthritis was most painful. A retired Colorado radio announcer divided up his activities this way: 'I clean the house one room per day, working slowly and resting frequently. For exercise, I take three or four short walks per day rather than one long one. But when it comes to making love, there's just no way to do it a little at a time.'

Stick to Your Exercise Routine

The vast majority of survey participants exercised regularly and credit that activity with helping them function better than they otherwise would. 'Walking and swimming have given me the ability to continue to live relatively normally and with minimal pain,' wrote a hospital worker from Michigan. A New Jersey homemaker said that the hand exercises her doctor prescribed enable her to use her fingers better and therefore do more daily chores. Nearly all those who exercise stressed the importance of finding and maintaining a routine. 'You don't always see immediate results from exercise,' explained a retired New York executive, 'but you have to keep at it just to stay even.' For most people in the survey, exercise was not only helpful but enjoyable in itself, making it a very sweet-tasting medicine: 'It improves my mental outlook and gives me an exhilarated feeling,' a Tennessee newspaper reporter observed. (If you don't already have an exercise program or a practitioner who can help you create one, please see Chapter 17 for specific exercise advice.)

Ask for Help If You Need It

'When I need help,' a twenty-nine-year-old Texas teacher has learned, 'I ask and don't care if they call me a weakling or whatever. I just laugh at their ignorance and let them assist me.' Not everyone can be so cavalier about needing the assistance of others, but if you do need help, you owe it to yourself to say so.

The help may take the form of a hired housekeeper, if you can afford one – or can receive the services some other way. A sixty-eight-year-old resident of a low-income high rise in Seattle has a welfare house helper spend twenty hours per month at her apartment, and, she said, 'Having the hard household tasks done for me is a blessing.' A person to help with the yard work or odd jobs makes good sense, too, unless you can rely on a little extra effort from members of your own family, as most of our survey participants do. One homemaker, in fact, put her 'sympathetic husband' first on the list of the most useful items she's discovered for people with arthritis. Similarly, a thirty-seven-year-old insurance agent said, 'My wife and I work together. She is aware of my condition and helps if needed. No, neither she nor I tolerate pity and sympathy. Understanding is the key in our relationship.'

Rest Periodically

Rest, the number-one self-help strategy for pain relief, was what made it possible for many survey participants to accomplish their day's work. They took periodic breaks, either for a short nap in bed or time in an easy chair, relaxing with their feet up – or in some other comfortable position. A forty-seven-year-old California store owner who's had rheumatoid arthritis since childhood said he managed to keep working by being 'up and active two hours, prone two hours.' Experiment to determine the amount of rest you need, and then do your utmost to make sure you get it. 'When I entertain,' said a freelance writer from New Mexico, 'I tell people when I invite them what time I expect them to leave.'

Don't Overdo Any Activity

Moderation is the best policy, survey participants have found, as almost any activity may lead to trouble if done to excess. How do you know when you've done too much? You learn the hard way, at least once, and then you use that experience to guide you in the future. A retired family counsellor in our survey group who couldn't seem to pull herself away from a job unfinished now avoids the overdo syndrome by setting a kitchen timer before she begins any physically stressful task. If she gets too engrossed to stop when she should, the buzzer is there to remind her.

Another way to keep from overdoing one activity is to alternate chores periodically, as this California housewife does: 'I avoid several days of repeated activity, like yard work, or several hours of any uninterrupted, intense similar activities as was my pattern before the arthritis set in ten years ago.' Here's how a homesteader in Wisconsin uses a similar ploy: 'When I wash dishes I only wash a few, then I dry them and put them away. If I just stay at the sink for a long time, it really brings on the pain.'

Listen to Your Body

When something you are doing becomes too physically stressful, heed your body's danger cries right away. Stop, stretch, rest, change activities – do whatever the situation seems to require. If you push through a sudden sharp pain, you may injure yourself seriously. This goes for exercise, too, where the athlete's trendy motto, 'No pain, no gain,' has been exposed as a foolish philosophy. 'In cleaning house or making love,' suggested a Pennsylvania salesman, 'do only what and how much your body tells you you can do – and believe me, it tells you!'

Use Good Body Mechanics

Be mindful of your affected joints and spare them any undue strain. In daily activities, including your exercise routine, it's best to avoid quick jerky movements that can give your joints a jolt. Try to maintain good posture when standing (not military attention, but a comfortable relaxed stance), and think about your posture when you're seated, too. If you can identify certain actions that tend to bring on pain, try to avoid them or work around them. An aircraft designer from New York said he performs what he calls 'motion study' before tackling new tasks. 'I don't rush into anything,' he explained. 'I try to think it out before starting, foreseeing the safest and easiest positions as much as possible.'

Participants with special hobbies were particularly inventive on this score. For example, a Kansas county sheriff who loves to build and fix things was having trouble using a screw-driver for a long enough time to accomplish much. Then he discovered that it helped to tighten with his left hand and loosen with his right, so that he was always turning the screw-driver toward his arthritic thumbs instead of away from them.

Try Sitting Down on the Job – or Anywhere Else

Several of the participants lived by the credo, 'Never stand when you can sit, and never sit when you can lie down.' Many of them managed to continue at their regular jobs because they could carry out their responsibilities from a chair. An Indiana factory worker explained, 'I am fortunate to have a job where I can sit most of the time and run my machine. This takes the load off my back and knees.'

A high bar stool at the kitchen counter enabled many of our participants to cook for themselves. They sat while preparing food, while ironing, and while doing the laundry. A thirty-nine-year-old Florida housewife has had rollers put on her most comfortable chair so she can sit while vacuuming and mopping the floor. In low-down work such as gardening, a small short-legged stool or a low stool with wheels can be a tremendous help.

Although the majority of participants preferred sitting, a small percentage of them could not sit comfortably even for a short time, including a draughtsman who worked standing at an easel instead of leaning over a table, and a budget analyst who wrote while standing at a podium rather than sitting at a desk.

Avoid Heavy Lifting

There are many definitions of 'heavy.' For a sixty-four-year-old retired typist, 'heavy' meant anything over five pounds. For a forty-one-year-old registered nurse, 'heavy' meant a patient's body, as she could no longer lift one by herself. Whatever your definition of 'heavy,' don't tax yourself by lifting more than you can handle. Here's the strategy favoured by a thirty-seven-year-old electronics technician from Virginia: 'I lift smaller loads and make more trips, rather than try to lift one large load.'

When you do lift, remember to keep the item close to your body instead of holding it with outstretched arms, so as not to strain your back.

Save Steps – and Stairs, Too

With a little forethought, you can save yourself a lot of extra running around that may sap your energy. For example, a Nevada accountant planned his errands by geographical area so he could accomplish several chores at once instead of needing to make repeated, separate trips. An interior decorator from Ohio wrote, 'When I shop, I stop in the entrance and look over the store, thinking how I can save steps before I venture in. At shopping malls, I sometimes use a wheelchair.' Others skipped as many trips to the store as they could by shopping from mail-order catalogues.

At home, too, especially if you have stairs to climb, try to plan your activities to minimize the number of trips you make from one part of the house to another. You may want to keep an upstairs and a downstairs supply of inexpensive cleaning and grooming supplies so you'll always have what you need at hand. 'I make as few trips as possible to the basement,' said a nurse from Michigan, 'and once I'm in the basement doing my laundry, I stay there until the wash is finished.'

Participants who mentioned stairs urged extreme caution in using them: Take them one at a time, hold on, and don't fall. If it's easier for you to go downstairs backward, then by all means do so.

Change Positions Often to Avoid Stiffness

Don't get stuck standing or sitting in any one position for too long a time. Try to switch positions periodically, or at least move around from time to time to loosen up. In the car, too, remember to stop *at least* once every two hours on long trips to get out and walk around.

'Taking stretch breaks is the best technique I've found to keep me going,' said a thirty-seven-year-old Californian with osteoarthritis. 'I have a typing business, and I've learned to get up every hour and stretch, no matter what!'

If only they could follow this rule while sleeping, many of the survey participants said ruefully, they would be able to start the day with much greater ease. Since they can't, they do the next best thing, which is to find a comfortable position for sleeping. The two favourites are (1) on the side in a foetal position, with a pillow *between* the knees, and (2) on the back with a pillow *under* the knees. Pillows used in these ways help keep the lower back in line. You can find many styles of specially shaped knee wedges and neck pillows, or you can use standard bed pillows, folding or stacking them under your knees to suit your needs. A fifty-eight-year-old Texas woman said the best pillow for between the knees is a child's float ring, covered with a flannel pad.

Here are some other suggestions for smoothing the way out of bed.

- Do some gentle stretching exercises in bed before you try to get up.
- Keep some milk in a thermos at bedside, and set your alarm for half an hour to an hour before your wake-up time so you can take your medication, go back to sleep for awhile, and reawaken less stiff.
- Take your medication with a late snack just before you go to bed at night to allay nausea and morning stiffness.
- To rise, position yourself near the edge of the bed, on your side. If you're lying on your right side, use your left hand and arm to steadily push yourself up to a sitting position as you swing your feet down, then stand up.

Relax Your Cleaning Standards a Little Bit

Learning to look past the dust makes housekeeping much easier. Changing the sheets less often helps, too. (And if you have fragile hands, choose flat sheets over fitted ones.) Accepting something short of perfection from yourself, though difficult, comes highly recommended by survey participants.

'My goal is to be as pain-free from arthritis as I can,' reasoned a crafts instructor from Ohio, who has both rheumatoid and osteoarthritis, 'so housecleaning takes a backseat in my schedule. I do such work when I'm feeling well enough to do so. My family and friends must accept this, as I must accept my limitations.'

'I'm less particular about the house,' conceded an Iowa housewife. 'I do what I can and I don't fret about what I can't.'

A soil tester from Wisconsin quipped, 'If your guests don't like your housekeeping, hand them the broom.'

Set a (Flexible) Schedule

Many participants found that arthritis pain or fatigue (or both) ebbed and flowed over the course of the day, creating a pattern of can-do and can't-do times, and they scheduled themselves accordingly. 'I rise early and do almost all my housework and cooking before noon,' said a retired teacher from New York State. 'By 1 p.m., I am too tired to do much.' Accepting of this framework, they figured out which activities deserve top priority, and then tried to do those things during their best time of the day. 'Early afternoon is the best time for making love,' noted a Connecticut homemaker, 'after the morning stiffness is gone and before the evening tiredness sets in.'

Several participants emphasized the importance of keeping a regular schedule to make sure they got enough rest, took their medications at the proper times, and exercised for a certain number of minutes or hours each day. A well-planned schedule can enhance your self-care program, as long as it *serves* you and doesn't *drive* you. Or, as a retired Florida car salesman put it, 'Schedule – and then reschedule when necessary.'

Let One Joint Compensate for Another

At the beginning of this chapter, we mentioned the yarn loops tied on cabinet doors that let a North Dakota social worker use her wrists and arms to do what her hands cannot. Many participants have found ways to let one joint compensate for the disability in another. For example, you can use your feet to wipe spills from the floor with a cloth or sponge, work an electric can opener with your forearm, and seal the lids on plastic containers with your elbow. You can use your hips, shoulders, elbows, or rear end to push doors open or shut. You can also operate the foot pedal of a sewing machine with your hand. You can pick up your child, as one Kentucky mother did, with your wrists. 'Just favour the aching parts,' advised a retired electrical engineer from Texas. 'They're not always in the same places.'

Here's a related rule from a communications consultant in North Carolina: 'Never use one hand if you can use two. It reduces the wear.' Other participants who followed her advice noted that they always use two hands to push/pull the vacuum cleaner, to lift, and to carry.

Speak Out to Spare Your Hands

When someone wants to shake your hand in greeting and you are afraid the contact may harm you, what do you do? Several of the participants said they avoided handshaking altogether, and explained as much to any new acquaintances at the first introduction, as this artist from Pennsylvania does: 'When meeting people, smile gently and say, "I'm afraid my arthritis is acting up."' If that kind of frankness doesn't appeal to you, there are several more subtle escapes. Depending on the social situation, you may be able to get around a handshake, if need be, with a quick hug, a touch on the arm, or a pat on the back. Sometimes it's friendly and painless to take the other person's hand with both of yours.

Many participants solved the problem of *hand* writing by using a word processor, but some find typing just as difficult as holding a pen. These people keep up their correspondence by telephone or by dictating letters into a tape recorder and sending the cassettes through the mail.

Protect Your Joints from Injury

When you can't avoid using your affected joints, you can guard against injury with many kinds of protective coverings. These range from back braces and cervical collars to splints and simple elastic bandages. Most people who used them did so only at specific times or for specific tasks. A Rhode Island homemaker wore a cervical collar while doing housework, for example; a Tennessee secretary put splints on her wrists when typing or playing golf; and a California composer with rheumatoid arthritis, mindful of how he uses his hands all day, found he needed to give them extra protection at night: 'I try not to bump my fingers or let them bend suddenly or too far, as it can be very painful. I avoid jobs that require too much flexing, as that also makes the pain worse, and I drop things a lot. Sometimes, I splint a finger before going to bed, because if I roll over and bend it too far, the pain is intense.'

Bend from the Knees – or Avoid Bending Altogether

Many of the survey participants who suffered back pain from arthritis said they stooped down rather than bent over when they had to reach to the floor, letting their legs do the work instead of straining their spines. This is sound practice for the back, but if your knees are arthritic – and there were more sore knees than bad backs in the survey group – stooping may be difficult, if not impossible. Some individuals said they must avoid stooping or bending altogether. 'The only thing I have changed is that I can no longer stoop,' said a seventy-one-year-old Pennsylvania saleslady who has had arthritis for forty-seven years. 'Stooping is very hard on the knees, and once I'm down, it's very difficult for me to get up.'

One solution is to use a long-handled spring action tool that extends your arm's reach by about three feet and has a hand with magnetic fingertips that are quite good at picking up dropped coins, paper clips, and the like. Almost everyone who uses this item has his own name for it. Participants called it by turns a reacher, a gripper, an extender, a long-lifter, a pick-up stick, a grab-it, and tongs, but they all meant the same thing. You can buy one for about eight dollars by mail order or try to make something similar yourself out of a clothes hanger or other materials: 'A helpful homemade tool to reach things too high or too low can be made from a broomstick,' wrote a seventy-four-year-old copy editor from Oregon. 'Cut off the broom and cut the head off a nail. Then pound the nail into the end of the stick.' She added, 'You could even clean up litter in the park with this gadget.' A Montana ranch wife made her 'picker-upper' by screwing a cup hook on the end of a thirty-six-inch pole.

Prepare Yourself for Extra Exertion

Anytime that you're planning on being more active than usual or are about to do something that has brought on pain in the past, you may be able to ward it off by trying a pain-relieving strategy in advance. 'When you are going to do something that usually causes more pain,' wrote a homemaker from Utah, 'use medication and precautions *before*, not after the pain starts. Some problems can be avoided or at least minimized by using caution and good sense.' Use whatever works for you. Some participants favoured two aspirin (or other medication), a warm bath, a nap, or a massage. A Georgia accountant said, 'I find that making love *after* a hot bath or shower lessens the pain in my hip.'

In Making Love, Strive for Open Communication with Your Partner

Finding a comfortable position for lovemaking takes inventiveness and the willing cooperation of both partners. It also calls for 'more talk' and 'frank communication,' survey participants said, which may actually enhance closeness and enjoyment. 'My husband is so caring and loving,' wrote a thirty-four-year-old Florida housewife, 'that we have a very good sexual relationship, no matter how bad the arthritis is. We do sometimes have to adjust positions depending on where I hurt, but being creative makes lovemaking even more exciting.'

Among those survey participants who favoured a specific position for intercourse, the first choice was to have the woman on top, no matter which partner is the one with arthritis. In this position, a man need not support his own weight on his knees, wrists, or elbows, and a woman need not support a man's weight. Some couples were more comfortable making love on their sides, either face-to-face or with the man facing the woman's back. 'Lying on one's side is easier on the back than the missionary position,' explained a California homemaker, 'and is quite pleasant to both parties.' But the majority of those who commented about sex said that they tend to vary positions from one time to the next. And in *any* position, they avow, the idea is to concentrate on the lovemaking and not on pain and stiffness. 'If you don't love your lover,' observed a photographer from Massachusetts, 'it will hurt whether or not you have arthritis. If you are both crazy about each other, you find ways to please each other and spare yourselves pain.' Some of the ways survey participants mention included more caressing and foreplay, oral sex, and mutual masturbation.

Several participants candidly conceded that they have to made love less frequently, less energetically, or abstain altogether because of arthritis pain, age, other health problems, or a combination of these factors. 'Make love at seventy-five and seventy-eight?' asked a Kentucky housewife with a serious heart condition and a thirty-year history of osteoarthritis. 'Well, no pain in saying "I love you" and kissing him on the nose.' Others claimed that sex actually had a positive effect on their pain. 'Sex is good therapy,' said an executive recruiter from Texas who's had rheumatoid arthritis for twenty of his forty-five years. 'It releases endorphins – the body's own painkillers!' A Wisconsin practical nurse wrote, 'Making love regularly seems to have a carryover effect in lessening pain.' And a Michigan factory worker found, 'It limbers up everything and makes you feel good!'

A few survey participants praised their water beds for making sex less painful and therefore more enjoyable. Many more were content with a few well-placed pillows to support their hips or knees during sex.

Meet Life's Little Challenges with the Proper Tools

Elaborate plastic food packages, medicine bottles with child-proof lids, and soft-drink cans with ring-pop tops were just a few of the items that bedevilled survey participants' attempts to carry on with business as usual. They fought back by arming themselves with pliers to open bottles, a crescent wrench to turn the car key, scissors to slit sealed bags, and ingenuity to use everyday utensils in creative ways, such as cleaning the bathtub with a floor mop instead of kneeling down and leaning over to do the job in the usual way with a sponge. If you can't handle the tops on aluminum drink cans, turn them over to your electric can opener, or purchase a 'tab grabber' made for the job. If your medication comes in a childproof container, put it in a different bottle as soon as you get it home so you'll be able to get at it when you need to. If you hate the one-finger pressure needed to push the small nozzles on aerosol cans, you can get a spray-handle kit that converts an aerosol can to a spray gun.

Some participants got a lot of help from the cane or crutch that they have to carry anyway, using it to make the bed, to push couch pillows in place, to close the drapes, or open the windows. Most have discovered some small or inexpensive item, from a long-handled shoehorn to an oversize felt-tip pen, that makes a big welcome difference in getting things done. 'The feather duster is the greatest invention since the can opener,' wrote an insurance secretary from Texas. 'It helps keep furniture clean and I don't have to rub the furniture with a cloth, move knickknacks around, or worry about bumping my fingers while dusting.' (Many other convenience items recommended by survey participants are described in Chapter 19.)

Let Your Furniture Help You Up

When getting out of a chair or up from a kneeling position, use your arms to pull yourself upright – and spare your knees. Several participants said they arranged their furniture with this idea in mind, setting their chairs near something very sturdy, such as a wall divider or solid cabinet, which they could grab hold of to pull themselves up. 'I can't get up from a low chair or couch,' explained a writer from Texas, 'so the low couch that I have – because I can't afford to buy a new one – is close to a table, which I pull up on.' Others have installed special grab bars or railings in key locations about the house. And a lithographer from California, disabled by both rheumatoid and osteoarthritis, helped himself up with ropes hung from the ceiling of his apartment.

Stay Warm

Dress for warmth in layers of comfortable clothing that let you keep your body at your ideal temperature as you go through the day. From the comments we received, this rule applies not just in cold climates but to warm ones as well, where air conditioners can create misery-provoking draughts. Many participants selected soft loose clothes that have elastic waists instead of buttons and zippers. They like long underwear, sweat suits, leg warmers, knee socks, and natural fibres such as cotton and flannel.

Certain painful joints just seem to work better with the benefit of a special extra layer to help retain warmth. Gloves were a frequently mentioned favourite, and so were socks with the feet cut off to make a cozy knit tube that slips easily over an elbow or knee. 'To keep the body heat in my hands at night,' wrote a sixty-six-year-old home health-care aide from Florida, 'I rub on Vaseline and wear cotton gloves to bed.' A thirty-nine-year-old housewife from Pennsylvania used terry-cloth bands (such as the ones tennis players wear) to hold warmth in her wrists, and a sixty-one-year-old motel maid from Ohio frequently wrapped her knees or ankles with clear plastic wrap in on-two-hours/off-two-hours cycles.

Everybody hangs pot holders near the stove, but if your hands are extremely sensitive to cold, you need a pair of 'oven mitts' by the refrigerator and freezer, too. And when you make yourself an iced drink, try covering the lower half of the glass with an elastic slip-on coaster or a folded washcloth.

Carry What You Need – Comfortably

Big pockets, baskets, tote bags, plastic grocery bags with handles that loop over the wrists – even shirttails, in a pinch – made it easier for participants to carry miscellaneous items about the house, off to work, or home from the store. Several women noted that they have traded in their handbags for a roomy lightweight backpack. This makes sense for basic comfort and is especially useful for those who need to carry a back-support pillow or other special aids wherever they go.

If there *is* an item that can help you do your day's work more comfortably, whether it's a cushion, a splint, or a folding footrest, do find a way to carry it with you so it's there when you need it. For example, a sixty-five-year-old secretary from California said she always wears a scarf, and that way, if her shoulder acts up, she simply ties the scarf into a sling. At the same time, try to lighten your load by not dragging along the things you really don't need.

Wheeled carts are reliable helpers for toting laundry, groceries, or garbage. And several women said they use a tea cart at home for transporting cleaning supplies or meals from one room to another.

Get a Power Assist

Depending on the availability of human help at your house and the amount of money you can spend, you may want to find a motorized way to accomplish certain tasks. Several of the participants relied on snowblowers to clear their walks, rider mowers to cut the grass, and a host of indoor labour-saving devices, from electrically powered vegetable peelers to self-propelled vacuum cleaners. (Vacuuming, by the way, was cited most often as the chore most likely to cause pain, so a lighter-weight, easier-to-use model may be well worth its cost.)

Although there is a well known power-assist way to take care of dirty dishes, there were more participants who advocated hand-washing than ones who recommend using an automatic dishwasher. 'Washing dishes feels *good*,' said a retired teacher. 'Between the warmth of the water and the exercise of squeezing the sponge, it's practically therapy.' (If squeezing a sponge is painful, try flattening it with your palm. You may want to try a mitten-shaped bath sponge that you can *wear* for washing dishes and wring out by pressing against the sink.) Several participants said they intentionally left their dinner dishes in the sink overnight, because dish washing was the best antidote they've found for morning hand stiffness.

While you're at the kitchen sink, please be careful not to strain your other joints with the position you assume. If your knees or feet bother you, try sitting on a high stool. If it's your back that's the problem, you can (1) spread your legs slightly and bend your knees to relieve the pressure; (2) open the undersink cabinet and rest one foot inside it; or (3) rest one knee on a chair.

Summary of Tips on Keeping Up Your Everyday Activities

Pace yourself.
Break one big job into several small chores.
Stick to your exercise routine.
Ask for help if you need it.
Rest periodically.

Don't overdo any activity.

Listen to your body.

Use good body mechanics.

Try sitting down on the job – or anywhere else.

Avoid heavy lifting.

Save steps – and stairs, too.

Change positions often to avoid stiffness.

Relax your cleaning standards a little bit.

Set a (flexible) schedule.

Let one joint compensate for another.

Speak out to spare your hands.

Protect your joints from injury.

Bend from the knees – or avoid bending altogether.

Prepare yourself for extra exertion.

In making love, strive for open communication with your partner.

Meet life's little challenges with the proper tools.

Let your furniture help you up.

Stay warm.

Carry what you need – comfortably.

Get a power assist.

Part 2
Arthritis: What Exercises Really Work

Introduction

The US and UK surveys conducted revealed that exercise is the single best treatment for the pain and disability of arthritis. Not only does exercise often succeed where drugs, braces, and surgery have failed to relieve pain, but exercise can also help restore the normal appearance and full function of the joints.

The book you have in your hands fully explores the types of exercise that benefit people with arthritis. These range from overall aerobic activities, through strengthening (isometric and isotonic) exercises, to range-of-motion workouts that increase the mobility of each individual joint.

Most of the exercises in this book were derived from the original survey participants' experiences, and were then reviewed and refined with the help of two exercise experts, Dr. Willibald Nagler and Dr. Irene von Estorff of the Department of Physical Medicine and Rehabilitation at The New York Hospital – Cornell Medical Center in New York City. The book also contains additional exercises contributed recently by readers who found the original book helpful and wrote to share their positive experiences with exercise.

This book contains:

- Self-evaluation checklists to help you determine a safe level of activity and set reasonable exercise goals
- Strategies for devising your own individually tailored beginner's exercise program
- Explanations of the different types of exercises, with directions on how to combine them for maximum benefit
- Instructions on how to increase your activity levels over time
- Guidelines for modifying your exercise regimen during an arthritis flare-up or when specific joints become inflamed and swollen
- Suggestions on how to integrate exercise routines into your everyday activities

- Tips on how to make simple exercise equipment with materials you can find around your house, and
- Advice from others with arthritis on how to get motivated to start an exercise program. (You needn't worry about keeping motivation high once you get rolling. Your own pain relief and increased activity will surely keep you going then!)

Section 7, 'The Life-Enhancing Value of Exercise for Arthritis,' will guide you in constructing your own exercise program from the book's large assortment of suggested activities. Section 8, 'Mental Gymnastics,' covers relaxation techniques that will complement your exercise regimen, as well as give you tips on how to warm up and cool down. The aerobic exercises – such as walking, swimming, cycling, and dancing – are discussed in Section 9, 'Aerobic Fitness Exercises for Arthritis.' Stretching and strengthening exercises appear in Section 10, 'Exercising Away Pain from Head to Toe'; individual exercises are grouped into chapters by joint – from neck and jaw to ankles and feet. In Section 11, 'Exercising under Special Circumstances,' you'll find advice on particular situations – including safe exercise during a flare-up, precautions for pre- and postsurgery exercise routines, and ways to modify arthritis exercise to accommodate other health problems.

We hope you will show this book to your doctor, physiotherapist, or exercise instructor, and anticipate that these professionals will welcome the information it contains, especially if they themselves have not had detailed instruction in prescribing exercise for arthritis.

Indeed, many of the original survey participants said that they had been told to exercise – but were never told how! – presumably because their doctors didn't know or didn't have time to explain. Some were given the wrong exercises – and made to suffer needlessly – by practitioners who should have known better.

This book combines documented-safe exercises with cookbook-style directions and illustrations, based on the accumulated experience of many people with physical problems similar to yours – people who understand firsthand the challenge and the value of regular exercise in the treatment of arthritis.

We encourage you to begin at once by starting to move more today. Why wait until you feel better to begin, when beginning to exercise can help you to feel better now? Ready? Let's proceed together. We want to help you every step of the way!

Section 7
The Life-Enhancing Value of Exercise for Arthritis

The weakest and oldest among us can become some sort of athlete, but only the strongest can survive as spectators, only the hardiest can withstand the perils of inertia, inactivity, and immobility

— Drs. J. H. Bland and S. M. Cooper from
Seminars in Arthritis and Rheumatism.

Chapter 20
The Miracle 'Drug' That You Can Give Yourself

What to expect from your own arthritis exercise program

Truly, the value of exercise in fighting arthritis cannot be over-stated. Its effectiveness is demonstrated beyond question, both in the Arthritis Survey results and in numerous medical studies conducted at hospitals. Rest, which was long touted as the best treatment for arthritis, has proved to be a poor and often destructive substitute for activity.

As was discovered in the arthritis survey exercise helped ninety-five percent of those Arthritis Survey participants who tried it. No other approach to arthritis – no drug, no surgical procedure – matches exercise for high rates of improvement. Nor can any other treatment modality boast exercise's low risk of serious complications or unpleasant side effects.

Exercise figures in every good comprehensive treatment plan for arthritis. It is the all-purpose adjunct therapy for individuals at every stage of ability and disability. *Whatever else people do for their arthritis, they do better if they exercise as well.*

Many problems that are usually attributed to arthritis itself, such as poor posture and hesitant gait, are really the result of inactivity. Exercise is the key to better body mechanics – to feeling and doing better.

According to the US study, the chief benefits that you stand to gain from exercise are (1) increased flexibility of your affected joints, and (2) pain relief. Many Arthritis Survey participants also reported that regular exercise (3) improved their general health by lowering high blood pressure and cholesterol levels, and even

(4) helped those with diabetes to gain better control over their blood-sugar levels.

In addition to these results, or perhaps in part because of them, respondents also credited exercise with (5) lifting their spirits, (6) helping them fight stress, (7) giving them more energy during the day, and (8) ensuring better sleep at night. Thus, it (9) improved the overall quality of their lives.

Sounds like a miracle drug – and it is.

Arguments in favour of exercise only increase as one gets older. Among individuals between the ages of fifty-five and eighty-eight, a recent study at Scripps College revealed, regular exercise (10) rendered people better able to reason, remember, and solve problems. In Dallas, investigations with thousands of men and women at The Institute for Aerobics Research and the Cooper Clinic showed that even moderate exercise would (11) significantly reduce a person's chance of dying of heart disease or cancer.

Since exercise can also help keep weight in check, it can (12) retard or altogether prevent the development of arthritis in certain joints. A very encouraging study supported by the National Institutes of Health showed that overweight women who drop roughly a pound a year for ten years can often avoid osteoarthritis of the knee.

The motion of exercise nourishes the joints: with motion, fluids are squeezed in and out of the joint space, delivering nourishment to the cartilage, getting rid of waste products. Without motion, this vital exchange cannot take place. The cartilage covering the ends of the bones where they meet has no blood supply of its own. The only way for the cartilage to take in needed nutrients and oxygen is via the motion of the joint. (In osteoarthritis, the cartilage is particularly vulnerable to destruction.)

We trust that if you've read this far, you're fairly well convinced that you want to begin an exercise program. Great. Now the question is: What kind of exercise should you do?

Arthritis exercise comes in three prescription strengths:

- *Aerobic activities*, such as walking and swimming, that build stamina and boost cardiovascular fitness
- *Stretching, or 'range of motion' exercises*, such as leg raises and finger curls, that keep the joints mobile

- *Strengthening exercises*, including lifting light weights, that prevent muscle atrophy.

Each type plays a role in maintaining and improving your overall flexibility, as well as in preventing the deformities that arthritis can cause.

This book offers instructions in all three types of arthritis exercise. Please don't be discouraged by the range of options available to you. No one is expected to work through all the manoeuvres at any one time. Rather, we hope you'll use the book the way you'd consult a menu at a restaurant: you choose what suits you from the many available possibilities. The rest of this section, like a helpful waiter, provides explanations, suggestions, and sample combinations.

Aerobic exercises tend to be everyone's favourites because they are intrinsically enjoyable, or can be made that way. Many of them can be done in the company of others, and therefore provide opportunities for pleasant social contacts. Walking is our favourite aerobic exercise since it is safe and effective, and can be done virtually anywhere. Walking can be easily adapted to your level of fitness by adjusting the speed and duration of the activity. For example, some people can put their sneakers on every day, and walk at a rapid clip for forty-five minutes to an hour, covering as much ground as three or four miles. Less-fit beginners will want to start off slowly, with the goal of doing just a little bit more walking than they've been used to. If you're starting from zero, you might begin with a walk from one room to another right in your own home, or around the block once or twice.

Aerobic exercise will increase your general level of fitness and endurance over time. It will also give you relief from much of your pain and stiffness by increasing the blood flow to your affected joints and muscles. To guarantee the flexibility of individual joints, however, you need range-of-motion exercises that stretch every single joint, every day. You will no doubt want to concentrate on those joints that are most in need of attention because they ache or fail you in your regular activities. You may want to help yourself further by giving some exercise attention to your smoothly functioning joints as well, to ensure that they will continue to function dependably. Don't worry about doing this extra work right away however, especially at the outset, when you can easily get overwhelmed by a program that is too time-consuming or confusing.

The strengthening exercises that build up your muscles give your joints the best possible protection from injury and deformity. Strengthening exercises may be isotonic or isometric. The *isotonic* ones involve motion against resistance. For example, when you raise and lower your arm hefting a can of tomatoes, the can's weight provides the resistance that makes your arm work hard and get strong. (The same movement without the can would be a range-of-motion stretch.) The *isometric* exercises involve no movement of the joint, just force against resistance. Pushing against a wall, for example, is another way to strengthen your arm. The wall never moves, of course, but your muscles are still working. The lack of motion makes such exercises do-able even on days when your joints hurt too much to engage in isotonic activity. Isometric exercises promise considerable gains in strength and pain relief, but the gains disappear quickly if you drop the exercises.

Now that you know the general types of exercises you will be doing, it's time to assess your own abilities and preferences in order to determine your exercise prescription. Please turn to the next chapter, and get a pen or pencil ready to answer some questions about yourself.

Chapter 21
Only You Can Write the Right Exercise Prescription

How to gauge your physical condition and exercise readiness

Many medical and nonmedical practitioners, from rheumatologists to yoga instructors, advise exercise, but not all of them can prescribe it effectively. Our aim in this chapter is to guide you to the best possible exercise help – and also to encourage you to become your own reliable expert in the matter of arthritis exercise.

The practitioners who enjoy the most success in teaching beneficial exercise, according to our research, are physiotherapists with a special interest in arthritis. These individuals provide a variety of treatments that temporarily relieve arthritis pain, such as ultrasound, diathermy, and massage, but they get their best long-term results by devising personally tailored exercise programs and by encouraging people in their care to exercise daily. Physiotherapists, unfortunately, are in short supply: according to some estimates, people with arthritis outnumber physiotherapists by more than one thousand to one.

Although physiotherapists rarely failed to help Arthritis Survey participants in their care, a few did cause harm by being incompetent or insensitive. If you feel the advice or the treatments you get from a physiotherapist are not helping – or worse, are harming – you, then stop them immediately.

Another potentially excellent source of exercise advice is your doctor. But if he or she has not yet recommended exercise, then we urge you to raise the subject as soon as possible. Please discuss your exercise plans on your very next visit to the doctor's office – and take this book along with you to break the ice.

If your doctor resists the idea of exercise, which is unlikely, then please seek a second medical opinion. The types of doctors who provided the most help to Arthritis Survey participants – and the best exercise advice – were rheumatologists (arthritis specialists), orthopaedists (also called orthopaedic surgeons), and doctors of physical medicine and rehabilitation.

Exercise instructors at local gyms and fitness centres also helped many of Arthritis Survey participants. If you seek advice from one of these experts, however, please make certain that the instructor understands the special needs of people who have arthritis, and has experience working with them.

Ultimately, you will become your own best exercise expert, because only you can judge the difficulty of any given manoeuvre, the pain it causes you during or after your exercise session, the improvement it brings to your condition, and the change in your strength and endurance over time.

A great many step-by-step instructions are provided in this book, because we know how daunting it can be to undertake a new self-treatment. You may rely heavily on the instructions at first, until you master the material you need to pursue your own exercise prescription. Soon you will be using it only occasionally, to refresh your memory or give you ideas for more advanced routines.

Osteoarthritis vs. Rheumatoid Arthritis

The exercises in this book are intended for people who have either osteoarthritis or rheumatoid arthritis, which are the two most common forms of arthritis. They differ from each other in their cause and effect.

Osteoarthritis is a 'wear and tear' condition in which the cartilage protecting the ends of the bones flakes off, leaving rough edges and preventing the joints from functioning smoothly. Most often, the joints affected by osteoarthritis are the 'weight-bearing' joints, especially the knees, hips, back, and neck. It is not uncommon for disabilities to make themselves felt on one side of the body and not the other, so that the left knee is extremely stiff and painful while the right knee feels fine.

Rheumatoid arthritis is an autoimmune disease, in which the body's own agents attack the tissues of the joints, often making them feel hot and swollen. The joints most commonly affected by rheumatoid arthritis are the hands, wrists, ankles, and feet, and the pain tends to be symmetrical on both sides of the body.

All the participants in the Arthritis Survey had received a diagnosis of either osteoarthritis, rheumatoid arthritis, or both. In general, rheumatoid arthritis tends to set in at a younger age, and to grow alternately better and worse for no apparent reason over the course of time. People with rheumatoid arthritis also experience fatigue that limits their stamina, although they can increase their stamina through exercise.

Exercise is beneficial for everyone with arthritis, regardless of type. What differentiates your exercise program from someone else's will have more to do with your level of fitness and the number of affected joints than with the form of arthritis you have.

Know Your Limits – And Potential

Exercise programs differ because people differ so vastly in their abilities and needs. Start to assess your basic exercise level with the following simple quiz. Circle one answer to each question.

Quiz 1: Exercise Readiness
I consider myself:

1. very active
2. moderately active
3. inactive by choice – a 'couch potato'
4. inactive because of pain or disability

When I get up in the morning, I feel:

1. hardly any pain or stiffness
2. a fair amount of pain and stiffness that lasts up to twenty minutes
3. pain and stiffness that persists for an hour or longer
4. severe pain and stiffness that seems never to go away completely

As I go through the day, I find that I:

1. can keep up my normal activities pretty comfortably, at work and/or at home

2. manage well but need to rest at least once during the day
3. need to modify the way I do things and need to rest periodically, but still manage on my own
4. need help to do most things

My experience with exercise in general, and arthritis exercise in particular, is:

1. extensive
2. moderate
3. limited
4. nonexistent

My age is:

1. forty or younger
2. forty-one to fifty-five
3. fifty-six to sixty-five
4. over sixty-five

Now we'd like you to place yourself in one of four categories, depending on the way you answered the above questions. Look at the numbers of the answers you circled. If you circled all ones, for example, or mostly ones, then you can begin with a Level 1 exercise program, which is quite physically demanding. Likewise, if you circled all twos, then begin with a Level 2 program, which is a little less taxing. If you circled some twos and some threes, begin with the Level 3 for safety's sake. (You can always advance yourself more quickly later if you find the Level 3 is too simple for you.) If you skipped around with your answers, from one to four, then the safest course for you is to begin with a Level 4 program, then modify it accordingly.

The next quiz will help you assess the condition of your joints, so that you can determine the areas that need the most attention in your exercise program. No doubt you have several affected joints, and some are more painful than others. Thus, your personal exercise routine might include very gentle motions for your fingers, for example, but more vigorous shoulder and elbow movements.

Quiz 2: Joint Condition
Grade each of your joints according to the following scale:
1 = little or no pain, good range of motion
2 = moderate pain, adequate range of motion
3 = extreme pain, very limited range of motion
4 = inflamed (hot and swollen)
R = surgically replaced joint, painful or pain free, at any level of
mobility

Jaw _____	Back _____
Neck _____	Hips _____
Shoulders _____	Knees _____
Elbows _____	Ankles _____
Wrists _____	Feet/Toes _____
Hands/Fingers	

As in the Exercise Readiness quiz, the grades you give yourself
determine the level of activity for each joint. You can then select
the relevant stretching and strengthening exercises keyed to your
level, knowing you will be able to perform them safely.

If you have a surgically implanted replacement joint, please
consult your surgeon before attempting any of the exercises recommended for that part of your body. When selecting aerobic
exercise, remember that certain precautions apply to artificial
hips and knees, and you need to respect these if you want the
joint to last as long as possible.

Every exercise program includes all three types of exercises:
1) aerobic conditioning that has become so highly regarded for
its beneficial effect on the heart and lungs, 2) range-of-motion
exercises that stretch each individual joint to the fullest extent
possible, and 3) strengthening exercises that build up muscle to
give the joints strong support. Even the simplest program will
combine all three types for best results, because each one com-
plements the other.

Aerobic exercise will benefit your heart and lungs, and relieve
pain and stiffness by improving the blood circulation throughout
your body. When you read the chapters on the various forms of
aerobic exercise in section 9, just select the one that appeals to
you most. Feel free to cross train by combining aerobic activities,

or pursuing different ones on different days. You may enjoy your exercise program more if you swim three days a week and walk four, for example, or ride a bicycle in the summer and walk through shopping malls in the winter. These activities are easily tailored to your time and tastes. Many people find that variation is the spice that keeps motivation cooking.

When you begin to select range-of-motion and strengthening exercises, you'll want to focus on the joints that hurt, function poorly, or appear obviously affected by arthritic changes. Your other joints can also be put through their paces each day, as a preventive measure – quickly and easily after exercising the problem joints.

You can gauge whether you're doing just the right amount or going too far by the way you feel after you exercise. Pain is a reliable measure of joint strain and muscle overuse. Don't be too alarmed if you feel some discomfort for up to about one hour after your initial workout. If you do the same amount the next day, you should feel less discomfort, and even that will be short-lived. However, if you are considerably sore, or the soreness lasts beyond the one-hour point, your body is telling you to cut back. Please heed the advice.

You can use the guidelines in the next chapter to assemble your own individualized exercise routine, and then fine-tune it as you grow stronger and more flexible. Remember, you don't have to stop there – you can keep modifying your regimen indefinitely, to meet your changing needs. As you become expert in judging the motions that work best for you, you may even want to create your own exercises, combining them with the ones offered here, and devising creative strategies for working exercise into your schedule every day, wherever you are, whatever else you may be doing. Then you'll have mastered your exercise prescription and dosage schedule.

To hasten that day, let's begin to assemble your individually tailored program right now by consulting the advice in the next chapter.

Chapter 22
How to Develop a Tailor-Made Exercise Routine

How to combine the three types of exercise into an arthritis exercise program that works for you

Now that you know the kinds of exercise you need, the level of exercise you can safely attempt, and the specific joints that you will emphasize in your daily routine, you can assemble your own exercise program.

It's easier than you think. All you have to do is consult the sample routines laid out beginning below, and then use the blank forms on the following pages to construct your own.

Let's suppose, for example, that you are quite limited by pain, have no significant experience with exercise, and feel too tired to attempt much that is novel or challenging. Your first exercise routine can be one that you carry out in bed, before you even get up to face the day. (In fact, you'll probably find that going through the routine gets you ready – and raring – to start the day!)

Sample Routine 1 (Level 4: In-Bed)
Start with the exercise preparation in chapter 23 and the deep breathing and relaxation exercises in chapter 24.

Slowly and gently proceed through the range-of-motion exercises listed below. (Each one is explained step-by-step in chapters 30–38, and the numbers in parentheses after each exercise name tell you where to find it.) At this point, you need not worry about repeating the movements any set number of times. Just see how it feels to stretch your body.

A-E-I-O-U Shout (p. 403)
Left-Right (p. 405)
Shoulder Shrug (p. 409)
Swinging Pendulum (p. 410)
Elbow Limber-up (p. 430)
Elbow Twist (p. 430)
Wrist Assist (p. 435)
Wrist Twist (p. 436)
Wrist Rotator (p. 439)
Finger Spread (p. 444)
Okay All Around (p. 445)
Pelvic Tilt (p. 456)
Knee-to-Chest (p. 456)
Leg Spread (p. 467)
Leg Roll (p. 468)
Straight Leg-ups (p. 468)
Lift backs (p. 470)
Knee Push (p. 482)
Ankle Twist (p. 493)
Foot Circles (p. 493)
Toe Curls (p. 494)

At first, you may achieve only rough approximations of the movements as they are described. Be patient with yourself. Improvement comes with practice, and you have the rest of your life to perfect your form. If any movements seem wrong for you, however, or cause you sudden pain, then by all means stop them or modify them to suit you.

Later in the day, perhaps after a rest period, repeat the sequence outlined above, and add to it these strengthening exercises:

Bed Head (p. 404)
Bodybuilder (p. 412) [This *can* be done lying down.]
Alternate Elbow Builder (p. 431)
Praying Hands (p. 438)
Finger Push-ups (p. 445)
Squeeze Play (p. 447)
Bent-Knee Sit-ups (p. 457)
The Squeeze (p. 472)

Knee Press (p. 482)
Toe Helper (p. 494)

* WARNING: Be especially gentle with any joint that is hot and swollen. Although it helps to move even inflamed joints through their range of motion, it hurts to do any more. Too much motion can actually cut off the blood circulation to an actively inflamed joint. This is the one case where rest takes precedence over motion. Do very little with your inflamed joints until the flare-up passes. (See chapter 39 for more information about exercise and arthritis flare-ups.)

For your aerobic exercise, try walking (see chapter 25). At first, you may not get true aerobic benefit from the activity, as it's unlikely you'll be able to walk quickly enough to do so. Just concentrate on walking a little farther each day and a little more vigorously than you did the day before.

No doubt you will feel some muscle fatigue in the aftermath of these exercises. That's only natural, and the feeling will gradually disappear as you become more accustomed to the movements. But persistent pain that lasts for more than one hour is different: it's a danger sign of joint overuse. Be kind to yourself: do less the next time. You're better off building up slowly rather than rushing things and suffering a setback.

As you become accustomed to exercising, you can pay more attention to the number of repetitions of each movement. You started with one, and can gradually build up to three or five, then ten, and eventually as many as thirty.

Sample Routine 2 (Level 2: Moderately Active)

You, too, can begin with the Section 8 Preparation and Relaxation exercises. You could also use the first sample routine as a morning stretch, even though you are probably capable of more strenuous activity.

Take your pick of the aerobic activities in Section 9, and try to pursue one of them for forty-five minutes, at least three times a week. You may vary the activities if you like, so that you walk twice a week, for example, and ride a bicycle twice.

Here is a suggested list of range-of-motion exercises, each of which you can probably repeat three times. But be careful not to push through pain, and if pain following exercise persists for more than one hour, cut back on the number of repetitions. When you can do these easily, you can add more repetitions.

A-E-I-O-U Shout (p. 403)
Yes-No (p. 406)
Head Roll (p. 405)
Shoulder Roll (p. 410)
Butterfly Stretch (p. 411)
Crisscross (p. 413)
Wing Tuck (p. 429)
Chop Wood (p. 430)
Wrist Twist (p. 436)
Wrist Rotator (p. 435)
Finger Lifts (p. 444)
Typist's Warm-up (p. 444)
Pelvic Tilt (p. 456)
Knee Drops (p. 457)
Leg Lifts (p. 471)
Lift backs (p. 470)
Knee to Chest Plus (p. 481)
Knee Kicks (p. 482)
Foot Circles (p. 493)
Soft Shoe (p. 494)

Feel free to add to the list if you want to give extra attention to specific joints that need more exercise. Here are some isometric and isotonic exercises to strengthen your muscles:

Neck Push (p. 406)
Wallflower (p. 414)
Push-offs (p. 416)
Elbow Builder (p. 431)
Wrist Rise (p. 437)
Finger Skids (p. 447)
Sit-downs (p. 458)
Hip Strengthener (p. 472)
Ballet Bends (p. 483)
Ankle Builder (p. 496)

You can use the following forms to record your own exercise plan, and then keep track of additions and changes. This is a good way to mark your progress and to troubleshoot for the causes of later soreness, but if it seems like too much paper work for you, by all means just move on to the next chapter and start moving.

ARTHRITIS EXERCISE PROGRESS CHART

Week #   Day #

Aerobic activity _____   Length of time _____

Range of Motion Exercises

Joint	Exercise#	Number of Repetitions
_____	_____	_____
_____	_____	_____
_____	_____	_____
_____	_____	_____
_____	_____	_____
_____	_____	_____
_____	_____	_____
_____	_____	_____
_____	_____	_____
_____	_____	_____
_____	_____	_____
_____	_____	_____

ARTHRITIS EXERCISE PROGRESS CHART

Week #   Day #

Aerobic activity _____   Length of time _____

Joint	Exercise#	Number of Repetitions
_____	_____	_____
_____	_____	_____
_____	_____	_____
_____	_____	_____

_____	_____	_____
_____	_____	_____
_____	_____	_____
_____	_____	_____
_____	_____	_____
_____	_____	_____
_____	_____	_____
_____	_____	_____
_____	_____	_____
_____	_____	_____
_____	_____	_____

Section 8
Mental Gymnastics

There are many misconceptions regarding meditation. A common one is that the process of meditation is austere. Another is that meditation is boring. Sometimes meditating is viewed as passive, a withdrawal from the world, for wimps, not productive people. Exercise, in contrast, is seen as active, macho, getting out there and really doing something.

– Dean Ornish, M.D.

Chapter 23
Preparation for Exercise

How to get yourself mentally and physically ready to begin your arthritis exercise program

The commitment you're making to give yourself the benefit of regular exercise is one of the most important steps you can take to improve your arthritis. It's like turning over a new leaf, or making a New Year's resolution. Now, while you're feeling motivated and confident, is the time to build in safeguards for your exercise program.

You can make the program inviting and therefore effective by the way you set it up and go about it. The right music played in the background, for example, can increase the pleasure you derive from your exercise period, and help to make you feel good about the time spent exercising, even before the activity becomes its own reward.

Here are some reminders of the promises exercise can fulfill:

Pain relief
Greater stamina
Increased range of motion
Added strength
Improved joint function
Extra energy
Heightened self-sufficiency
Brighter outlook
Better sleep
Normalized blood pressure and cholesterol levels
Loss of excess weight

Starting an exercise program is a way of taking control of your future. By exercising, you give your body the best possible chance of beating the odds arthritis has stacked against you. Planning and sticking to an exercise regimen shows you care about yourself. Your actions prove that you refuse to give in to the feelings of helplessness and depression that often accompany arthritis.

Setting the Stage

You may do your first exercises of the day in bed, as part of the routine that helps you arise feeling limber. Later on in the day you'll probably need to choose a different setting for your aerobic, stretching, and strengthening exercises. The time and place are important determinants of success.

You may have noticed a particular hour in your daily routine when you seem to have more than your usual vim and vigour – and the least possible pain. People with rheumatoid arthritis frequently find that their pain tends to be worse in the mornings, and so prefer to exercise in the afternoons. In contrast, people with osteoarthritis tend to feel best in the morning, and then notice an increase in pain as the day progresses.

If you're free to exercise at your peak-energy time, by all means seize the moment. If not, then look for an opportunity when you can rest for fifteen or twenty minutes before starting to exercise. A catnap or brief period of quiet meditation may recapture some of the bounce and enthusiasm that will smoothe your way.

If you take pain medications, please be mindful of how you schedule the timing of your drug prescription and your exercise prescription. The two don't really mix well. If you begin to exercise at the moment your pain medication reaches its peak of power, your body may miss important pain messages. You may be unable to sense the twinges that would normally signal you to abandon an activity beyond your ability. You want to feel as comfortable as possible when you begin exercising, but not so comfortable as to be oblivious to danger.

Warming Up

Preheating your muscles for exercise helps you avoid strain. Many people think of warm-ups as activities in themselves, such as stretching the legs before running. However, there are safe, effective warm-up techniques that can *precede* even the simplest actions.

In bed, for example, sleeping under an electric blanket or down comforter gets your whole body toasty. This warmth is the ideal prelude for an in-bed exercise routine.

Later in the day, you may warm up for an exercise period by dressing in extra layers of clothing, or by taking a warm bath or shower, followed by an application of liniment. This form of passive warm-up is all that is needed for most stretching and strengthening exercises. In fact, numerous exercises can actually be done while you are lying in a warm tub or standing under a hot shower. Similarly, you can facilitate your hand and foot exercises with a sink or basin of warm water.

Active warm-ups for aerobic activity involve motion, but we don't want you to overdo it. The best way to warm up for walking, for example, is to start walking slowly. After about ten minutes, as your body heats up through increased blood circulation, you can pick up your pace with confidence. Elaborate stretches before walking may actually involve more muscle exertion – and danger of injury – than a series of slow, steady steps. Your regular arthritis exercise stretching and strengthening routine, however, would no doubt serve as excellent preparation for your aerobics, provided you have the time and energy to do everything in one fell swoop.

Cool-down after exercise is just as important as warm-up before. Slowing your pace as you come to the end of your aerobics is part of cooling down. So is a graceful flourish to your final stretch, accompanied by a few deep breaths. Many people like to relax with an ice pack for about ten minutes in the afterglow of a good workout. You will probably need at least ten minutes to return your heart rate to normal.

Motivational Strategy

No one knows better than you do what strategies will work to keep your motivation high. Are you a persevering sort who never waivers after making a decision? Or are you likely to lose interest in this new endeavour during the several weeks it may take to see real results? Are you a loner who will happily strike out for an early-morning walk before going to work? Or do you prefer a social setting for exercise – walking with a group of friends, say, or working out in a gym?

Taking stock of yourself now and planning what to do if and when you lose the urge to exercise can help you over the hard spots.

Here are some suggestions that may help keep you on track:

- Keep a log of your exercise progress, and the improvements in your condition.
- Set aside a place for your exercise, with everything you need handy – exercise equipment, mats, music, a special warm-up suit, etc.
- Arrange to exercise regularly with a friend or in a group, to put your exercise in a social context.
- Schedule a time of day that you can devote to exercise, and don't let anything else cut into that time. Exercise is *important*.
- Ask your doctor to help you compile a list of vital statistics, including weight, blood pressure, cholesterol level (including the percentage of high- and low-density lipoproteins), and sedimentation rate (for rheumatoid arthritis). After two months of regular exercise, take the profile again and see how the numbers have changed.
- Sit down and write yourself a letter, explaining your goals and hopes. Put it away somewhere. You may never need to look at it again, but if you find yourself looking for excuses to avoid exercise, take out the letter and read it.

Chapter 24
Relaxation Exercises

How to tap the energizing power of meditation and other techniques that focus the mind

All physical exercises tend to benefit the mind as well as the body, by invigorating the spirits. The emphasis in this chapter, however, is on thought exercises that relax the mind and thereby relieve the body of the negative effects of stress.

Relaxation exercises require no physical exertion. They include deep breathing, progressive relaxation, imagery (visualization), and meditation. A time investment of as little as ten or twenty minutes a day spent in one of these quiet activities may result in a significant degree of pain reduction. What's more, these exercises can result in other positive physical effects, such as decreased blood pressure and heightened immunity to disease, as documented in medical studies.

Stress aggravates arthritis pain for 670 of the 1,051 US Arthritis Survey participants – fully sixty-four percent of the survey group. It isn't that their ailments are caused by emotional problems, to be sure; it's just that stress can make arthritis symptoms flare. By the same token, the relief of stress may quiet those symptoms. For this reason, hundreds of the survey respondents relied on the relaxation exercises outlined here to get arthritis relief.

Deep Breathing

Meditation and other formal relaxation techniques all begin by focusing the attention on breathing. This ploy takes your mind off external concerns and helps you gain active control over your body. When you breathe deeply you slow the rate of your breathing by taking a few big breaths instead of many small ones. Deep breathing often works quickly to block the more unpleasant aspects of stress, such as the painful pounding of a racing heart or tight muscles that are cramped with tension.

Inhale through your nose for several seconds, letting your chest expand fully. Try not to raise your shoulders as you inhale, as this motion does not help the lungs fill with air. Concentrate instead on widening the girth of your chest, picturing it inflating like a balloon. Your abdomen will expand, too, as your diaphragm drops down to increase the influx of air into the lungs.

Hold your breath for just a moment or two, and then slowly, slowly let it out through your mouth. As you exhale, picture your diaphragm rising and your chest contracting, as though squeezing the air out of your lungs. Picture physical tension leaving your body with each exhalation.

Once you become accustomed to deep breathing, and experiencing the comfort it brings, you may use it periodically throughout the day, any time something unpleasant jars you. Also try deep breathing as you go to sleep and again upon awakening.

Progressive Relaxation

This technique helps you achieve relaxed muscles by first reminding you how it feels to be all tensed up. The goal is to work and then relax all your muscles in order – starting from the face and proceeding down, or beginning at the feet, according to your preference.

Start by lying in a comfortable position with your eyes closed. Wriggle around a bit, then lie still and breathe deeply. If you are working with your feet first, tighten the toes and arches of one foot as hard as you can, hold briefly, and then let the muscles go limp. Do the same with the other foot.

Now tense one whole leg, straightening the knee and lifting the leg slightly to add to the tension. Then let the leg relax and slump back into place. Do the same with the other leg.

Continue on up your body, first tensing your abdomen and buttocks, then relaxing them completely. Clench each fist before you let your hands relax. Tense each arm and lift it and then let it fall limp at your side.

You can tense your neck by raising your head slightly, then lying back again. The muscles of your face can screw themselves into a sneer, fabricate an exaggerated grin, and knit your eyebrows to wrinkle your forehead.

When you have completed all these movements, lie still and concentrate on your breathing.

Imagery

Positive images, perhaps of beautiful places that you conjure up and elaborate upon in your mind, can have a powerfully soothing effect. Just as you can work yourself into a state of agitation by, for example, imagining an angry confrontation with your spouse, you can create the experience of deep relaxation by picturing a scene by some pleasant mountain stream, for example, smelling the grass and feeling the warm sunshine on your back as you watch the deer gather to drink there. Some people are able to use just such an imagined haven as a refuge from pain.

Many 'guided imagery' tape recordings are available that can help you paint the details of pleasant scenes, in case you feel your own imagination isn't up to the task.

Meditation

With its long history in Eastern traditions, meditation has won new converts among medical doctors in recent decades because of its boon to health and well-being. Meditation brings on what Dr. Herbert Benson of Harvard Medical School has called 'the relaxation response.' This is a physiological state of deep rest. People experiencing the relaxation response are wide awake, but calm and refreshed. They may continue to feel the positive effects of twenty minutes' meditation throughout the day. You can, too.

Many books describe meditation techniques and practices. The basic outline here is drawn from one of Dr. Benson's books, called *Your Maximum Mind*.

• Begin by choosing a word or phrase that you can use as a focus for the meditation exercise. This could be a pleasant thought, such as 'peace,' or the opening of a prayer, or even a soothing sound that has no real meaning.
• Seat yourself in a comfortable position with your eyes closed and your muscles relaxed.
• As you breathe deeply, repeat your focus word or phrase to yourself with each exhalation.

- If worries or other thoughts come into your mind, calmly shoo them out again by repeating your focus word or phrase.
- Continue in this fashion for ten or twenty minutes.

These are the basic steps of meditation. Don't let the simplicity fool you into thinking that there's nothing much to it. Total concentration and the relaxation it brings will improve with practice, and may improve your quality of life significantly. If you want to make more of it, set aside a special place for meditation, where you keep a few favourite items that evoke positive feelings. Set aside a particular time of day, too, when you are least likely to be distracted. Ask your family and friends not to call you at this time. Take the telephone off the hook, or let the answering machine pick up, just to be safe.

We have considered each of these relaxation exercises separately, but they are easily combined. You may find, for example, that you can introduce a favourite image into your meditation, replacing your focus word or phrase with pictures. Deep breathing figures importantly in meditation, and also facilitates imagery.

Now that you are completely relaxed, you're ready to start your aerobic exercise.

Section 9
Aerobic Fitness Exercises for Arthritis

Walking has a global effect on the entire person. It adds hours to one's day and years to one's life. Walking is a superior way to handle stress, and provides the isolation needed for meditation. Not the least of its benefits is the opportunity it gives for creative thinking and solving life's problems.

If these rewards seem similar to the claims made by runners and cyclists and adherents of other activities, it is because they are. Exercise is the generic drug.

— George Sheehan, M.D. from the preface to *Walking* by Casey Meyers

Chapter 25
Walking

How to turn an activity you've done all your life into a safe, beneficial aerobic exercise

Walking is the oldest and best of the weight-bearing exercises for people with arthritis. We recommend it over jogging. More than half of the participants in the US Arthritis Survey reported that they walk regularly for fitness and to maintain maximum mobility.

Jogging causes so many injuries that even young, athletic exercisers often choose to walk or swim instead. People with arthritis must be extra careful about any exercise that bounces and shocks the joints the way jogging does. And yet, some aerobic activity is crucial in the treatment of arthritis because it helps all the muscles and joints by increasing the blood flow to affected areas.

Luckily, numerous activities other than jogging can give the heart and lungs the necessary workout to improve circulation and stamina. Walking, generally considered the best aerobic exercise for people with arthritis, is easy, accessible, effective, and enjoyable. It can be geared to any level of fitness, and pursued by people of all ages.

Hospital studies show that walkers accrue the same cardiovascular benefits as runners, and with far fewer injuries. More to the point, clinical investigations document the fact that walking decreases arthritis pain. One hundred and two individuals with osteoarthritis recently participated in a study to test the benefits of walking, conducted at New York's Hospital for Special Surgery. The walkers in the group, who trekked for thirty minutes, three times a week for two months, experienced such significant levels of pain reduction that many were able to decrease the amount of medication they used.

Walking makes an ideal arthritis exercise because it is low-impact yet high-endurance once individuals build up to relatively long walks several times a week. Many formerly sedentary arthritis sufferers from the original survey group reported that they had transformed themselves into inveterate and hardy walkers. One woman, after many years spent in an extremely limited life-style, turned over a new, more active leaf by walking fifty feet a day.

A fitness exercise such as walking offers particular advantages to women because it can help prevent osteoporosis by strengthening the bones. Some researchers have found that exercise, coupled with calcium supplements, can even help prevent osteoporosis among women who are already past menopause.

No exercise could be more convenient than walking. You need no special equipment and no special clothing, other than comfortable shoes. You don't have to travel to the tennis court, the gym, the pool, or the golf course, you just get up and go. You can easily fit walking into your daily activities. Sometimes you can even fit your daily activities, such as shopping or doing errands, into your walk. And although walking will quicken your heart rate and get your body into condition, it won't make you perspire enough to require a shower or change of clothing immediately afterwards.

The number of times per week that you walk and the length of time you spend walking during each aerobic exercise session will depend on your level of exercise readiness. If you have been extremely limited in your activities because of pain or disability, your first goal may be to walk five minutes at a time in your own home, or around the block.

If you have fallen into inactivity by habit instead of being forced into it by pain, you may be able to start out by walking – slowly at first – for twenty minutes at a time, four times a week. Then you can increase the distance you walk, or the time you spend walking, or both, each week, until you are up to three or even four miles in an hour, five to seven days a week.

Remember, though, that persistence is more important than pace. No matter how slowly you walk, your joints will reap the benefits of exercise, and your heart will, too. A recent study at the famed Cooper Institute for Aerobics Research in Dallas demonstrated this surprising fact.* Dr. John Duncan recruited women who had been leading sedentary lives, and put them on one of several walking programs. Once they got up to snuff, the three groups of walkers all showed up at the track five days a week and covered the same amount of ground, but in different periods of time: aerobic walkers finished the three-mile course in thirty-six minutes, brisk walkers took forty-six minutes, and slow strollers required a full hour to go the whole distance. Reporting his results in the *Journal of the American Medical Association*, Dr. Duncan said that although the aerobic walkers huffed and puffed the most and burned the most oxygen, all three groups showed the *same* healthful changes in their cholesterol levels.

Dr. James Rippe, director of the Exercise Physiology and Nutrition Laboratory at the University of Massachusetts School of Medicine, offers this sage advice to new walkers on how fast to step: 'Walk as though you have someplace to go.'

Dress for comfort and according to the weather. A good formula for cold weather is to dress in layers. These tend to hold in warmth, and you can always remove a layer or two if you feel too warm. In summer, even when you dress in light clothing, be alert for signs of heat stroke if you are a fast walker. The symptoms of this dangerous overheating include dizziness, headache, nausea, and cramping.

Give careful thought to the place you go for your walk. At first, select a round-trip route that you can complete in a reasonable amount of time. Later, as you walk more, you may want to change your destination. If you have a path or trail near you that promises the added bonus of beautiful scenery, so much the better.

* The Cooper Aerobics Center, founded by Ken Cooper in Dallas in the early 1970s, is comprised of the Cooper Clinic, a preventive and rehabilitative medicine facility; the Cooper Institute for Aerobics Research, where researchers study the role of exercise and other lifestyle factors in the maintenance of health; the Cooper Wellness Program, which provides a supportive, live-in environment where participants can focus time and attention on the challenging task of how to make positive lifestyle changes; and the Cooper Fitness Center, a health club in which all members' exercise efforts are supervized by a well-trained staff of health professionals.

Some people prefer to walk on grass or the soft surface of an artificially surfaced indoor track, as they feel it reduces the impact on the joints in their feet and ankles. Others find they can manage well on a sidewalk, so long as their walking shoes provide good cushioning.

Once you get out and about, you will notice the exercise habits of other walkers, many of whom dress in elegant sweat suits and fancy walking shoes. You'll see that some of them walk with one finger pressed against the side of the neck, or the opposite wrist, to check their pulse and make sure they've got their hearts pumping at the ideal rate. A few very serious walkers may even sport sophisticated wrist meters, with enough tiny dials to satisfy a jet pilot, on which they monitor their vital functions. You can take the exercise as far as you like for maximum fitness, but the primary goal in arthritis care is simply to keep your body moving and bearing its own weight.

If you have an uneven gait, or walk with a limp, make sure that walking for aerobic exercise does not exacerbate your condition. Try to walk at a slow pace, taking smaller than usual steps, if necessary, so that you maintain as even a stride as possible. Otherwise, you may place undue strain on several joints. When walking with a cane, hold it in the hand opposite the affected leg. (If it's your right hip or ankle that pains you, hold the cane in your left hand.)

Breathe deeply and evenly as you walk, and swing or pump your arms. Also, try to maintain your best posture, looking straight ahead of you, with your head up, chest out, shoulders back but relaxed, hips tucked under, and tummy in.

As for time spent walking, any amount of time is better than no time. According to an earlier, larger study at the Cooper Clinic, headed by Dr. Steven N. Blair, walking as little as half an hour a day can increase a person's longevity by warding off two of the leading killers – heart disease and cancer.

Walking works wonders. But how can you make yourself undertake the work of walking? Try walking one or more of the following ways:

- Around the track at your local high school
- On a beach or through the woods where beauty surrounds you

- On a treadmill while reading the newspaper or watching the television news
- Along a sidewalk looking at the passersby and the store window displays
- Through a shopping mall in any weather
- With a friend or family member
- With your pet
- To and from work
- On your errands
- Listening to music on a portable radio
- Listening to taped lectures or talking books on a small tape player with headphones
- Letting your mind run free to dream up creative ideas
- Even on days that aren't balmy, sunny, and bright
- At dawn, to start the day off right
- During lunch hour, as a break from the day's other activities
- In the evening, when the full moon can be your night light

Because walking came naturally to you in childhood, you may take it for granted now. All the fuss made over it in books and magazines may seem misplaced, but keeping the activity's advantages in mind can help you adhere to your exercise regimen. Remember, brisk walking gives you a good workout that will benefit your heart as much as your joints. What's more, since most people can walk for a longer time than they could run or play tennis, walking tends to build muscular endurance while it burns calories. And walking is so accessible and easy to do that you're far less likely to quit this exercise regimen than any other you might try.

Chapter 26
Swimming and Water Exercises

How to find your way to healthy workouts in the water – even if you can't swim a stroke

Water's buoyancy makes swimming virtually a no-impact aerobic activity. If you don't know how to swim, you can learn now, taking advantage of the many courses offered at health clubs, YMCAs/YMHAs, and schools. If you don't care to take the plunge, remember that being a nonswimmer need not stop you from venturing into the shallow end of a warm pool and doing your range-of-motion exercises there, or splashing around to give your joints a good workout. You may also find that just being in the water relaxes you and further reduces your pain, especially if it's in the comfortable range of 86 degrees Fahrenheit.

Even jogging becomes a safe, sane exercise for people with arthritis when they jog in waist-deep water! It's well-nigh impossible to sustain an impact injury while jogging in a swimming pool. Your bones don't take a pounding when you water-jog, even when you vary your pace from a slow gait to a faster one. The deeper you submerge yourself in the water, the less you stress your joints as you jog or walk. Try these activities first in waist-level water, then in water up to your shoulders to see the difference for yourself. You can also run in the deep water, where your feet will never touch the bottom of the pool, but your arms and legs will have to pump and cycle, respectively, to propel you forward. You'll be in good company: remember that superstar runners maintain fitness while recovering from injuries by running in water.

Swimming counts as an ideal aerobic exercise because it makes both the arms and the legs work hard, and gets the heart pumping.

Some experts, however, argue that swimming is no match for walking or running as a weight-bearing exercise. While it's true that the water provides a virtually stress-free environment for the bones and joints, swimmers have been shown to have thicker, stronger bones than people who perform no exercise.

Perhaps you used to be a good swimmer, but arthritis has cramped your style, making it hard for you to turn your head in proper form for breathing while swimming the crawl. Try using a snorkel – the kind skindivers wear – so you can breathe easily without overexerting your neck muscles. Even though this technique has been used with great success in hospital studies, some people find that the sidestroke, with its more gentle action, works better for them than the crawl. You can experiment with different strokes until you find the one that suits you best. You can also combine a variety of strokes to add interest to your swimming. By alternating between difficult and simple strokes, you can pace yourself, getting a good workout while avoiding rapid fatigue.

If your legs are in great shape but your arms or shoulders are too weak to swim yet, you can still start out in the pool by using a kickboard. This aid allows you to kick to your heart's content and propel yourself across the pool while your arms do hardly any work at all.

Warm up for swimming by performing a few range-of-motion exercises at the side of the pool before you break into your laps.

More than 200 of the original US Arthritis Survey respondents made the effort to get to a pool regularly, even if it meant travelling by bus at considerable inconvenience. The return on their time investment paid off in terms of decreased pain, they reported. Those who had to pay for pool time by joining a health club reasoned that they were saving money in the long run – by cutting their monthly costs for pain medications.

We encourage you to try out the pool at the club before you join. If the water is too cold, or if there are too many people swimming laps at the hours you hope to exercise, you will not be able to fulfill your needs. More than likely, you'll have several pool facilities to choose from, and can find one that suits you perfectly.

Another advantage of water is that it makes exercise a virtually no-sweat proposition. The reason is that water is much more efficient than air at dissipating heat – four times as efficient, to be exact. The result is that your body doesn't get overheated and you can continue to feel comfortable even though you're working hard in hot weather.

If you perform your stretching and strengthening exercises in a pool, you'll find that the water gives just enough resistance to add an extra degree of muscle building to many of these manoeuvers. Some movements, on the other hand, actually become easier. For example, you'll find that a standing knee-to-chest stretch or a straight leg-up raise can be performed with reduced effort when your legs are buoyed by water.

When you first begin aquatic exercise, or whenever you need a little added support, you can wear a buoyancy vest or belt to help you stay upright as you work out in the water.

At the pool, as on the walking paths, you'll encounter the advanced equipment of enthusiasts, such as water dumbbells and weighted benches for transferring bench or step aerobics to the water setting. Depending on your level of ability (and income!), you may want to try some of these exercise aids, but the water itself suffices for most people. Given the popularity of exercise and the increased availability of swimming pools, more and more people are pursuing aquatic aerobics.

Chapter 27
Cycling

How to use bicycles, indoors or out, in a low-impact aerobic exercise program for arthritis

Cycling is a good aerobic activity for people with arthritis because it involves an even lower level of impact than walking. We're talking about the normal leg motion here, of course. If you fall off the bicycle, the impact is stunning!

Cycling enthusiasts say that this sport is so gentle on the body it can even be pursued by people who can't walk. Some doctors, however, counter that cycling is great for the hips, but not so great for the knees. From what we can determine, some knee problems attributed to cycling are really due to riding bikes with pedals set at improper heights, or to overexertion in cycling that pushes the legs too far, too fast, before muscles adapt to the exercise. Do exercise with caution: cycling may aggravate *your* knees.

Numerous clinical studies have demonstrated the benefits of bicycling in the overall treatment of arthritis. One study involved twenty-three women with rheumatoid arthritis who exercised with stationary bicycles, but at different levels of difficulty and for varying periods of time. Even those women who exercised for just fifteen minutes per session found that they developed greater strength and endurance, and that fewer of their joints felt painful and swollen. In another study, the subjects who rode stationary bicycles achieved the same overall flexibility as another group who did only flexibility (range-of-motion) exercises – and increased their endurance as well. In yet another study that included cycling as part of an exercise regimen, most of the subjects felt so much improved by the time the research program ended that they continued to follow the routine on their own.

Equipment becomes an important consideration in cycling, as bicycles with many gears offer the most options to people with arthritis. Riding a bike gets you out and about, making it an appealing pastime. Do be sure to pay close attention to safety, however. Now that the pattern of injuries incurred while bicycling is well-known, every cyclist needs to wear a helmet. Even top pros who have never fallen off a bike in their lives avow that head protection is essential, whether riding on special bicycle paths or on streets shared with autotraffic. Night riders need reflectors on the bicycle itself, as well as on their clothing and helmet. It's also a good idea to equip your bicycle with head- and taillights.

The racing bike, which requires the rider to assume a near-fetal position and then crane his neck up to see straight ahead, has at last given way in popularity to the upright touring and all-terrain bikes. This trend is a real boon to people with arthritis. You will be much more comfortable sitting straight up than hunching over for the sake of reducing air resistance on your body. When you are riding to gain exercise and fresh air, as opposed to winning first place in the *Tour de France*,* sitting up is the position of choice.

A bicycle has to fit its rider for comfort and efficiency. This is generally true, but especially important for people with arthritis, to avoid added stress on any joint. A reputable bicycle dealer will ask you to sit on the bike before you buy it, and then adjust the seat so that you can almost but not quite straighten your leg when you have pushed the pedal as far down as it will go. Also, you need an optimal distance between the seat and the handlebars, or you will develop back pain from overreaching. This distance is defined by the length of the rider's forearm, from the elbow to the tips of the fingers. (Sometimes the handlebar distance looks right on purchase, but will need adjusting later, either by tilting the seat or changing the bars so that they extend farther back.)

The gears on the bicycle function to give you an energy advantage. Used properly, they improve your pedalling efficiency, so that you can keep up the same rate of leg work whether you're on a hill or a level surface. They have nothing to do with speed, so you need not be scared away from a ten-or-more-speed

* The *Tour de France* is a three-week bicycle race that covers more than 2,000 miles.

bicycle just because you're not planning to go very fast. A 'ten-speed' bicycle should really be called a 'ten-gear' bicycle. After all, no bicycle can go faster than you can pedal it, no matter how many gears it has.

Most adult bikes come equipped with hand brakes. If you have the hand strength to operate these brakes, do check to see that your hands can comfortably span the distance (called the 'reach') between the handlebars and brake levers. If you have trouble using your hands, you may want to try to find a bicycle with foot brakes instead.

When you ride, put the balls of your feet on the pedals.

Cycling can now be enjoyed as an indoor as well as an outdoor sport. Exercycles rooted to one spot in your home can be adjusted to offer minimal resistance when easy riding is required. You can reduce the tension to zero, if need be, or raise it to mimic the steepest hillside imaginable. These indoor bicycles go by many names, such as 'stationary cycle,' for obvious reasons, and 'bicycle ergometer,' which is the term physiotherapists prefer, because it emphasizes the point that you can measure the amount of work you're doing as you spin your wheels. (The hospital studies mentioned above were all performed with bicycle ergometers.)

We think of cycling as legwork, and it is, but some stationary cycles include activities for the arms as well. As you pump the pedals with your feet, you grasp handles that you push/pull back and forth with your arms. There are even cycle ergometers designed expressly for upper-body work, and these offer an alternative to people whose legs can't take the strain of most aerobic activities.

Seat comfort is an all-important consideration. Whether you ride indoors or out, you need to remain seated throughout your workout. Some people will experience nothing more annoying than a mild soreness the first few days of getting used to a bicycle seat. Others find the pain in their buttocks never goes away. If you are in this latter category, cycling is not for you. Before you give up the advantages of the sport, however, try to make your bike seat as comfortable as you can with a padded seat cover, or even by changing the seat (to one often called a saddle) altogether until you find one that you can tolerate.

Add another level of comfort to your riding by wearing padded gloves. These bicycle gloves, which are perforated for use in warm weather, were originally introduced to give serious racers a better grip and greater comfort during long rides. If you don't like them or find them too expensive, then by all means build up the grips on your handle bars with foam padding. You can purchase large, soft grips at bicycle stores, or you can make your own out of layers of foam.

Stationary cycling combines itself easily with other activities. Many people find their exercise period the ideal time to read a book or magazine, watch the news on television, or see a movie on the VCR.

Chapter 28
Dancing and More

How to set your aerobic workout to music and step through it with rhythm and pleasure

The best exercise regimens are often the ones that provide a real recreational and social outlet, so that they not only improve your physical condition but put you in the swing of things and make you feel good to be alive.

Dancing provides this combination of good movements and good times with others. Ballroom dancing in particular, with its built-in opportunities to rest between numbers, is becoming a favourite exercise pastime. Folk dancing, even more than couples dancing, brings groups of people together for active recreation. There are even a few specialized dance schools that cater to people with arthritis.

At least one hospital study has shown that the rigours of aerobic dance, believe it or not, can be modified to make this popular activity low-impact enough for people with arthritis – and beneficial for them, too.

Dancing combines range-of-motion manoeuvres and strengthening exercises in the prescribed steps. When you dance to the music of a song set, continuing until the music ends, you get built-in repetitions of the movements, not to mention endurance training. What's more, dancing definitely drives depression away with its strong positive effect on the spirits. The chance to be with other people in an active form of recreation makes dancing virtually boredom-proof. People may abandon their exercycles and find excuses to avoid the swimming pool on a chilly day, but dancing retains its appeal over the long haul. It's really a fun way to rediscover how much your body can do.

Health experts consider dancing a reasonable alternative to other aerobic activities, including walking, swimming, cycling, and jogging.

'Ya gotta keep dancing!' several Arthritis Survey participants maintained.

One of the chief benefits of dancing is the relaxed style of movement that comes from mastering steps to music. As dancers become accustomed to rhythmically positioning their bodies in space, they find that they develop dancelike ways of doing other activities. Their motions may become more fluid, so that they stop walking with a stiff-legged gait. Instead of striking rigid poses while they stand at the kitchen counter or sit at a desk, for example, they bring the good body mechanics of dancing to bear by adding a little motion. Some dancers gently dip and shift their weight from one leg to the other while working standing up, or perform a rock-and-roll stretch of the lower back while typing at the computer keyboard.

If you've never danced before, you'll want to do some at-home preparation before you take to the dance floor. Your regular range-of-motion and strengthening exercises, outlined in Section 10, will get your body ready for new moves. If you're worried about catching your breath while you're keeping step to the beat, remember that you can gain an aerobic advantage by starting to walk regularly.

In discussing your exercise plans with your doctor, check to see if there's any reason that dancing might cause a problem for you. Even if you have artificial joints in your hips or knees, or a tendency to accumulate fluid in these joints, you will more than likely be able to hit on safe ways to approach the dance floor.

The best way to determine the best type of dancing for you is by assessing your joint condition. Painful hands are best held gently by a ballroom partner – not allemanded left and right in a square dance setting where you can't control who will grasp your hand, or how vigorously. However, your toes will less likely get stepped on while folk dancing, where partners tend to hold each other at arm's length. You can keep an even greater distance from your fellow dancers by taking a class in modern dance or jazzercise. That way, you'll do the steps on your own, but you'll still be in a group of dancers where movement and music can improve your muscle tone and lift your spirits.

Ballet, especially in toe shoes, is generally considered too stressful for joints already stressed by arthritis. If, however, you can find a beginner's class with an understanding teacher, you may well find the disciplined, graceful exercises at the barre to be just what you need to improve your posture, muscle strength, and flexibility.

Should you decide to take formal lessons in social dancing, or dance/exercise classes, try to arrange a brief meeting with your instructor before classes begin, when you can talk candidly about your arthritis and any special concerns you might have. This gives you a chance to explain in advance that you may, for example, want to rest frequently at the outset, or avoid altogether any movements that seem to you to be too jarring. If you feel embarrassed about initiating such a discussion, you can always drop a note, but do let the instructor know what to expect from you in class.

Since you'll be on your feet and using them a great deal, you'll need supportive, comfortable dancing shoes. These can be of almost any variety, but low-heeled styles make the most sense. Classic saddle shoes, which were popular in the 1960s, are making a comeback these days – cushioning many dancing feet moving to the big band sound at swing-dance fests. The shoes fit right in with the period outfits that include full circle skirts and skinny ties. Their fit on the feet can be quite comfortable, too, given their good support, laces, and wide-toe box. Sturdy leather saddle shoes provide more protection from your partner's feet than any sneakers made of leather or canvas can!

Other Dancelike Disciplines

Some of the routinized movements from Oriental martial arts, such as karate and t'ai chi ch'uan, share the benefits of dance as a form of aerobic exercise. Karate, for one, includes stretching, isometric and isotonic strengthening, and aerobic activity. Just as dance combines these movement basics in a structure set to music, karate incorporates the elements of exercise in a technique with a long historic tradition and a philosophy of peace and harmony. Teachers of karate frequently speak of the discipline's emphasis on self-expression, and the way karate respects the needs and capabilities of each individual.

Movies have convinced many of us that karate is all about violence, or defending oneself against violence, but you can learn karate even if you have considerable physical limitation. More importantly, you can find arthritis relief in its movements.

Chapter 29
Exercise by Any Other Name

How to turn your chores and favourite pastimes into aerobic exercises that help keep you going strong

Everybody knows somebody who seems to be in great shape but swears that exercise is not the reason. These people can't be coaxed out for a walk, hate the idea of swimming laps, and equate exercycles with instruments of torture. Yet they carry themselves well, and can charge up the stairs without pausing to catch their breath. What's their secret?

They *are* exercising; they just don't know it. They pursue jobs, chores, or hobbies that confer all the advantages of aerobic exercise. They've been fooled into fitness by doing the things they have to do or the things they love to do.

In the original US Arthritis Survey group, for example, were waitresses who spent hours on their feet, trekking back and forth to some restaurant's kitchen, carrying trayloads of dishes. This activity, though it cannot boast the relaxation of walking in the woods, certainly gets the heart pumping and the muscles contracting.

Other survey group participants, however, physically exerted themselves in pursuit of a favourite pastime. These individuals enjoyed a workout *and* a wonderful time.

Gardening exemplifies the kind of activity that combines aerobic, stretching, and strengthening exercises with the pursuit of pleasure. Gardening has shown itself to be the aerobic equal of walking for those people addicted to digging and planting. The excitement of tending the growing shoots makes the activity so engrossing that there is no problem in building up to a fitness level of endurance. On the contrary, gardeners with arthritis must often be dragged indoors against their will before they overexert themselves. It is not unusual to find someone forgetting all about pain during a two- or three-hour stint of hoeing and weeding in the garden.

If this sounds like your kind of exercise, try to keep the fitness goals in mind as you plan your vegetable or flower garden. Each time you go outdoors to do your gardening, try to vary the activities as much as possible. If you spend your whole time crouched down between the rows, for example, you not only miss out on aerobic exercise, but you will no doubt exacerbate stiffness in your legs. If weeding is the order of the day, try pulling weeds for twenty minutes, and then getting up to carry each small load to a compost heap or other disposal site.

Aim to maintain an awareness of your posture and movements as you work. This means keeping your back straight and bending with your knees when you must get down to ground level. Stay loose by occasionally shrugging and rolling your shoulders as you work. Carry potted plants high and close to your body, so they don't force you to stoop over. For really heavy loads, use a wheelbarrow.

Equip yourself with any gardening tools that are specifically designed to make the job easier on your body. Some examples include:

- A soft pad to sit or kneel on while weeding
- A low stool as another comfort aid for weeding work
- A hose caddy
- Extra long-handled shovels, hoes, and rakes that enable you to stand up straight while working in the garden.

If you don't have a green thumb or any hope of developing one, you may find other aerobic-type physical outlets in and around your house. Yard work such as raking leaves qualifies. So do many aspects of home upkeep, including indoor and outdoor painting, polishing and refinishing old furniture finds, and giving your house a truly thorough cleaning. Laundry is another task that can be turned to aerobic advantage by ignoring a few modern conveniences and taking the wash outside to dry it on a clothesline.

Caring for and playing with your children – your own or someone else's – can give you an exhausting physical workout and much pleasure, too. Some people with arthritis fear that children will be too rough on them, or insist on playing active games that could tire out a young adult with no disabilities of any kind. However, even very young children can be taught to recognize and respect a caregiver's physical limitations. As long as they know they are getting an adult's full and willing attention, they are usually content to structure the play at the older person's pace.

Sexual activity also offers many of the same benefits as exercise, such as flooding the brain with endorphins that lift the spirits and quell pain. Sexual arousal also induces the body to release adrenalin and cortisone into the blood. These substances act as natural painkillers.

You may need to experiment with your partner to find the most comfortable positions for intercourse or other sex play. It goes without saying that aerobic activity will be the natural outcome of your enjoyment – not the primary goal!

As gerontologist Alex Comfort has remarked, 'Most people can and should have sex long after they no longer wish to ride bicycles.'

Section 10
Exercising Away Pain from Head to Toe

Stretching, because it relaxes your mind and tunes up your body, should be part of your daily life.

– Bob Anderson author, *Stretching*

Chapter 30
Neck and Jaw Exercises

Specific exercises for two prime locations of muscle tension and stress in the body

You can do your neck a lot of good by remembering that good posture starts at the head. As you go through the day, try to keep your head up and well aligned with the rest of your body. If you 'lead with your chin' as you walk or work, you'll be scrunching together the seven vertebrae in your neck. Instead, keep your chin tucked in, just as you tuck in your tummy to straighten your back.

Move your neck as much as you can to keep its muscles relaxed. Many of us have a tendency to apply stress and tension directly to our neck muscles, holding them rigidly and aggravating pain in the neck!

The Yes-No and Left-Right exercises described on pages 405–6 can be done anytime, anywhere, to loosen up a tight neck, as can parts of the Head Roll. Stress and tension may also express themselves in the jaw, through rigidly held 'tight-lipped' expressions and grinding or clenching of the teeth.

The first exercise in the following group stretches the jaw, while the rest concentrate on the neck. They are arranged according to starting position, so that the first few can be done as part of an in-bed routine upon awakening.

If you have rheumatoid arthritis, please approach these exercises with caution, as the disease can make the neck joints extremely unstable. You'll want to stretch and strengthen your neck muscles gently and wisely. The advice, 'Don't push beyond pain,' is especially relevant here.

A-E-I-O-U Shout
Type: Stretching
Starting position: This exercise can be done in virtually any position.

Steps:

1. Pronounce or mouth the vowel sound 'A' for several seconds, exaggerating the motion of your lips and jaw for maximum stretch. Your mouth should be wide open, as though you were cheering silently.
2. Say 'E,' drawing out the sound and baring your teeth like an angry cat.
3. Drop your jaw as far as possible to say 'I' with the stretch of a big yawn.
4. Sustain the 'O' sound, with rounded lips and raised eyebrows.
5. Push your lips far forward as you say 'U' with 'oomph.'

Shoulder Shrug

Type: Stretching
Starting position: You can do this exercise lying in bed, sitting, or standing, with your arms at your sides.
Steps:

1. Slowly and steadily raise your shoulders to a shrug.
2. Hold for a moment, feeling the effect on your neck muscles.
3. Keeping your head still, gently press your shoulders as far down as you can.
4. Hold, feeling the stretch in your neck.

Note: This exercise benefits the shoulders and appears in that section as well.

Bed Head

Type: Stretching and strengthening
Starting position: Lie on your back in bed or on the floor.
Steps:

1. Press your head straight back into your pillow or mat.
2. Hold for a moment, then release the pressure.
3. Lift your head above your pillow or mat as high as you can, without lifting your shoulders.
4. Hold, feeling the stretch in your neck, then release.

Note: Later in the day, you can repeat steps 1 and 2 of this exercise by pressing your head against your arm or a wall.

Head Roll (see page 407)
Type: Stretching
Starting position: Sit in a chair or stand with your feet at a comfortable distance apart. Hold your head high and look straight ahead.
Steps:

1. Tilt your head to the left as though you were trying to put your ear on your shoulder. *a*
2. Stop when you've stretched your neck as far as you can. Don't try to bring your shoulder up to meet your ear.
3. Roll your head forward and down, as though trying to touch your chin to your chest. *b*
4. Continue the roll toward the right, as though trying to place your right ear on your right shoulder. *c*
5. Come full circle by tilting your head back, but not too far. *d*
6. Return to starting position.
7. Repeat these steps, circling your head to the right this time.

Note: If you have been advised not to tilt your head back, simply omit Step 5 of this exercise.

This exercise can be done in bed by modifying it slightly to omit the forward and backward motions. Simply slide and tilt your head to the left, then back up to the center, then to the right and back to center.

Left-Right
Type: Stretching
Starting position: You can do this exercise lying in bed, sitting, or standing, with your arms at your sides.
Steps:

1. Keeping your head level, turn to the right as though trying to see behind your back.
2. Return your head and your gaze to center.

3. Turn your head to look toward the left as far as you can.
4. Return to starting position.

Advanced variation: After you have turned your head as far as possible, tilt it down as though trying to touch your chin to your shoulder.

Yes-No
Type: Stretching
Starting position: You may sit or stand virtually anywhere.
Steps:

1. Nod your head yes, slowly, several times. Keep your neck still but relaxed, moving only your head.
2. Turn your head side-to-side, as though making an exaggerated 'no' gesture. Again, keep your neck still and move only your head.

Head Pull
Type: Stretching
Starting position: Sit in a chair with your back straight and your hands clasped behind your head.
Steps:

1. Gently pull your head forward and down to stretch the back of your neck.
2. Hold for a moment.
3. Return to your starting position.

Neck Push
Type: Strengthening
Starting position: Sit or stand comfortably.
Steps:

1. Press the palm of one hand against your forehead, and your forehead against the palm of your hand.
2. Hold for a moment, keeping the pressure on your hand and head without moving either one.
3. Repeat with the other hand.

Note: If your hands and wrists are particularly painful, you may apply the pressure with your forearm. Another possibility is to press your head against a wall.

Head Roll (Illustrated)

Tilt your head to one side, then forward, then to the other side in a slow, continuous roll that gently stretches your neck muscles.

Try to move only your head and neck, keeping your shoulders level. (In other words, resist the temptation to raise your shoulder to your ear!)

The full circle includes a tilt back, too, but this part of the stretch is a problem for some people. If your neck hurts in this position, or if you have rheumatoid arthritis, leave out this stop.

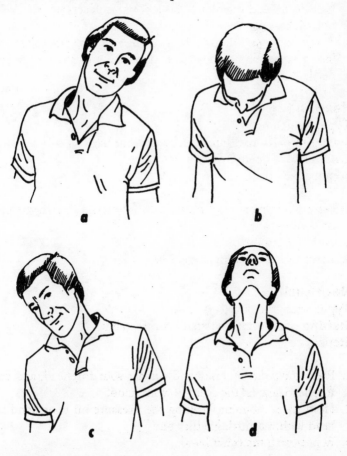

Chapter 31
Shoulder Exercises

How to shrug, roll, stretch, and strengthen the joints that carry the weight of the world

You really do carry the weight of the world on these body parts, lifting them (and consequently tensing your neck) to shoulder life's stresses and strains.

Your shoulders bear the distinction of being the most flexible joints in your body, when they are functioning smoothly. Since they are capable of so many kinds of motion, your exercise regimen will combine several movements to work your shoulders to their full potential.

Most shoulder exercises can be done one shoulder at a time, or both together, whichever way suits you better. Many of them also exercise the neck, arms, and hands.

If you use a cane to assist you while walking, you'll find that it makes an excellent baton for shoulder stretches. A few other simple aids to exercise that you may already have around the house include a clothesline for shoulder stretches and a couple of rice cartons or canned goods to be used as one-pound weights.

The most difficult shoulder exercises are those that ask you to extend your arms out straight at shoulder level, as in the Semaphore and the Crisscross.

Shoulder Shrug
Type: Stretching
Starting position: You can do this exercise lying in bed, sitting, or standing, with your arms at your sides.
Steps:

1. Slowly and steadily raise your shoulders to a shrug.
2. Hold for a moment, feeling the effect on your neck muscles.
3. Keeping your head still, gently press your shoulders as far down as you can.

Note: This exercise benefits the neck and appears in that section as well.

Swinging Pendulum

Type: Gentle stretching
Starting Position: In bed, lie face down near the edge of your bed, with one arm hanging free over the edge. (You'll need to roll to the opposite edge to repeat the exercise with your other shoulder.)

In a sitting or standing position, lean forward and let one or both arms hang down, straight but relaxed. You may work the shoulders individually or together.
Steps:

1. Swing your arm(s) gently to and fro, parallel to your body.
2. Swing your arm(s) gently out and back, perpendicular to your body.
3. Swing your arm(s) in small circles, first to the left, then to the right.

Shoulder Helper

Type: Very gentle range-of-motion exercise
Starting position: Sit in a chair.
Steps:

1. Put your right hand on your left shoulder and gently lift the shoulder as far as it will go.
2. Still using your right hand, press the left shoulder down as far as you can.
3. Pull your shoulder forward to its limit.
4. Push your shoulder back as far as possible.
5. Using your left hand on your right shoulder, repeat the above steps.

Shoulder Roll

Type: Stretching
Starting position: You may sit or stand with your shoulders relaxed. Try to proceed through the steps in one fluid motion, making a circle with your shoulder(s).

Steps:

1. Raise your shoulder(s).
2. Bring your shoulder(s) forward.
3. Push your shoulder(s) down.
4. Pull your shoulder(s) back.
5. Return to starting position.
6. Circle your shoulder(s) in the opposite direction (reversing the order of Steps 1–4).

Wall Walker
Type: Stretching
Starting position: You may stand or sit about two feet away from a wall, with your left side to the wall, arms at your sides.
Steps:

1. Let your left hand slowly 'walk' up the wall, as though your fingers were the legs of an insect. *a*
2. 'Walk' about shoulder level if you can, but try not to raise your shoulder or lean away from the wall. 'Let your fingers do the walking.' *b*
3. Turn and 'walk' your right hand.

Note: This exercise is also included in the Hands/Fingers section, as it benefits those joints as well.

Butterfly Stretch
Type: Stretching
Starting position: Sit in a chair or stand at ease, arms at your sides.
Steps:

1. Clasp your hands behind your head.
2. Open your elbows out to your sides as far as you can.
3. Bring your elbows together in front of you, making them meet, if possible.
4. Return to starting position.

5. Place your fingertips on your shoulders, elbows pointing out to the sides.
6. Pull your elbows back as far as you can.
7. Push your elbows forward and try to touch them together.
8. Return to starting position.

Semaphore (See pages 417–18)

Type: Stretching
Starting position: You may sit in a straight-back chair or stand at ease, arms at your sides.
Steps:

1. Extend your arms straight out to the sides at shoulder height. *a*
2. Keeping your arms straight and at shoulder height, touch your hands together in front. *b*
3. Move your arms back out to your sides. *c*
4. Still keeping your arms at shoulder height, move them as though you could touch your hands together in back. *d*
5. Extend your arms out to the sides again. *e*
6. Raise both arms straight up, biceps close to your ears. *f*
7. Lower your arms and let them hang at your sides.

Circling

Type: Stretching
Starting position: Sit in a straight-back chair or stand at ease.
Steps:

1. Extend your arms straight out to the sides, like a child pretending to be an airplane.
2. Move your arms so that your hands make tiny forward circles in the air.
3. Gradually make the circles larger.
4. Stop, then circle in the opposite direction, starting with small circles progressing to larger ones.

Bodybuilder (See page 420)

Type: Stretching and strengthening
Starting position: Sit in a straight-back chair or stand at ease, arms at your sides.

Steps:

1. Raise your arms straight out to the sides with your palms up, and make your hands into fists.
2. Bend your elbows to bring your fists over your shoulders, raising as big a bulge as you can in your biceps. *a*
3. Straighten your elbows to put your fists in the air, over your head. *b*
4. Bring your fists back down over your shoulders, then straight out, then drop them down at your sides.

Circle Twist
Type: Stretching
Starting position: Sit in a straight-back chair or stand at ease.
Steps:

1. Extend your arms straight out to the sides, with your palms facing the floor.
2. Clench your hands in fists and move your arms so that your fists make tiny forward circles.
3. Gradually make the circles larger.
4. Stop and rotate your arms in the opposite direction, starting with small circles and gradually enlarging them.
5. Twist your arms so that your palms (still clenched in fists) face the ceiling.
6. Now make circles, from small to large, first forward, then backward.

Crisscross (See page 421)
Type: Stretching
Starting position: Stand at ease, arms at your sides.
Steps:

1. Extend both your arms straight out in front of you at shoulder height.
2. Keeping arms straight, cross the right one over the left, then left over right. *a*
3. Move your arms out to the sides.

4. Lower your arms and try to cross your wrists in back, right over left, and left over right. *b*
5. Return to starting position.

Straight Edge (See pages 422–3)

Type: Stretching
Starting position: You may sit in a chair or stand at ease. You will need a cane (or a yardstick, broom handle, or exercise baton). Have your arms hanging relaxed, one end of the cane in each hand.
Steps:

1. Lift the cane as high over your head as possible. (If you have more mobility in one shoulder than the other, then your cane will make a diagonal line, instead of a horizontal line, above you.) *a*
2. Lower the cane and rest a moment.
3. Hold the cane straight out in front of you, about shoulder height.
4. Using both arms, move the cane to the right and then to the left. Try to keep your back and hips still as you do this, concentrating on moving your shoulders. *b*
5. Holding the cane out front at shoulder level, and keeping both hands on it, lift and lower first one end of the cane, then the other. (Rest here again, if you need to.) *c*
6. Lift the cane over your head and then bring it down to shoulder height behind your head. (You may bend your head forward.) *d*
7. Return to starting position.

Wallflower (See page 424)

Type: Strengthening
Starting position: Stand next to a wall, with the right side of your body about six inches from the wall.
Steps:

1. Lift your right arm out to the side until your forearm is pressing against the wall. *a*
2. Continue to exert pressure for a few seconds at a time.
3. Relax your arm.
4. Turn and repeat the exercise with your left arm.

Weightlifter
Type: Strengthening
Starting position: Sit in a straight-back chair or stand at ease, holding one-pound weights.
Steps:

1. Lift the weights straight out in front of you.
2. Lower the weights, then lift them straight out to the sides, to shoulder height if possible.
3. Lower the weights, then try to lift them in back, to a height of about one foot.

Pulley Pulls (See page 425)
Type: Stretching and strengthening
Starting position: Sit or stand under your pulley rig, with one end of the rope in each hand, arms straight. (You can use a real clothesline pulley, hung up for this purpose, or make do with a length of clothesline hung over an open door or on a plastic hook.)
Steps:

1. Pull down with your right hand, letting the motion carry your left hand up as high as possible. *a*
2. Pull down with your left hand, so that your right hand rises on the rope. Experiment with rope length and your grip position to get maximum stretch.
3. Repeat, and return to starting position.

Note: If it's hard for you to hold the rope, make loops of the ends and slip them over your hands. Then you can pull with your forearms.

Rowboat
Type: Strengthening
Starting position: Sit in a large rubber tube, with your legs dangling over the rim. Your arms should be free to paddle.
Steps:

1. Using your arms and hands as oars, extend your arms behind you for each stroke and propel yourself across the

pool. (Your hands will push the water and send you sailing backward.)

2. Now stroke in the opposite direction, extending your arms ahead of you to begin each stroke. (This time, your hands will pull the water, and you will travel in the direction you are facing.)

If you have access to a swimming pool, try this shoulder-strengthening water exercise. (You need not be a swimmer to attempt it, since it can be done in shallow water.)

Push-Offs (See page 426)

Type: Strengthening
Starting position: Stand facing a wall, with your feet apart and about twelve inches away from the wall. (After you try this exercise, you may find you're more comfortable standing a little closer or a little farther away.) Rest your palms on the wall at about shoulder height. This exercise is a standing push-up.
Steps:

1. Lean in toward the wall as far as possible without touching your forearms to the wall. Keep your legs and back straight. *a*
2. Push yourself back to the starting position. *b*

Note: The farther from the wall you stand, the greater the shoulder effort needed to accomplish the Push-off. As you advance, increase your distance, but don't exceed two feet.

Fan Belt (See page 427)

Type: Strengthening
Starting position: You may sit or stand in a comfortable position. You will need a rubber exercise belt, or a homemade substitute made from an elasticized belt or bungie cord.
Steps:

1. Slip the belt over your forearms.
2. Spread your foreams as far apart as possible, pushing against the resistance of the exercise belt. *a*

3. Relax.
4. Keeping your arms straight, move the left one up and the right down, again pushing against the resistance of the exercise belt. *b*
5. Move your right arm up and the left down, still pushing against the resistance of the exercise belt.
6. Relax.
7. Take the belt in your hands and pull on it as though you were shooting an arrow, first with your left hand, then your right. *c*

Semaphore (Illustrated)

If you put a couple of signal flags in your hands, these stretching motions might well send important messages!

Remember to keep your elbows straight and your arms at shoulder height as you do your flag-waving.

Note: *Figure d is shown from a different perspective to show the full stretch from behind. You are not expected to change positions.*

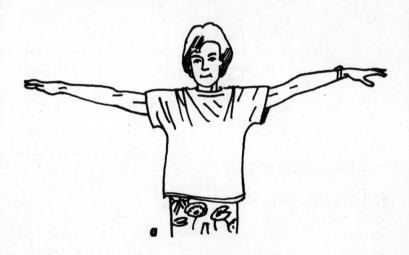

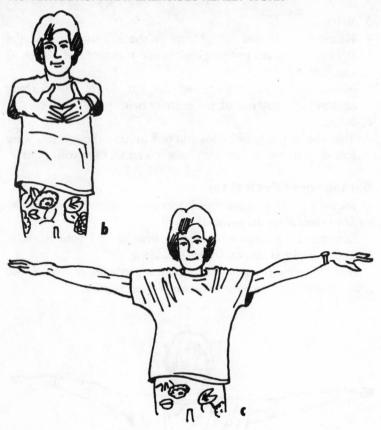

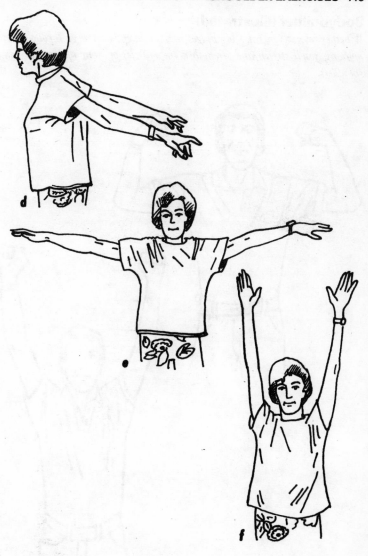

Bodybuilder (Illustrated)

Whether or not you raise big bulges in your biceps as you go through these motions, you'll stretch and strengthen the muscles of your upper arms and shoulders.

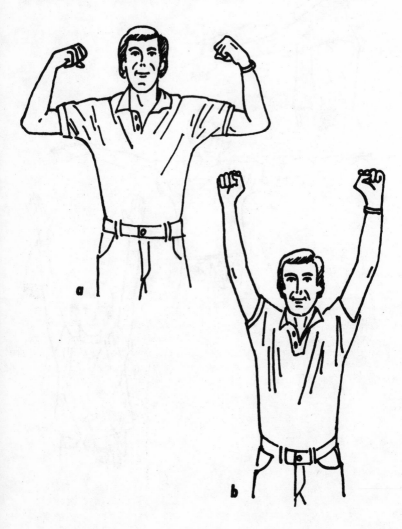

Crisscross (Illustrated)

With your arms in front, you may well be able to cross them at the elbows and perform a scissors-like motion the first time you try this exercise.

When you reach behind yourself, you'll find you get enough of a stretch by crossing your arms at your wrists.

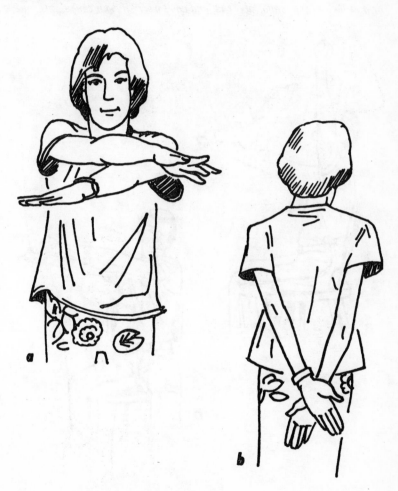

Straight Edge (Illustrated)

Try to keep your cane at shoulder height for maximum benefit as you go through these motions. (You may need to start at a lower height than shown in the illustration.)

If one of your shoulders is more restricted than the other, then just raise that arm as high as you comfortably can, and don't worry if your cane slants.

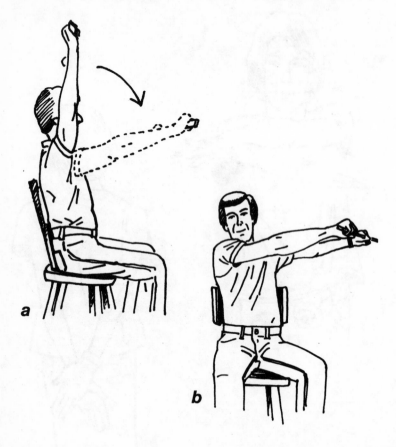

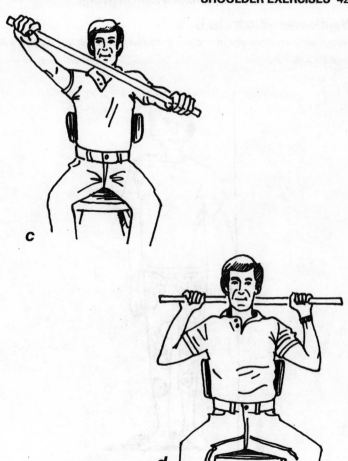

c

d

Wallflower (Illustrated)

Strengthen your arms, one at a time, by pushing hard against a wall in this isometric exercise.

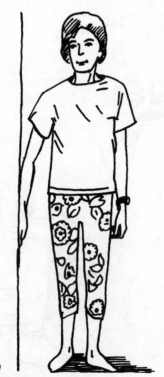

a

Pulley Pulls (Illustrated)

Work your arms alternately with this simple machine rig, so that each arm allows itself to be raised by the other. This is a shoulder exercise, not a hand exercise, so if you have pain in your hands, feel free to make loops at the ends of your rope and exert the pull force with your forearms.

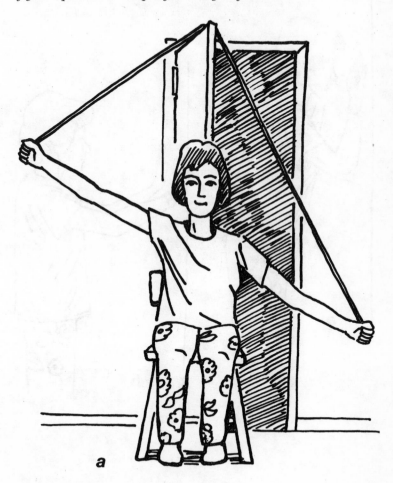

a

Push-Offs (Illustrated)

These stand-up push-ups are easier than the military kind. Nevertheless, they build up strength in the arms and shoulders.

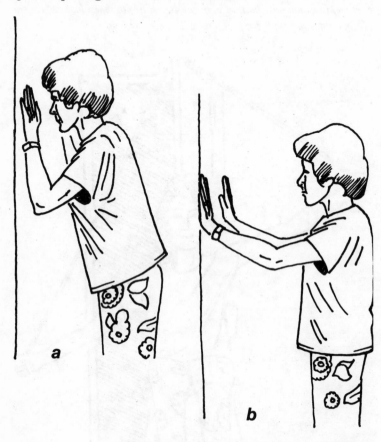

Fan Belt (Illustrated)

Working your arms against the resistance of an exercise belt or bungie cord can help build shoulder strength.

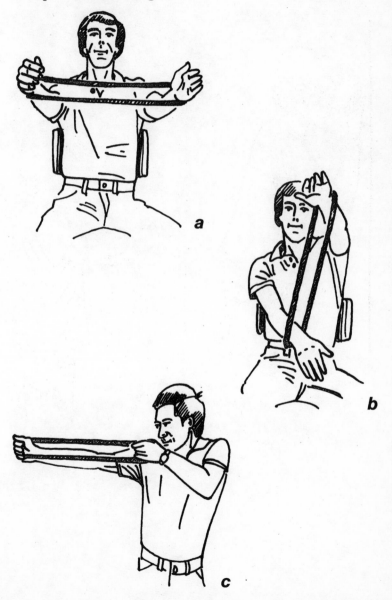

a

b

c

Chapter 32
Elbow Exercises

How to elbow your way into greater arm strength and range of motion

Many of the exercises recommended for shoulder stretching and strengthening also benefit the elbows, and vice versa. Although the exercises presented in this chapter differ from the shoulder movements in the previous chapter, both sets of exercises tend to benefit both sets of arm joints.

These descriptions call for exercising both elbows together, but of course you may work one elbow at a time if that's easier for you. Ordinary kitchen or living room furniture make ideal gym equipment for these exercises.

Elbow Macaroni
Type: Stretching
Starting position: You may sit in a straight-back chair or stand at ease, with your arms at your sides.
Steps:

1. Bend your elbow to bring your hand near your shoulder.
2. Move your hand away from your body, down and around to make a circle. Try to keep your upper arm and shoulder still. Return to starting position.
3. Bend your elbow again and circle your hand in the opposite direction, moving it toward your body and around.

Wing Tuck (See page 432)
Type: Stretching
Starting position: You may lie on your back, sit in a straight-back chair, or stand at ease, with your arms at your sides, palms facing in.
Steps:

1. Bend and raise your elbows until you can tuck your hands into your armpits. *a*

2. Flap your 'wings' down, catching your hands or thumbs under your arms. *b*
3. Raise your elbows again, then return to the starting position.

Elbow Limber-Up #1

Type: Very gentle stretching
Starting position: You may perform this exercise lying in bed, sitting in a straight-back chair, or standing at ease.
Steps:

1. Extend your arms straight out in front at shoulder height, palms facing each other.
2. Bend your elbows and touch your hands to your chest.
3. Reach straight out again.

Elbow Limber-Up #2

Steps:

1. Put your hands on your shoulders so that your elbows point out to the sides.
2. Open your arms, elbows straight, hands extended out as far as you can reach.
3. Return your hands to your shoulders.

Elbow Twist

Type: Stretching
Starting position: You may lie in bed, sit in a straight-back chair, or stand at ease.
Steps:

1. Extend your arms out to the sides, palms facing up.
2. Keeping your arms straight, twist your elbows so that your palms face down.

Chop Wood (See page 433)

Type: Stretching
Starting position: You may lie on your back or stand at ease.
Steps:

1. Clasp your hands and hold them close to your left shoulder, as though resting an axe there. *a*

2. Gently swing the axe by straightening your elbows and moving your hands toward your right thigh. *b*
3. Raise your clasped hands to your right shoulder, and swing the axe toward your left thigh.

Free Hand (See page 434)

Type: Stretching
Starting position: You may sit in a straight-back chair or stand at ease, arms at your sides.
Steps:

1. Bend and lift one elbow to shoulder height, leaving your hand dangling free, as though your elbow had been pulled up by a puppet string. (Remember to raise your *elbow*, not your shoulder.)
2. Make circles with your hand, moving your arm below the elbow, first toward the body, then away from the body.
3. Slowly straighten your elbow to return your hand to your side.
4. Repeat with your other elbow.

Elbow Builder

Type: Strengthening
Starting position: Sit in a straight-back chair at a heavy table or desk.
Steps:

1. Put your forearms under the table, with your elbows bent and palms up.
2. Push your forearms up as though trying to lift the table.
3. Hold for a moment, feeling the resistance, then relax.

Alternate Elbow Builder

Type: Strengthening
Starting position: You may sit or stand, with your arms at your sides.
Steps:

1. Cross your right forearm over your left, both palms facing up.
2. Press down with your right forearm and up with your left, without moving your arms in either direction.

3. Hold for a moment, feeling the resistance of one arm against the other.
4. Repeat with your left forearm over your right.

Wing Tuck (Illustrated)

Experiment to find the most comfortable way to tuck your hands under your arms — thumbs in or thumbs up. You can achieve the proper stretch either way.

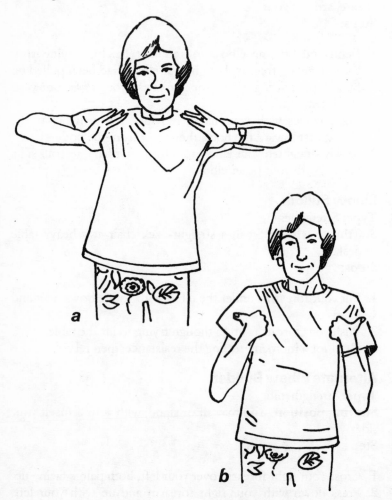

Chop Wood (Illustrated)

Since you're not really wielding an axe as you swing from shoulder to thigh, you needn't make these movements choppy or jerky. Just aim for maximum stretch.

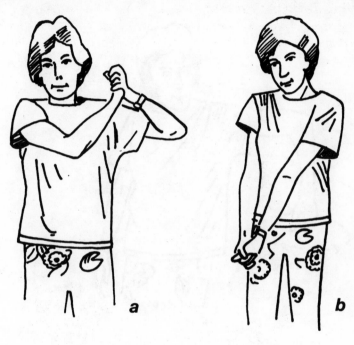

a

b

Free Hand (Illustrated)

Imagine you are a marionette and that the puppeteer has pulled up the string connected to your elbow. This leaves your hand dangling free and swinging in circles.

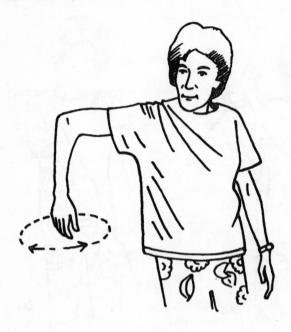

Chapter 33
Wrist Exercises

How to gain strength and flexibility from a twist of the wrist

Since most wrist exercises can be done from virtually any starting position – lying in bed, sitting in a chair, or standing at ease – we won't specify a position unless we have to. The only essential requirement is that you allow your wrists enough room to move.

In most cases, the choice is yours whether you wish to exercise both wrists together or work one at a time.

If you have severely affected wrists that have been set at a new angle by arthritis, please be careful to exercise *against* the drift only. Your goal is to regain lost ground.

Wrist Assist (See page 438)
Type: Very gentle stretching
Steps:

1. Using your left hand to help the right, gently bend your right wrist so that your right hand drops forward. *a*
2. Bend your right wrist the opposite way, so that your left hand is raised. *b*
3. Repeat the movements to exercise the left wrist.

Wrist Rotator (See page 439)
Type: Stretching
Steps:

1. Rest your forearm and hand on a flat surface. Rotate your wrist so that your hand slides in a clockwise direction as far as it can go. Try not to lift your fingers, or move your elbow, but just work your wrist. *a*
2. Hold for a moment, feeling the stretch, then rotate your wrist to make your hand slide counterclockwise. *b*

Wrist Twist

Type: Gentle stretching
Steps:

1. Rest your forearm and hand with your palm down on a flat surface. Twist your wrist so that your palm is turned toward the ceiling.
2. Twist back so that your palm rests on the flat surface.

Stop and Go

Type: Stretching
Steps:

1. Bend your wrist to raise your hand as though signalling 'Stop.'
2. Bend your wrist the other way so that your hand drops forward as far as it can go.

Note: For extra stretch, try the Stop and Go with your forearm resting on a flat surface, and your wrist at its edge. As you make each motion, use the other hand to push your wrist a little farther than it wants to go.

Swaying Palms

Type: Stretching and strengthening
Steps:

1. Clasp your hands in front.
2. Push your right palm against the left, bending the left wrist back.
3. Push your left palm against the right, bending the right wrist back.

Figure Eights

Type: Stretching
Starting position: You may rest your forearm on a flat surface, with your wrist extending free over the edge. Another way is to extend your arms, and pretend you are conducting an orchestra.

You can also let your arms hang at your sides, or bend them at the elbows.

Steps:

1. Trace a figure-eight pattern in the air with your hand, so that your wrist executes twists and turns through its full range of motion. Your fingers may assume any relaxed position you like. *a*
2. As you become comfortable with this exercise, exaggerate the motion by bending your wrist more sharply through these twists and turns.

Wrist Builder

Type: Stretching and strengthening
Steps:

1. Hold a light saucepan out as though trying to catch drips from a leak.
2. Using your wrist to make the motion, twist the saucepan over as though dumping it out.

Wrist Rise (See page 440)

Type: Strengthening
Steps:

1. Sitting at a table, reach your hand under it, with your palm facing the floor.
2. Press the back of your hand against the table, feeling the pressure in your wrist. *a*

Variation:

1. Put your left hand on the surface of the table, palm down.
2. With the heel of your right hand, push down on your left hand while simultaneously trying to raise the left hand against the pressure. *b* Here again, motion is not the goal; developing strength through isometric exercise is.
3. Repeat with the left hand over the right.

Praying Hands (See page 441)
Type: Strengthening
Steps:

1. Put the palms of your hands together as though in prayer, with your elbows out and wrists bent at right angles. *a*
2. Press your palms together, allowing no movement in either direction.
3. Hold, feeling the push in your wrists.

Wrist Assist (Illustrated)
Let one hand help the other to achieve this very gentle stretch of the wrists.

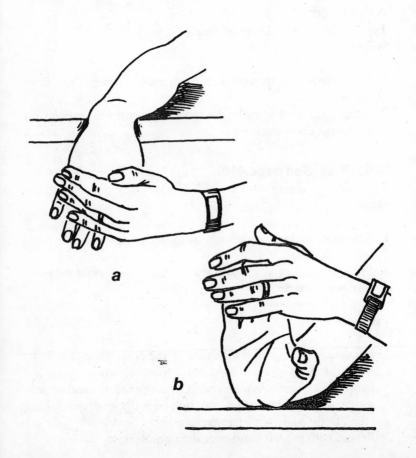

Wrist Rotator (Illustrated)

Slowly swivel each hand from side to side, swivelling your wrist. Your hand should move like a windscreen wiper on slow speed.

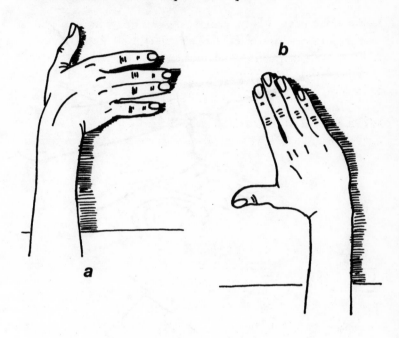

Figure Eights (Illustrated)

Trace the pattern of a figure eight in the air. The many twists and turns will put your wrists through their full range of motion.

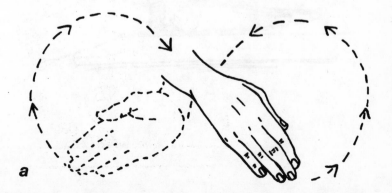

Wrist Rise (Illustrated)

Here's another way to strengthen your wrists by trying to lift each one against the opposing pressure of a table, or your other hand.

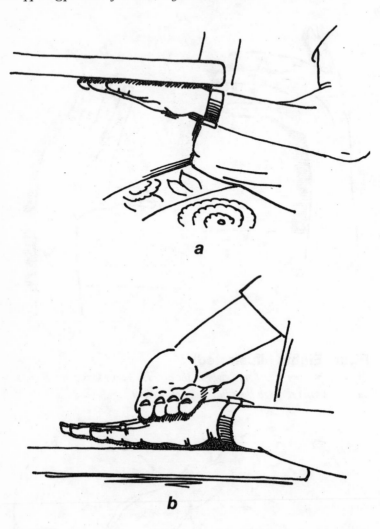

a

b

Praying Hands (Illustrated)

Although no movement is visible in this isometric exercise, the pressure of one hand against the other safely strengthens the wrists.

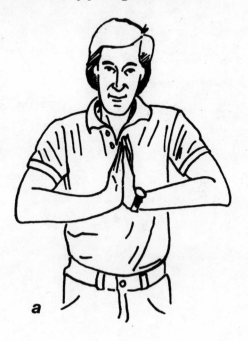

a

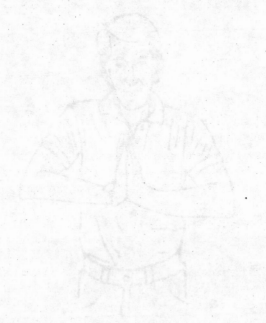

Chapter 34
Hand and Finger Exercises

*How to help prevent hand and finger deformities with exercises that preserve
your manual dexterity*

Hand and finger exercises can fit into the busiest schedule, virtually anywhere. Since they often involve fine movements that require effort and concentration, you may find that you prefer to exercise one hand at a time. Your hands are well worth the individual attention, as each one contains fifteen joints – not counting the wrist!

If you have rheumatoid arthritis, you may have one or another of the hand and finger deformities that frequently accompany this disease. The deformities may result from weakness in the muscles and ligaments that allow the joints to bend at odd angles. In ulnar deviation, for example, the fingers appear tilted sideways at the knuckles, and thus seem to slant away from the thumbs. If you have this condition, avoid any exercises that might aggravate the drift. Try to exercise in the opposite direction only, in an effort to correct the deformity.

The swan's neck and boutonniere deformities involve the joints closest to the fingertips and the middle joints of the fingers, freezing them in characteristic positions. In swan's neck, the fingertip bends down, following the normal direction of motion, but the middle joint bends up, as though broken. This gives the finger the appearance of a swan's arched neck. The boutonniere deformity is just the opposite: the fingertip bends up, while the middle joint bends down. Exercise can help prevent and sometimes even correct these deformities. For example, the Okay All Around and Typist's Warm-up exercises support normal motions of the fingers, and the Squeeze Play exercise strengthens the muscles, ligaments, and tendons of the hands.

People with osteoarthritis may develop excess bony growths in their finger joints. These are called Heberden's nodes when they occur at the joints nearest the fingertips, and Bouchard's nodes when they occur at the middle joints. The nodes may cause pain, swelling, or redness as they develop, but most discomfort soon subsides. In any case, the nodes need not limit hand function to any great extent. Regular exercise will make sure of that!

Many people find that exercise goes more swimmingly in water. All of the following movements can be done in a sink or basin of warm water. (You'll need to modify the Wall Walker a bit, by walking up the sides of the basin, and do the Finger Curls without raising your hand in greeting.) If you decide to immerse your hands, then arrange your exercise space so that you can keep the rest of your body comfortable while you give your hands a workout.

Finger Spread
Type: Gentle stretching
Steps:

1. With your palm resting on a flat surface, spread your fingers as widely apart as possible.
2. Slowly draw your fingers together again, still keeping your palm flat.

Typist's Warm-Up
Type: Full stretching
Steps:

1. Make fists of both hands.
2. Relax your hands.
3. Wiggle your fingers up and down.
4. Circle your wrists.
5. Rub your hands together, as though you were rubbing lotion on them.

Finger Lifts
Type: Stretching
Steps:

1. With your hand resting on a flat surface, lift your thumb as high as you can and then rest it.

2. Lift your index finger as high as you can, without raising any of the other fingers, and then rest it.
3. Lift your middle finger in turn, then rest it.
4. This is the hardest part for most people: lift your ring finger as high as you can, and then rest it.
5. Lift your little finger, then rest it.

Okay All Around (See page 448)
Type: Gentle stretching
Steps:

1. Make the 'okay' sign by joining the tips of your index finger and thumb. Hold for a few seconds, keeping your other fingers as straight as you comfortably can. *a*
2. Straighten your index finger and join the tip of your middle finger to your thumb. *b*
3. After straightening your middle finger, join your ring finger and thumb. *c*
4. In the same fashion, touch the tip of your little finger to your thumb. *d*

Note: You can add strengthening to the stretch of this exercise by pressing your fingertips lightly together for a few seconds each time you join your thumb to another finger. Since the joints don't move with the pressure, this is an isometric exercise.

Finger Push-Ups
Type: Strengthening
Steps: Follow the same steps as for Finger Lifts above, but move each finger against pressure. You can do this by sliding your hand under your buttocks in bed, by pushing against the underside of a desk or table, or by exerting counterpressure with your other hand.

Wall Walker (See page 450)
Type: Stretching
Starting position: You may stand or sit about two feet away from a wall, with your left side to the wall, arms at your sides.

Steps:

1. Let your left hand slowly 'walk' up the wall, as though your fingers were the legs of an insect. *a*
2. 'Walk' above shoulder level if you can, but try not to raise your shoulder or lean away from the wall. 'Let your fingers do the walking.' *b*
3. Turn and 'walk' your right hand.

Note: This exercise is also included in the Shoulder section, as it benefits those joints as well.

Finger Slides (See page 451)
Type: Stretching
Steps:

1. With your hand resting on a flat surface, slide your index finger as far as it will go toward your thumb.
2. Still keeping your hand flat, move the middle finger to meet your index finger. *a*
3. Slide the ring finger over, too. *b*
4. Your little finger has no doubt followed the movement of your other fingers. Let it go the rest of the way now. *c*
5. Beginning with the little finger, slide your fingers one by one away from your thumb. *d*

Thumb Wrestle (See page 453)
Type: Stretching
Steps:

1. With your hand open and fingers straight, extend your thumb away from your other fingers as far as you can. *a*
2. Move your thumb forward so it is perpendicular to your palm. *b*
3. Reach your thumb across your palm and try to touch your little finger. *c*
4. Circle your thumb in the opposite direction.

Finger Curls (See page 454)
Type: Difficult stretching

Steps:

1. Hold your hand up, as though greeting someone, with your fingers as straight as possible.
2. Slowly curl the index finger by bending the joint nearest the fingertip *a*, then the middle joint *b*, until the tip of your index finger touches the uppermost part of your palm. You may move the finger with your other hand, if need be.
3. Uncurl your index finger.
4. Attempt the same manoeuvres with the middle finger.
5. Curl and uncurl the ring finger the same way.
6. Curl and uncurl the little finger.
7. Moving all four fingers simultaneously, curl and uncurl them.

Finger Skids (See page 454)
Type: Strengthening
Steps:
Follow the same steps you did for Finger Slides, but use the tip of your index finger to resist, for a few seconds, the movement of each finger.

Note: Since the tendency in rheumatoid arthritis is for the fingers to slant away from the thumb, it's best to perform this strengthening exercise *toward* the thumb.

Squeeze Play
Type: Strengthening
Steps:

1. Squeeze and work a small rubber ball or therapeutic putty in each hand.

Finger Straighteners
Type: Corrective (The goal of this exercise is to help straighten fingers affected by swan's neck and boutonniere deformities.)
Steps:

1. Rest your left hand, palm down, on a table top.
2. Flatten your hand and fingers as much as you can.

3. Using the heel of your right hand to exert pressure, gently push the left finger joints flat.
4. Repeat the steps for flattening with your right hand.

Okay All Around
Stretch all your fingers with these variations on the 'okay' theme. Make the 'okay' sign with each one in turn.

Strengthen your fingers, too, by pressing the thumb and each finger together with a little extra pressure.

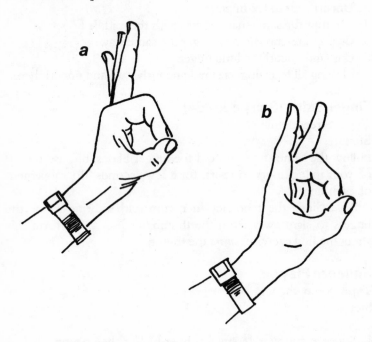

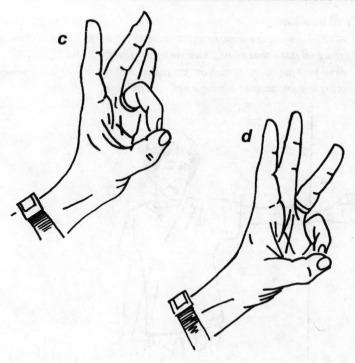

Wall Walker

Walk your fingers up a wall, letting them do all the work. Think of them as a five-legged insect that found its way into your house.

Send your fingers up as high as they can go, without raising your shoulder to help them and without leaning away from the wall.

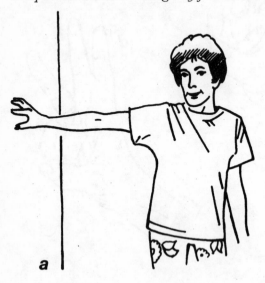

a

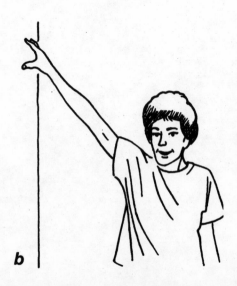

b

Finger Slides

It takes control and concentration to stretch your fingers by moving each one individually in this fashion. The real challenge comes in holding the rest still while one moves.

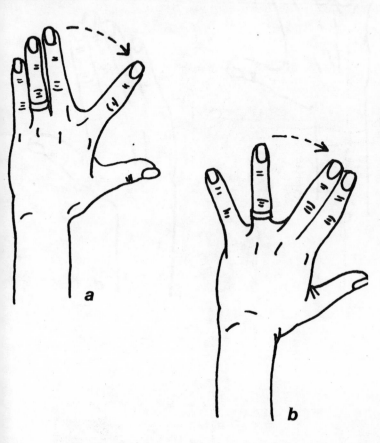

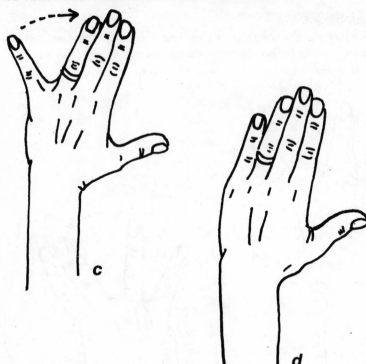

Thumb Wrestle

Put your thumbs through their full range of motion by acting out this prelude to a thumb-wrestling match.

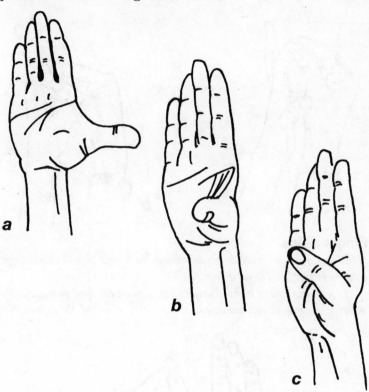

Finger Curls

One joint at a time, bend and then straighten each finger. You'll definitely need the help of the opposite hand to accomplish this unusual movement.

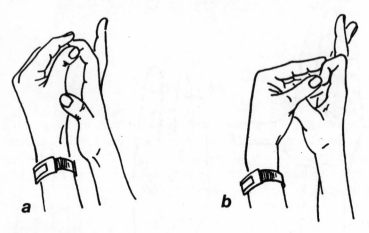

a   b

Finger Skids

By adding resistance from the opposite hand, the Finger Slide stretch changes into the Finger Skid strengthener.

If your hands are turned outward, as is often the case in rheumatoid arthritis, exercise in only one direction — against the drift of the deformity.

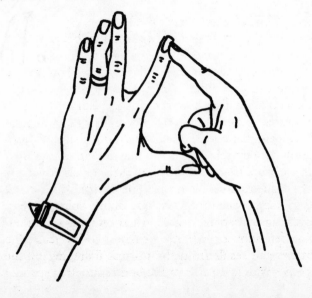

Chapter 35
Back Exercises

How to exercise away back pain by stretching and strengthening your abdominal muscles

The exercises in this section are called back exercises, but as you'll see, the place you really feel them is in your gut. Performing them faithfully will stretch and strengthen the abdominal muscles you need to maintain good posture and a normal level of activity. As a bonus, you'll probably wind up with a flatter tummy.

We recommend the starred exercises as an essential part of every exercise regimen. Even if you feel no pain or stiffness in your back, you will no doubt find that these manoeuvres increase your general muscle tone and flexibility. They will also help keep back pain at bay.

Probably the most common, serious mistake people make with regard to back exercise is attempting sit-ups with the legs straight. This position is risky for the back. You can achieve the same good effects – better effects, in fact, because you won't be using your hip muscles as much – by keeping your knees bent as you sit up and lie back down. Another approach, as you'll see, is to reverse the usual order by performing Sit-downs instead of Sit-ups.

Anyone can have back pain, with or without arthritis. Even people who know they have arthritis may suffer back pain from other causes. Given this possibility, get prompt treatment for any back pain that comes on suddenly and sharply. This is likely the result of a muscle strain, and may require a couple of days' rest to clear up. If the pain in your back travels down your legs, it may be due to a problem with one of your discs – the cushioning tissue between the vertebrae of the spine. Bulging discs can press against spinal nerves, often bringing on a tingling or burning sensation or extreme weakness in the legs. The same symptoms can result from the normal flattening of the discs that comes with age, or from the bone spurs that sprout on the vertebrae as a result of osteoarthritis. Check with your doctor. Whatever the cause of the discomfort, exercise – especially gentle stretching and strengthening – invariably plays a role in any back-pain treatment plan.

Knee To Chest (*) (See page 460)

Type: Stretching
Starting position: Lie on your back, knees bent and feet flat, arms relaxed at your sides.
Steps:

1. Lift your right knee toward your chest as far as you can. *a*
2. Lower knee to and through starting position, so your right leg is extended straight on the bed (or floor). *b*
3. Wobble your leg to relax the muscles.
4. Return to starting position.
5. Repeat for your left leg.

Advanced addition: If you can move your knee easily toward your chest, try pulling it with your hands to bring it still closer.

Pelvic Tilt (*)

Type: Stretching and strengthening
Starting position: Lie on your back with your knees bent so you can keep your feet flat. Leave your arms relaxed at your sides.
Steps:

1. Tighten your buttocks and pull in your abdominal muscles. Exhale as you do this. The movement will cave in your abdomen and flatten out the curve in your lower back.
2. Relax your muscles as you inhale.

Knee to Chest Rock (See page 461)

Type: Stretching
Starting position: Lie on your back, knees bent and feet flat, with your arms at your sides.
Steps:

1. Pull both knees to your chest, one at a time, and hold them in this position. *a*

2. Curl your head and shoulders forward and gently rock from side to side in this position for a few seconds. *b*

Simplified version: If you can't bring your knees very close to your chest, raise them as high as you can and grasp the backs of your thighs with your hands, instead of trying to clasp your knees in your arms. *a*

   Advanced addition: Bring both knees up together and clasp your arms around them. *b*

Knee Drops (See page 462)
Type: Stretching
Starting position: Lie on your back with your knees bent and feet flat.
Steps:

1. Keeping your knees together, drop both of them to the left as far as you can. Try to keep both shoulders touching the bed (floor) as you do this. Your right hip and buttock will necessarily rise off the floor as your knees drop to the left. *a*
2. Return to the starting position.
3. Drop both knees to the right.

Bent-Knee Sit-Ups (See page 462)
Type: Stretching and strengthening
Starting position: Lie on your back, knees bent and feet flat, arms relaxed at your sides.
Steps:

1. Exhaling, pull in your abdominals and raise the upper part of your body toward your knees. You need not come very far up (just far enough to see your navel), and you may lead with your outstretched arms. *a*
2. Hold the position, but don't hold your breath, for a few seconds. Be conscious of breathing in and out.
3. Inhaling, relax your muscles slowly as you lower your head and shoulders.

Advanced addition: Instead of leading with your arms, try doing this exercise with your arms folded across your chest.

Sit-Downs (See page 463)

Type: Stretching and strengthening
Starting position: You may sit on an exercise bench or the edge of your bed. Fold your arms across your chest, or extend them out in front of you.
Steps:

1. Exhaling, use your abdominal muscles to lean your body backward several inches – about as far as you lift up for a sit-up. (As you advance, you may be able to lean farther back.) *a*
2. Hold the position, but don't hold your breath, for a count of three. Be conscious of breathing in and out.
3. Inhaling, return to a straight sitting posture and relax your muscles.

Cat Stretch (See page 463)

Type: Full stretching
Starting position: Get down on the floor on all fours with your back flat and your weight evenly distributed. *a*
Steps:

1. Slide your hands forward, letting your elbows bend and touch the floor. *b*
2. Lower your head and raise your rear end.
3. Smoothly sink back on your haunches, so that you are almost sitting on your ankles. (Your elbows will straighten out as you do this step.) *c*
4. Return to the starting position. *d*
5. Drop your head and pull in your abdominals to curve your back like a Halloween cat. *e*
6. Relax your muscles and roll your head back. *f*

Roller Blades

Type: Stretching
Starting position: You may stand in a comfortable position or sit on the edge of a chair. (Steps 1 and 2 may also be done while lying down.)

Steps:

1. Squeeze your shoulders together for a few seconds in an effort to make your shoulder blades meet in the middle of your back.
2. Relax.
3. Again, try to make your shoulder blades meet, this time by pushing your elbows together behind you.

Twists and Turns (See page 466)
Type: Stretching
Starting position: Sit in a straight-back chair or stand at ease.
Steps:

1. Rest your hands on your hips and lean the top of your body to the left. Try not to bend forward as you do this. Also, try to keep your feet, legs, and hips steady. *a*
2. Straighten up slowly.
3. Repeat these motions to the right.
4. Twist the upper half of your body to the left, as though trying to see behind you. Keep your lower body still. *b*
5. Return to face front.
6. Repeat these motions to the right.

Back against the Wall
Type: Strengthening
Starting position: You may sit in a straight-back chair, or on the floor with your back literally against the wall.
Steps:

1. Exhale as you press the upper part of your back against the chair back or wall – as though you could push your shoulder blades through it.
2. Hold the position without holding your breath.
3. Inhale as you relax.

Knee to Chest (Illustrated)

Pulling the knee to the chest gives the lower back a gentle stretch. You'll feel the curve in your lower back straighten out as you do this.

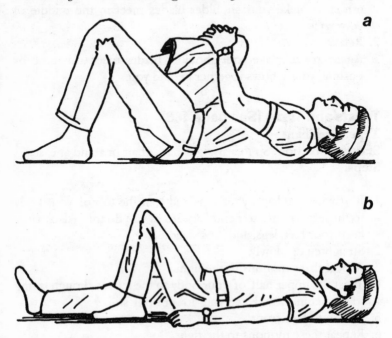

Knee to Chest Rock (Illustrated)

Depending on your degree of flexibility, you can achieve this rocking motion by grasping your legs at different places.

If you are new to exercise, make this easy on yourself by grasping the backs of your thighs; that's the easiest way. Holding your knees in the intermediate position, while clasping your arms around both knees gives the greatest stretch and is the most difficult way to approach this exercise.

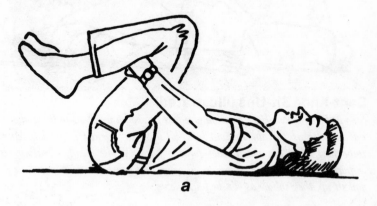

a

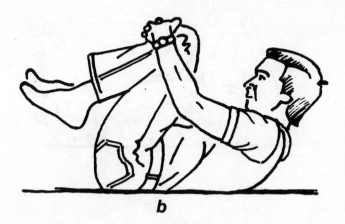

b

Knee Drops (Illustrated)

Try to keep both your shoulders on the bed (or floor) as you drop your knees first to one side, then the other. If you can't get your knees all the way down, don't worry. You'll build up to that in time.

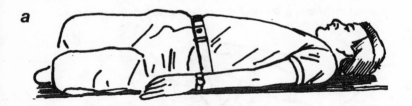

Bent-Knee Sit-Ups (Illustrated)

Sit-ups from a bent-knee position give just as good a workout to the abdominal muscles as the old straight-knee sit-ups you learned in school. More important, they are much safer for the back. While steady breathing is important during any exercise, you'll get a real boost here if you exhale as you sit up, then inhale as you lie back down.

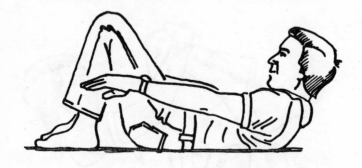

Sit-Downs (Illustrated)

These reverse sit-ups provide yet another way to stretch and strengthen the abdominals.

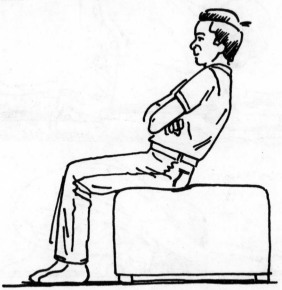

Cat Stretch (Illustrated)

The several steps of this exercise mimic the motions cats make with their supple spines as they awaken from one of their famed catnaps.

The completed series gives you a full yet gentle stretch in all directions.

a

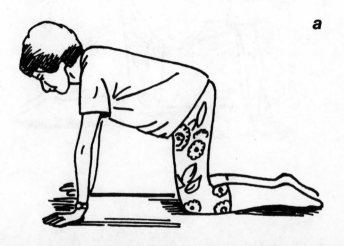

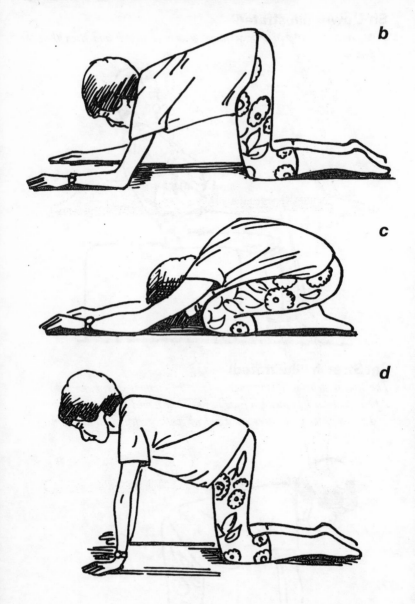

b

c

d

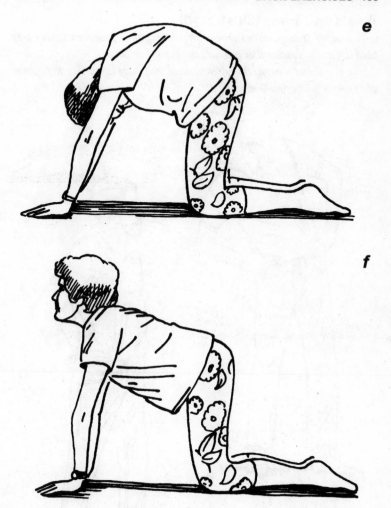

e

f

Twists and Turns (Illustrated)

Give yourself a maximum sideways stretch with these manoeuvres. Try very hard not to bend forward as you lean to the right or left.

For the second part of this stretch, twist your body to the side to find out what's going on behind you.

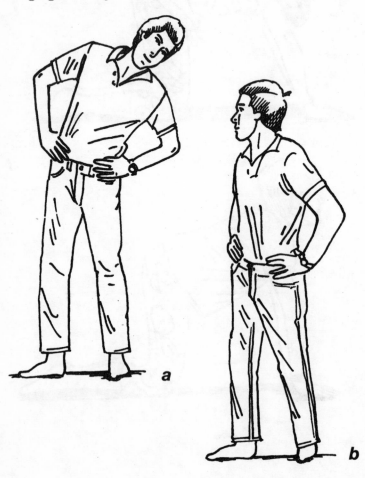

Chapter 36
Hip Exercises

How to perform effective hip exercises standing, sitting, or lying down – even in the pool

The hips boast a wide range of normal motion that enables us to do everything from walk forward to slide sideways on a bench – not to mention pedal backwards on a bicycle and bend down to tie a shoelace. Individual exercises stretch and strengthen different muscles that control the hips. In your exercise program, you will want to incorporate at least one exercise for each type and direction of hip motion. For example, a beginner's program might include the Leg Spread, the Straight Leg-ups, the Simple Knee Cross, and the Liftback. Each one emphasizes a different movement.

Many exercises for the back also benefit the hips, such as the Knee to Chest. Sometimes, people with low back pain have trouble attempting certain hip exercises, and need another way to accomplish the same stretch. For example, the Simple Knee Cross is a variation of the Knee Cross intended specifically for people suffering from back pain.

Leg Spread
Type: Stretching
Starting position: Lie on your back with your legs out straight.
Steps:

1. Spread your legs as far apart as you can to give your hips a sideways stretch.
2. Bring your legs back together.

Caution: If you have back pain, move one leg at a time, keeping the inactive leg bent at the knee.

Advanced addition: Lift your legs slightly before spreading them, so they glide through the air instead of sliding on the bed (or floor).

Note: You can turn this stretch into a strengthening exercise by looping an exercise belt over your ankles, calves, or thighs and then spreading your legs against the resistance of the belt.

Leg Roll (See page 474)
Type: Stretching
Starting position: Lie on your back, with your right knee bent and your left leg straight.
Steps:

1. Flex your left foot so that your toes point to the ceiling.
2. Rotate your left leg counterclockwise so that your toes point to the side, away from your body. (Feel the twist in your hip.) *a*
3. Rotate your left leg in the opposite direction, pointing your toes toward the ceiling again, and then toward your right side. *b*
4. Relax your left foot.
5. Switch position so your right leg is extended and your left leg is bent at the knee.
6. Repeat the rotation movements with your right leg.

Straight Leg-Ups
Type: Stretching and strengthening
Starting position: Lie on your back, with your knees bent and feet flat, arms relaxed at your sides.
Steps:

1. Straighten your right leg so it lies flat.
2. Lift your right leg, keeping your knee straight, as high as you can.
3. Lower your leg slowly.
4. Bend your knee to return to the starting position.
5. Repeat the movements with your left leg.

Simple Knee Cross (See page 475)
Type: Stretching
Starting position: Lie on your left side, with your legs extended.
Steps:

1. Bend your right knee and pull it up toward your body so that your right foot is near your left knee. *a*

2. Press your right knee across your left leg, down toward the floor (or bed). *b*
3. Raise your right knee toward the ceiling, keeping your right foot on your left knee. *c*
4. Return to the starting position.
5. Turn to your right side and repeat the movement with your left leg.

Knee Cross (See page 476)

Type: Stretching
Starting position: Lie on your back, with your knees bent and feet flat, arms relaxed at your sides.
Steps:

1. Cross your left thigh over the right. *a*
2. Press your legs together and tip your knees toward the left side as far as you can. (Your right hip will naturally rise as you do this.) *b*
3. Raise your knees and return to the starting position.
4. Repeat with your right thigh over the left, tipping toward the right.

Lateral Leg-Ups (See page 477)

Type: Strengthening
Starting position: Lie on your right side, with your legs straight. Prop your left hand in front of your body for support.
Steps:

1. Lift your left leg as high as you can, keeping it straight. *a*
2. Hold it at the height you reached for several seconds.
3. Lower it gently.
4. Repeat.
5. Turn over and repeat the movement with your right leg.

Forced March

Type: Stretching
Starting position: Stand in a comfortable position. You may use the back of a chair to lean on for support if need be.

Steps:

1. Bend and raise your left knee as high as you can, as though you were taking a step in an exaggerated military march.
2. Lower your left knee so your foot is on the floor where it started. (No need to march forward.)
3. Repeat the movement with your right knee.

Note: This exercise appears in the Knee section, as it benefits those joints as well.

Cancan (See page 478)
Type: Stretching
Starting position: Stand comfortably, giving yourself a chair or other sturdy support to lean on.
Steps:

1. Bend and raise your left knee – to hip level, if you can.
2. With your dangling left foot, make small clockwise circles in the air. (Though your knee may appear to circle, it's really your hip that facilitates the motions.) *a*
3. Make counterclockwise circles with your left foot.
4. Return to the starting position.
5. Repeat the movements with your right knee and foot.

Note: This exercise also appears in the Knee section, as it benefits those joints as well.

Hula Hoop
Type: Stretching
Starting position: Stand in a comfortable position.
Steps:

1. Slowly and gently, swivel your hips in circles to the left, as though you were trying to twirl a hula hoop.
2. Swivel your hips to the right.

Lift Backs
Type: Stretching

Starting position: You may lie face down or stand facing a chair that you can lean on for support. The standing position works better for people with back pain.
Steps:

1. Raise your right leg behind you as far as you can.
2. Lower your right leg.
3. Repeat with the left leg.

Note: If you stand during this exercise, make sure to lean your upper body forward to avoid arching your back.

Leg Lifts
Type: Stretching
Starting position: Stand to the side of a chair that you can lean on for support.
Steps:

1. Raise your left leg straight out in front of you.
2. Lower your left leg.
3. Repeat with the right leg.
4. Turn to face the chair support.
5. Lift your left leg out to the side and then lower it.
6. Lift and then lower your right leg out to the side.

Swordplay (See page 479)
Type: Stretching
Starting position: Stand facing the back of a chair, with both your hands on it for support.
Steps:

1. Move your right foot far to the side and put your weight on it. Bend your right knee as far as you can, keeping your left leg straight. *a*
2. Hold for a few seconds to feel the stretch.
3. Return to the starting position.
4. Make the same sort of fencer's lunge to the left side, keeping your right leg straight.

Hip Walkout

Type: Stretching and strengthening
Starting position: Stand where you have room to walk.
Steps:

1. Walk a few steps.
2. Turn out your feet, as Charlie Chaplin used to do, and walk a bit more.
3. Turn your feet towards each other, pigeon-toed, and walk on.

The Squeeze

Type: Strengthening
Starting position: You may do this exercise lying down, sitting, or standing.
Steps:

1. Squeeze your buttocks together as tightly as you can.
2. Hold for a moment, then release, and relax.

Hip Strengthener

Type: Strengthening
Starting position: Stand with a wall a few inches from your left side and a support chair to your right.
Steps:

1. Raise your left leg to the side, so that your leg is fully pressed against the wall.
2. Keep pushing your left leg against the wall's resistance.
3. Relax and return to the starting position.
4. Turn and repeat the motion with your right leg.

If you have access to a warm swimming pool or a large hot tub, you can incorporate the following water exercises into your regimen of hip exercises.

Scissor Kick

Type: Stretching
Starting position: Sit on the pool steps or the hot tub bench with both legs extended straight out in front.

Steps:

1. Spread your legs as far apart as you can.
2. Bring your legs together and scissor-cross them left over right.
3. Spread them far apart again.
4. Make a scissor-cross with your right leg over your left.

Flutter Kick
Type: Strengthening
Starting position: Face the side of the pool and hold on to it.
Steps:

1. Raise your legs behind you.
2. Slowly kick your legs up and down as though you were swimming.

Leg Circles
Type: Stretching and strengthening
Starting position: Stand in the water, with your left arm out to the side, holding the edge of the pool.
Steps:

1. Raise your right leg, and make a large, slow clockwise circle.
2. Still using your right leg, complete a large, slow, counterclockwise circle.
3. Turn and repeat the circles with your left leg.

Jumping Jacks
Type: Strengthening
Starting position: Stand in the water with your hands on your hips.
Steps:

1. Letting the water help buoy you, jump into a legs-apart position.
2. Jump and bring your feet together again.

Leg Roll (illustrated)

Make your hip do the work of rotating your leg first out, then in. Think of it as a log roll.

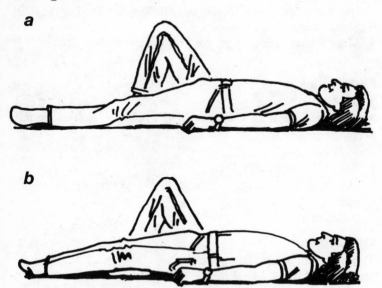

Simple Knee Cross (illustrated)

One knee crosses the other in this manoeuvre, but the hips do most of the work and get most of the stretch.

As you raise and lower your knee, picture the gentle motion of a butterfly's wing.

a

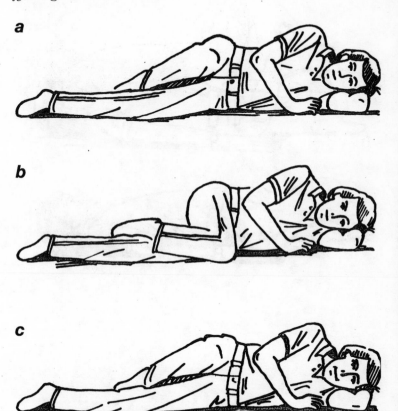

b

c

Knee Cross (illustrated)

This is a more difficult way to cross the knees — and stretch the hips. Remember, you can't be expected to make a touch-down the first time you try this.

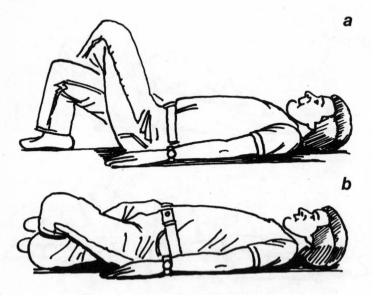

Lateral Leg-Ups (illustrated)

Raising your legs straight up from the side builds hip strength. Lift each as far as you comfortably can. To keep your balance as you go through this exercise, prop your upper hand in front of you.

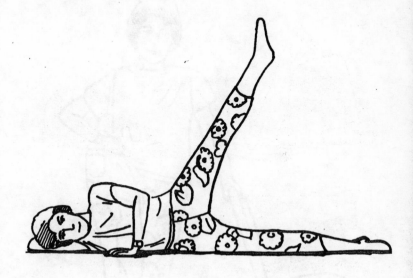

Cancan (illustrated)

Circle your raised foot in clockwise, then counterclockwise circles in the air — as those famed chorus lines of dancers did.

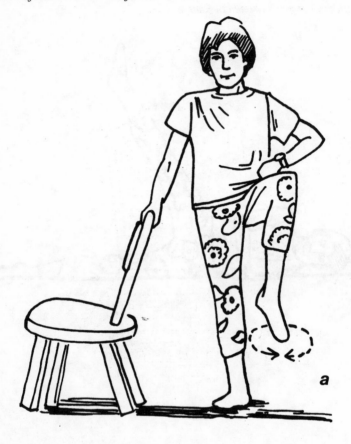

a

Swordplay (illustrated)

The stretch in this exercise comes from bending one leg and extending the other as though fighting a duel with make-believe swords. You need not make a sudden lunge to reap the benefits.

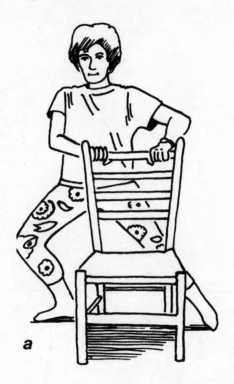

a

Chapter 37
Knee Exercises

How to bend and straighten the weight-bearing joints of the knees to best advantage

When functioning properly, the knees support us through a remarkable number of daily activities, absorbing the shock of walking and stair-climbing. Unfortunately, the hinge joints of the knees also are common targets for both osteoarthritis and rheumatoid arthritis.

Exercising the muscles that control the knee's opening and closing movements is the best way to maintain function and flexibility. You'll notice that many of the exercises in this section concentrate on perfecting the knee's ability to straighten all the way. It's easy to understand the importance of these manoeuvres when you remember that the knee becomes unevenly stressed if it tries to do everything from a half-bent position, and such stress eventually leads to further damage.

Some of the exercises in this section have been borrowed from the chapters on back and hip exercises, but most are specifically designed to straighten, stretch, and strengthen the knees, which you may work singly or together.

Knee to Chest Plus (See page 486)
Type: Stretching
Starting position: Lie on your back, knees bent and feet flat, arms relaxed at your sides.
Steps:

1. Lift your right knee toward your chest as far as you can. *a*
2. Lower your knee to and through the starting position, so your right leg is extended straight on the bed (or floor). *b*
3. Wobble your leg to relax the muscles.
4. Return to the starting position by bending your knee and sliding your foot back toward your body.

5. Continue sliding your foot back, bringing it as close to your buttocks as you can. (You may pull your foot with your hand.) Hold this position briefly. *c*
6. Return to the starting position.
7. Repeat for your left leg.

Advanced addition: If you can move your knee easily toward your chest, try pulling it with your hands to bring it still closer.

Knee Push
Type: Stretching
Starting position: Lie on your back, with your knees bent.
Steps:

1. Straighten your left leg so it rests full length on the floor (or bed).
2. Try to straighten your left knee even beyond straight – as though you could push it to bend the wrong way.
3. Return to the starting position.
4. Repeat the movement with your right leg.

Knee Press
Type: Stretching and strengthening
Starting position: Lie on your back with your legs extended.
Steps:

1. Press your heels into the mattress (or floor mat), keeping your knees straight.
2. Turn over and press your toes into the mattress, keeping your knees straight.

Precaution for people with back pain: When lying on your back, press one heel at a time, and keep the resting leg bent at the knee.

When lying face down, put a small pillow under your abdomen as a support for your lower back.

Knee Kicks (See page 487)
Type: Stretching
Starting position: Lie on your back with your knees bent and your feet flat.

Steps:

1. Bring your left knee toward your chest as you flex your left foot. *a*
2. Straighten your left knee and move your foot as straight upward as you can, so that the sole of your left foot faces the ceiling. Hold this position briefly, feeling the stretch. *b*
3. Bend your left knee again, near your chest. *c*
4. Straighten your left knee in an outward motion this time, as though trying to kick something away from you. *d*
5. Bend your left knee. *e*
6. Straighten your left knee once more, close to the floor. *f*
7. Repeat these movements with your right knee.

Forced March

Type: Stretching
Starting position: Stand in a comfortable position. You may use the back of a chair to lean on for support if need be.
Steps:

1. Bend and raise your left knee as high as you can, as though you were taking a step in an exaggerated military march.
2. Lower your left knee so your foot is on the floor where it started. (No need to march forward.)
3. Repeat the movement with your right knee.

Note: This exercise also appears in the section on Hips, as it benefits those joints as well.

Ballet Bends (See page 489)

Type: Strengthening
Starting position: Stand comfortably with your feet apart. You may use the back of a chair for support, or simply place your hands on your hips.
Steps:

1. With your feet a comfortable distance apart and turned outward, bend your knees. Try to keep your back straight and your knees over your toes. *a*

2. Straighten your knees to lift your body back to the starting position.
3. Turn your feet so that they are parallel to each other, but still a comfortable distance apart. *b*
4. Bend and straighten your knees as before. Remember to keep your back straight and your knees pointing directly over your toes.

Chair Bend (See pge 490)

Type: Stretching and strengthening
Starting position: Sit in a straight-back chair.
Steps:

1. Bend your left knee as far as you can, so that your foot moves under the chair.
2. Return to the starting position.
3. Repeat the movement with the right leg.

Cancan

Type: Stretching
Starting position: Stand comfortably, giving yourself a chair or other sturdy support to lean on.
Steps:

1. Bend and raise your left knee.
2. With your dangling left foot, make small clockwise circles in the air.
3. Make counterclockwise circles with your left foot.
4. Return to the starting position.
5. Repeat the movements with your right knee and foot.

Note: This exercise also appears in the section on Hips, as it benefits those joints as well.

Chair Lift (See page 491)

Type: Stretching and strengthening
Starting position: Sit in a straight-back chair with your feet flat on the floor.

Steps:

1. Lift your left foot out in front until your left knee is straight.
2. Slowly lower your left foot.
3. Repeat the movement with your right foot.

Advanced addition: Position your chair in front of a coffee table or a footstool. When you extend your leg, rest your foot on this support. Straighten your knee as much as you can. Then, for added stretch, lean slightly forward from your waist, keeping your back straight. You will feel the stretch in the backs of your thighs – your hamstring muscles.

Sack Race (See page 492)
Type: Strengthening
Starting position: Sit in a straight-backed chair with an exercise belt looped around your ankles.
Steps:

1. Extend your left leg forward and your right leg back, pushing and pulling against the resistance of the belt.
2. Relax.
3. Reverse, so that you extend your right leg forward and pull your left leg back.

Dig Your Heels In
Type: Strengthening
Starting position: Sit in a straight-backed chair with your feet on the floor and the backs of your heels touching the front legs of the chair.
Steps:

1. Push back with your left foot as hard as you can, feeling the driving force in your knee.
2. Relax.
3. Repeat with the right foot.

Knee To Chest Plus (Illustrated)

Knee workouts are all about bending and straightening. This extra step in the basic Knee to Chest exercise – bringing the heel right up to the buttock – adds a good knee bend to an otherwise excellent back stretch.

a

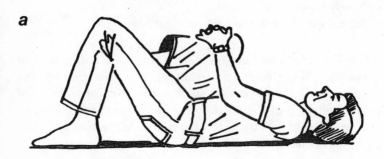

b

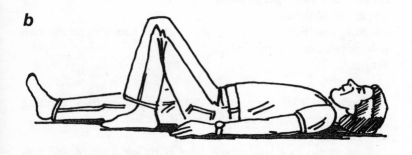

c

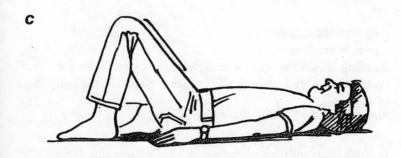

Knee Kicks (Illustrated)

Bending and straightening the knee at varying heights gives it a full stretch.

You'll feel the pull in the big quadriceps muscle that runs through each thigh.

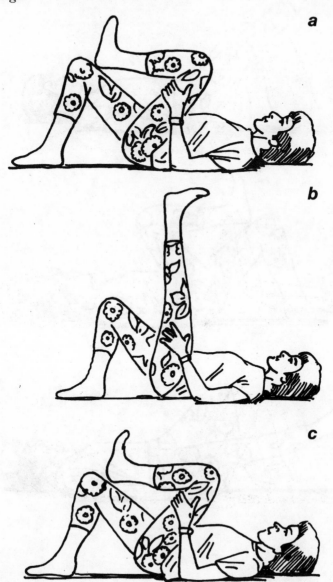

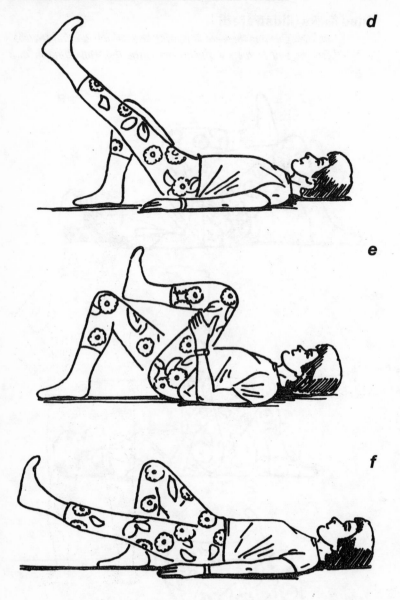

Ballet Bends (Illustrated)

These dancer's knee-bends are called pliés when done at the ballet barre. As you attempt them, remember to keep your knees directly over your toes.

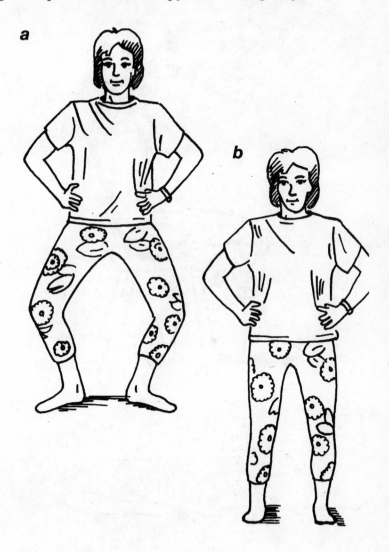

Chair Bend (Illustrated)

Strengthen your knees by bending each one individually, as far as you can, so that you bring your foot up under you as you sit in a chair.

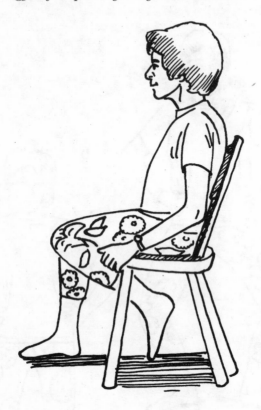

Chair Lift (Illustrated)

You can stretch and strengthen your knee by extending your leg straight out from a sitting position. Get the most extension you can, to keep your knee functioning at its best. For extra benefit, set your foot on a stool or coffee table. Then straighten your knee as much as you can and try to lean forward slightly.

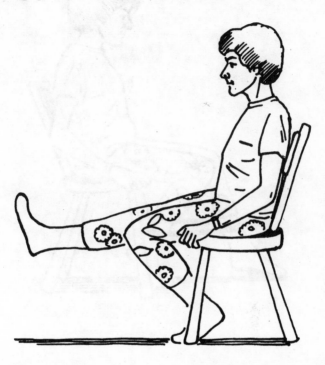

Sack Race (Illustrated)

An exercise belt or bungie cord will help strengthen your knees as you provide resistance by working one leg against the other.

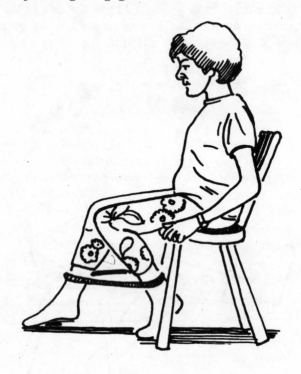

Chapter 38
Exercises for the Ankles and Feet

How to use exercise to keep you on your toes

Bearing the full weight of the body, the large and small joints of the feet need exercise and comfortable shoes to keep them functioning well. Stretching and strengthening will also bolster the tendons and ligaments, making them less likely to succumb to sprains and other injuries.

These exercises include some fancy footwork from soft-shoe dance routines – that can be done while sitting down.

Ankle Twist (See page 497)
Type: Stretching
Starting position: Lie on your back with your legs extended and slightly apart.
Steps:

1. Rotate your ankles so that your feet point in, toward each other. Hold this position briefly. *a*
2. Rotate your ankles in the opposite direction, pointing your feet out. Hold briefly. *b*

Foot Circles
Type: Stretching
Starting position: You may lie in bed with one foot hanging free over the edge of the mattress, or sit in a straight-back chair, raising one leg at a time to give each foot full freedom of movement.
Steps:

1. Circle your left foot in a clockwise direction.
2. Circle your left foot in a counterclockwise direction.

3. Repeat these movements with your right foot.

Toe Curls
Type: Stretching
Starting position: You may lie down or sit in a straight-back chair.
Steps:

1. Curl your toes tightly.
2. Straighten and spread out your toes as far as you can.

Toe Helper
Type: Gentle stretching and strengthening
Starting position: You may try this exercise while sitting or lying down.
Steps:

1. One at a time, put each toe through its full range of motion by moving it with your hand.
2. One at a time, try to exert pressure with each toe by pressing it against your fingers.

Ankle Stretch
Type: Stretching
Starting position: Sit in a straight-back chair with both feet flat on the floor.
Steps:

1. Raise your heels while you keep your toes on the floor.
2. Return to the starting position.
3. Raise your toes and arches, but leave your heels on the floor.

Soft Shoe (See page 498)
Type: Stretching
Starting position: Sit in a straight-back chair with both feet flat on the floor.
Steps:

1. Raise your heels off the floor, as in the Ankle Stretch. *a*

2. Swivel both heels to the right before bringing them back down. Your feet are now pointing at an angle. *b*
3. Raise your toes and arches, leaving your heels on the floor.
4. Swivel the fronts of your feet to the right.
5. Repeat steps 1–4.
6. Raise your toes and arches, and swivel them to the left.
7. Raise your heels, and swivel them to the left.
8. Repeat steps 6 and 7 – twice.
9. 'Dance' back to the starting position.

Foot Roll
Type: Stretching
Starting position: Sit in a straight-back chair. Place a rolling pin on the floor where you can reach it with your feet.
Steps:

1. Work the rolling pin with the bottoms of your feet to massage your arches and stretch your ligaments.
2. Work the rolling pin under your toes, curling and stretching them, too.

Side Stretch (See page 499)
Type: Stretching
Starting position: Sit in a straight-back chair with your feet flat on the floor and your knees slightly apart.
Steps:

1. Rotate your ankles and lift your arches so that only the outer edges of your feet remain on the floor. *a*
2. Return to the starting position.
3. Rotate your ankles and lift the outer edges of your feet so that your knees come together and the big toes and inner heels stay on the floor. *b*

Runner's Stretch (See page 500)
Type: Stretching
Starting position: Stand facing a wall with your hands on the wall at about shoulder height and your feet a few inches from the wall base.

Steps:

1. Extend your left leg behind you, keeping your left knee straight, your toes on the floor, and your left heel raised. You may bend your right knee. *a*
2. Try to lower your left heel to the floor, feeling the stretch in your Achilles tendon.
3. Return to the starting position.
4. Repeat the movements with your right leg.

Ankle Walkout (See page 501)

Type: Stretching and strengthening
Starting position: Stand where you have room to walk.
Steps:

1. Walk a few paces on tiptoe. *a*
2. Walk a few paces on your heels. *b*

Ankle Builder

Type: Strengthening
Starting position: Stand, holding on to a sturdy support.
Steps:

1. Rise up on tiptoe.
2. Come down slowly.
3. Raise your toes so that you stand on your heels.
4. Put your feet flat on the floor.

Stunt Work

Materials: Marbles, small dish or cup
Type: Strengthening
Starting position: Sit in a straight-back chair, with a small dish of marbles at your feet.
Steps:

1. Scatter the marbles on the floor, near your left foot, and set the dish or cup between your feet.
2. One by one, pick up each marble with your toes, and drop it into the dish.
3. Repeat with right foot.

Foot Piston (See page 502)

Type: Strengthening
Starting position: Stand, holding on to a sturdy support.
Steps:

1. Lift your left heel but leave your toes on the floor. *a*
2. Lift your right heel and lower your left. *b*
3. Repeat the motion, with one heel going up as the other is going down.

Ankle Twist

Bring your toes together, then apart, by moving just your ankles.

   This is a smooth rotation movement that makes your feet work like slow-speed windshield wipers.

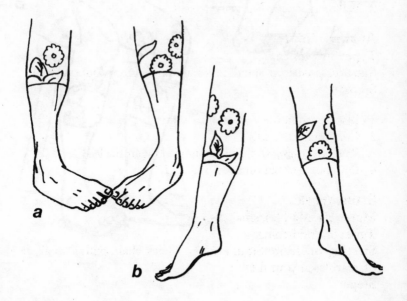

Soft Shoe

Use your ankles to swivel your feet, first on tiptoe, then on your heels. Tap dancers have incorporated this motion in many a dance routine.

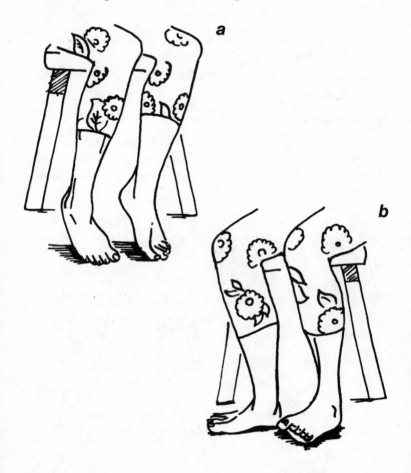

Side Stretch

Lift your arches, but don't lift your feet off the floor, so that the soles of your feet face each other.

Put your feet back on the floor and then roll onto your arches. Your ankles should be doing all the work.

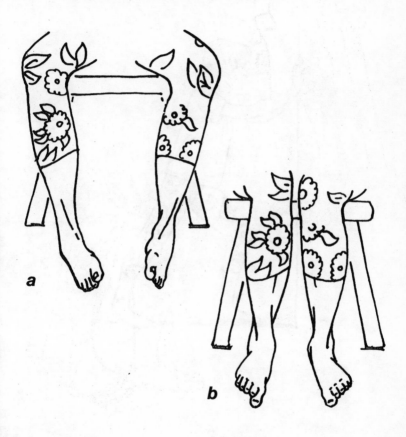

Runner's Stretch

Work the Achilles tendon at the back of your ankle the way runners prepare their feet for jogging — by leaning against a wall, extending one foot behind you and stretching your heel to the floor. Do this smoothly, without a jerk or a bounce.

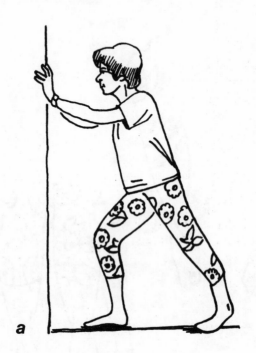

a

Ankle Walkout

Throw your weight into this ankle exercise by walking first on tiptoe, then down on your heels. Keep a sturdy chair handy for balance and safety's sake.

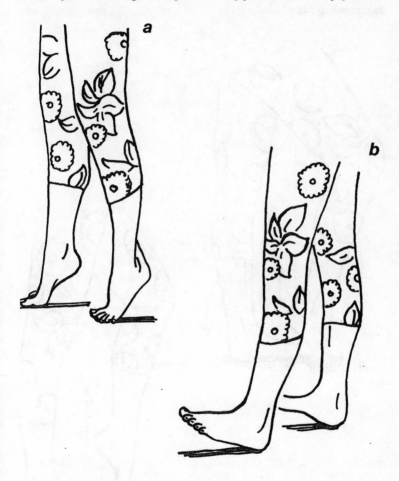

Foot Piston

As one heel goes up, the other one comes down.

  Neither foot ever fully leaves the floor during this exercise, but the ankles keep pumping like pistons.

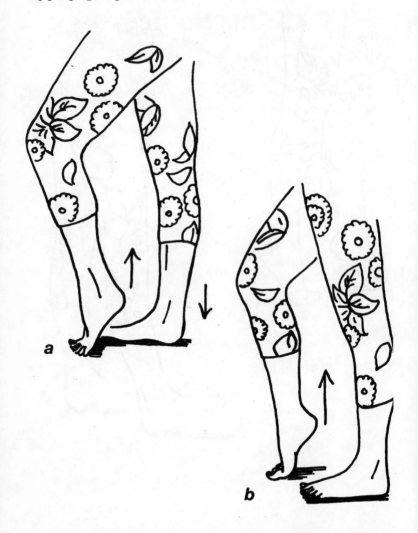

Section 11
Exercising under Special Circumstances

Since the activity of your arthritis may vary, your exercise program may vary as well. Do more when you're feeling well, less when you're not, but still do therapeutic exercises daily . . . In addition, it is important to get in as good shape as possible in preparation for a time when you may not be able to exercise as actively as you would like.

Fred G. Kantrowitz, M.D. author, *Taking Control of Arthritis*

Chapter 39
When Flare-Ups Interfere

How to modify your arthritis exercise program while coping with a sudden, dramatic worsening of your symptoms

Anyone who exercises outdoors has to lose a day occasionally on account of bad weather, but people with arthritis can encounter bad days even in full sunshine. Sometimes, joint pain or swelling may increase for no apparent reason, necessitating a change in routine.

Rheumatoid arthritis is a disease that goes in cycles. If you have it, you've no doubt found that you can experience long periods of general well-being, when your pain is under control. Then, for no apparent reason, a 'flare-up' will come along and aggravate your symptoms. You suffer from added pain and an increased number of stiff, swollen joints. You may even feel sick all over at these times – weak and feverish, so that you need to rest in bed.

People with osteoarthritis also recognize times when pain seems worse than usual, for reasons unknown.

Before you began exercising regularly, you may have reacted differently to flare-ups. You may have attributed them to the weather, to lack of sleep, a change in medication, or an increase in stress. Now the temptation may be to associate the flare-up with your exercise routine. You may have a whole new set of questions and concerns:

- Should I continue to exercise?
- What will happen if I exercise stiff or swollen joints?
- How can I balance rest and exercise during a flare-up?

First of all, be assured that exercise itself does not cause a flare-up. Some people fear that their increased activity may have aggravated their arthritis, when in fact the opposite is true. Exercise improves the overall condition of your body. Flare-ups may occur in any case because the normal course of arthritis is erratic. Please don't blame yourself for your suffering!

During an arthritis flare-up, you may need to curtail aerobic exercise, but you don't have to stop exercising altogether. It isn't even advisable to do so. Most joints, including the inflamed ones, reap benefits from moving through their full range of motion once or twice a day. Should you find that this amount of gentle stretching is impossible because movement hurts too much, isometric strengthening exercises that involve no motion may still be performed to good advantage.

If your first thought at the onset of the flare-up was of abandoning your exercise program, please put that thought out of your mind. Concentrate instead on how to modify your exercise program during the current crisis – with an eye toward getting back in full swing as soon as you feel well enough to do so.

Aerobic Adjustments

Depending on the extent of the flare-up, you may have to abstain from your regular aerobic activities for a while. No doubt, you'll find that you miss your daily walk or swim. You miss the chance to get out and the energy boost that exercise always gives you. Try not to fret over this change, but simply recognize it and realize how important exercise has become in your life – and will be again!

You may also find that you feel depressed. Pain alone can bring on depression, but lack of exercise in a person conditioned to its benefits often produces a mild downward mood swing.

Your body will definitely respond to the change. Exercising is a little bit like eating, in that you have to keep doing it regularly to stay healthy. As soon as you stop exercising, you start losing the edge you've gained. Your muscle bulk gets smaller and the ability of your muscles to perform work decreases. In other words, when you get back to your routine, you'll need at least a few days to build up to your preflare-up level of fitness.

Stretching

You can continue to perform gentle range-of-motion exercises even while confined to your bed. Move every joint every day – except, of course, those in which pain seems to be exacerbated by movement.

If the flare-up has forced you to cut back on aerobic activity or cut it out altogether, by all means use the extra time you have to put your joints through their range of motion more frequently. By keeping up the stretching routines as best you can, you help yourself maintain the progress you've made. You can't, of course, expect to greatly increase your flexibility during a flare-up.

Strengthening

Since your affected joints are exquisitely sensitive to motion during a flare-up, you may find the isotonic strengthening exercises – the ones that require you to move against an opposing force – too much of a strain. The isometrics, however, with their motionless, muscle-building pressure, may prove the perfect maneuvers for you at this time.

Isometrics can help you build strength in your wrists when you press the palms of your hands together, bolster your neck muscles when you press one palm against your forehead, improve your shoulder (or hip) condition when you work your arm (or leg) against a wall, strengthen your elbows when you push up from under a heavy table with your forearms, and brace your back by leaning hard against a chair-back or wall.

Chapter 40
Before and After Surgery

How to modify your exercise program to meet the requirements for joint replacement or other surgical procedures related to arthritis

Roughly one out of five members of the original US Arthritis Survey group went through surgical procedures to find relief from arthritis pain. If you are currently facing an operation, you will discover, as they did, that exercise is a crucial element of both preoperative conditioning and postoperative healing.

As anxious as you may be about the procedure, remember that surgery for arthritis is among the most successful treatments for severe, intractable pain and disability. Rest assured that performing the right exercises will improve the likelihood of a good outcome in the long run.

Your specific exercise prescription will be dictated by the type of surgery you face. The most popular forms are:

- *Arthroplasty* to partially or totally replace or resurface a damaged joint, usually the hip or the knee
- *Arthrodesis* to fuse the bones of a joint in order to stabilize it, typically the ankle or the wrist
- *Arthroscopy*, or the use of fibre optics and miniature tools inserted through small incisions, to remove cartilage or other damaged tissue, most frequently in the knee.

Before
If you are suffering enough pain and joint deterioration to require surgery, you may have very limited movement in your affected joint. Indeed, you may be unable to perform any exercise other than isometric strengthening or passive stretching – letting your physiotherapist carefully move the joint through its range of motion.

A muscle's natural state is motion, and enforced lack of motion will shrink the size of the tissue. Muscles may lose as much as thirty percent of their bulk in one week's worth of inactivity.

Your challenge during this preparation for the surgery period is to heed your body's pain messages while you get yourself in shape for the coming operation. On the one hand, you want to save the joint any unnecessary stress or pain. On the other hand, you want the rest of your body in tip-top condition for the combined stresses of anesthesia and prolonged rest. The more strength you amass before surgery, the speedier your recovery is likely to be.

We urge you to try to preserve your aerobic fitness as part of your preoperative preparation. If you're having surgery on your shoulders or hands, you may experience no difficulty sticking to your regular walking or cycling routine. But what if the surgery involves the weight-bearing joints of your hips or knees? Take heart – you can still find ways to work out. One solution is a hand-held bicycle called an arm-cycle ergometer, which should be available through the physical therapy department at your hospital. You'll find that you really have to spin the wheels with all your might to get the most out of this gadget, but it's probably worth the effort and definitely worth a try.

Such energy expenditure not only primes the heart and lungs, as you know, but can help you lose weight by burning calories and fat. If your upcoming surgery involves one of your weight-bearing joints, this may be the ideal time to try to shed extra pounds. Why give the weight-bearing joints any excess weight to bear?

The impending surgery may give you the incentive you've been lacking to do something about your weight. But don't opt for a crash diet that could leave you weakened by lack of important nutrients. You need your strength for surgery. You'll do best if you combine your aerobic exercise with a healthful diet, high in fibre but low in fat and calories.

As a safety precaution, you will probably be asked to drop your usual medications before surgery. If you take aspirin, your doctor will ask you to do without it beginning about two weeks prior to your operation. The reason is that aspirin interferes with blood clotting, and taking it could lead to unnecessary bleeding. One week before surgery, you may be asked to drop any other anti-inflammatory drugs you've been taking, for the same reason. (Your doctor may suggest that you rely on acetaminophen instead, best known by the name paracetamol, as this drug has no apparent influence on blood clotting.)

Any change in your regular medications may lead to a temporary increase in pain and may make it more difficult for you to exercise. As usual, it makes sense to heed the pain messages. Don't force your body to follow your regular exercise regimen under these circumstances. You'll get back to a full program soon – and then some.

After

A physiotherapist may be your first visitor after surgery. Indeed, the exercises you will be doing for rehabilitation are every bit as important as the surgery you went through. One cannot succeed without the other.

The exercise apparatus the therapist brings you for the start of your postoperative exercise program could be anything from a handful of therapeutic putty to squeeze with your new finger joints to a machine that will flex and straighten your new knee as though you were riding an automatic bicycle. The therapist will supervise you at first, and direct you as to how you should increase your activity as you grow stronger.

Try not to be discouraged if you discover that you feel less fit and have a narrower range of motion than you did beforehand. Remember how much time you've needed to rest, and that inactivity causes weakness. Slowly and steadily, you can regain the ground you've lost if you just keep up with your modified exercise regimen.

Among your cheeriest thoughts will be the realization that your pain in the affected joint has decreased dramatically or disappeared altogether. You may feel wobbly and out of sorts at first, but freedom from pain will enable you to pursue your rehabilitation program and return to full activity.

Find out from your doctor precisely what you can and cannot do during your recovery period. Make sure you understand how much time you will have to allow for full recovery. The surgery you've had should lead eventually to greater mobility and independence, but for right now, give yourself every chance to achieve the best possible long-term outcome by doing less than ever. Your family and friends will no doubt want to help you shop, cook, and do other errands and chores. Let them.

If you have received an artificial joint, be sure to ask about any special restrictions that may apply to it. Ask your doctor and your physiotherapist. Either one may tell you things the other forgets to mention. In the first few weeks of living with a new hip joint, for example, one has to be careful not to disturb the replacement by bending too much. Observe these precautions to guarantee yourself the longest possible life for your artificial joint.

Chapter 41
While Coping with Other Health Problems

How to balance an arthritis exercise program with the special demands created by other illnesses and medications

People with arthritis are not immune to other widespread health problems such as heart disease, high blood pressure, and diabetes.

Sometimes the coincidence of arthritis with another illness in the same body is just a run of bad luck. In many cases, however, arthritis medications may actually be the cause of the second condition. Ulcers, for example, are an all-too-frequent side effect of taking high doses of aspirin or other anti-inflammatory drugs. High blood pressure may develop with the fluid retention that often results from treatment with corticosteroids such as prednisone.* Diabetes may also follow in the wake of steroid drug use, and osteoporosis is yet another potential complication.

Proper exercise with proper precautions can benefit any or all of these conditions. As a person with two or more health issues to consider, you'll want to pick and choose your exercises with extra care.

The range-of-motion exercises you do for your arthritic joints are so gentle as to pose no risk to other body systems. Strengthening exercises, however, especially the isometric ones, are a different matter. Even though these muscle builders involve no motion, and are therefore painless enough to perform even during an arthritis flare-up, they may pose special problems for people with heart disease and high blood pressure. If you have

* Other corticosteroids prescribed for the original US Arthritis Survey group of 1,051 participants include cortisone acetate, methylprednisolone, dexamethasone, prednisolone, and triamcinolone.

either of these conditions, you will need your doctor's approval before attempting isometrics as they can cause brief interruptions in blood circulation.

Aerobic exercise is recommended across the board, as it has so much to offer. We've already ticked off the many advantages, including strength, flexibility, pain reduction, weight control, longevity, and a general feeling of well-being. In arthritis care, aerobic exercise helps preserve joint motion and prevent joint deformity. Let's look at its specific advantages in addressing other health problems.

Heart Disease

If you suffer from heart disease, aerobic exercise can help you strengthen the heart muscle itself. Aerobic exercise first became a household word for this proven positive effect on the heart. Indeed, it is often called cardiovascular exercise because it improves the function of the whole circulatory system.

The cardiologist who treats you for heart disease will want to have a say in your exercise program, and will determine how much of a workout is safe for you by means of an exercise treadmill test (see page 515). Without question, the prescribed activity will be walking. As Dr. Dean Ornish explains in his book, *Reversing Heart Disease*, walking is the preferred form of exercise because it provides the most health benefits and poses the lowest risk of injury or sudden cardiac arrest.

Dr. Ornish counsels the patients in his 'Opening Your Heart' program to walk at least thirty minutes every day, or one hour three times a week. If you have advanced arthritis in your weight-bearing joints, you may not be able to walk this much, at least not when you first start to exercise. But it's nice to know that you can stride for stronger legs and improve your heart's health while you do so.

We have not, up to now, discussed target heart rates or metabolic equivalent units – two subjects that pepper the conversation of exercise enthusiasts. Our reason? We merely want you to move, to find relief from pain, to gain flexibility, to extend the range of motion in your joints, and to discover pleasure in aerobic activity. We're not urging you to become a fitness freak or a marathon runner.

Now, however, in a discussion of heart problems, target heart rate becomes relevant.* In brief, you serve your heart best by exercising in a sustained fashion that makes your heart pump faster than when you're sitting still. The ideal, or target rate, is between forty-five and eighty percent of your heart's top speed. As you can imagine, pushing to the limit poses dangers, which is why doctors like to determine that limit in a controlled setting, where they can take care of you right away if something goes wrong. The exercise treadmill test, or an exercise cycle test, performed in a hospital or doctor's office, with electrocardiogram and blood pressure monitoring, meets all these conditions.

Once you've been informed of your target heart rate, you can easily determine, during your exercise sessions, whether you're pushing your heart hard enough. Simply place the flat of your fingertip on the inside of your wrist, near the base of your thumb, where you can feel your blood pulsing through the radial artery. Using a watch with a second hand, count how many beats you feel in a ten-second period. Then you can multiply the result by six to find your heart rate (pulse). Or, you can start with the target range and divide those numbers by six, so you know what your ten-second pulse should be.

The medications you take for your heart condition will no doubt influence the way you respond to exercise. Beta blockers (such as Inderal, Lopressor, and Tenormin) tend to slow down the heart rate and lower the blood pressure – just the way exercise does over time. Nitrates (including Minitran and Nitro-Dur), on the other hand, speed up the heart rate while they lower the blood pressure. By keeping your doctor informed of your exercise progress, you'll be able to make any needed adjustments in drug dosage as your body becomes more fit.

---

* Metabolic equivalent units, or METs, offer another way to measure the intensity with which you exercise. METs are expressed in amounts of energy used for energy production, per minute. You use one MET just sitting still. If your maximum MET value is 6, then your body consumes six times as much oxygen going at full tilt than it uses at rest.

Hypertension

If hypertension, or high blood pressure, is your problem, you may well be wondering what all the increased blood flow promised by exercise will mean for you. Won't your blood pressure rise even higher? The fact is, while your blood pressure may increase temporarily during an exercise session, it will drop to a lower level as a result of regular exercise. And the weight loss you may experience from all that brisk walking will help lower it even further.

By all means, check with your doctor about your exercise plans. It may turn out that you can decrease or even drop the medications you take for your high blood pressure once exercise becomes a regular habit.

Diabetes

Whether your diabetes traces from childhood or became a problem only recently, exercise offers one way to gain control over your blood sugar – with your doctor's advice and consent.

Like insulin, physical activity takes up blood sugar. This means that regular exercise will most likely change the amount of insulin you need to take. In fact, some people with Type II (adult onset) diabetes may reach a point where they no longer require any medication. Exercise and diet alone may provide all the necessary regulation of their blood sugar levels.

When you begin your exercise program, take careful note of your blood sugar at the start of each activity period, and again at the end. See whether you need to modify your insulin dosage, and discuss the changes with your doctor.

It's a good idea to time your exercise according to your insulin schedule to avoid problems. If, for example, you set out for a brisk walk during the peak of your insulin response, you may suddenly feel weak and dizzy due to hypoglycaemia. Be assured that you can find a way to coordinate your exercise prescription with your medicine prescriptions – it just takes a little time and careful consideration.

About the Research

The 1,051 participants in the US Arthritis Survey first learned of its existence from their favourite newspapers and magazines – *USA Today*, the *New York Times*, the *American Legion Magazine, Prevention, Popular Science, McCall's Needlework and Crafts, Field & Stream, Writer's Digest, Mother Jones, Medical Self-Care*, and others – where we placed advertisements and public notices inviting people with arthritis to fill out a detailed questionnaire.

Interested volunteers wrote to us or called our toll-free number to get a copy of the six-page Arthritis Survey questionnaire. In filling out the form, they told us about every doctor they had seen because of arthritis, from rheumatologists to clinical ecologists, and every non-M.D. practitioner as well, including chiropractors, physiotherapists, and nutritionists. They answered questions on the effects – and side effects – of a medicine-chestful of prescription drugs, injections, and professional treatments ranging from acupuncture to wax dips. A few of the participants were serving as research subjects in clinical trials of new arthritis treatments, and they gave us a fascinating glimpse of things to come.

They also told us about their operations and the long-term results of surgery. They ran through their exercise routines. They explained the ways they had changed their eating habits and how they had benefited from the change. They reported on over-the-counter treatments they had tried – and under-the-counter ones, too, such as DMSO and bee venom. And they told us what they did for themselves to relieve pain, raise spirits, and generally make life easier. (The text of the questionnaire comprises Appendix A.) In the vast majority of the 1,300-some responses we received, the detailed answers dispelled any doubts about the authenticity of the participants' experiences. However, we did have to reject about 150 questionnaires that were incomplete or otherwise unusable.

As a token of our thanks for the time they spent sharing their knowledge, we sent each participant a check for eight dollars.

As it turned out, a few of the checks came back to us, with notes saying that we should put the money toward the research – that participating in the survey had been a welcome chance to reach out and help others.

The money to conduct the survey (to cover advertising, printing, postage, payments to participants, long-distance telephone calls, and clerical help) came from our publisher, St. Martin's Press. This meant that we did not have to seek the financial support of any foundation or manufacturer. We are very pleased that we were able to work independently, without the pressure or influence of any organization's vested interest.

From among the 518 survey participants who volunteered to talk to us on the telephone (in addition to filling out the questionnaire), we chose 100 people to interview at length.

In talking about their complaints, several participants noted that they hate being called 'an arthritic' or 'an arthritis sufferer,' as though they were nothing more than the victim of their disease. They prefer to think of themselves as the people they really are – as husbands, wives, parents, friends, partners, and valued employees. They work, or have worked, as accountants, advertising directors, archaeologists, armed service members, army recruiters, artists, assembly-line workers, audiologists, auto mechanics, bankers, barbers, bartenders, beauticians, bookkeepers, bricklayers, budget analysts, cab-drivers, cafeteria servers, car dealers, carpenters, cartographers, chemists, childcare providers, chiropractors, choir directors, civil servants, college professors, composers, computer operators, construction workers, consultants, cooks, corporate executive officers, dairy farmers, dental hygienists, dentists, designers, detectives, dietitians, disc jockeys, doctors, dog breeders, draughtsmen, dressmakers, dry cleaners, economists, editors, educational administrators, electronics technicians, engineers, entertainers, family counsellors, farmhands, fire fighters, food brokers, foremen, forestry technicians, foundry workers, gardeners, guards, home health-care aids, hospital and nursing-home volunteers, househusbands and housewives, housekeepers, insurance agents, interior decorators, investors, janitors, lab technicians, laborers, lawyers, lecturers, letter carriers, librarians, locksmiths, loggers, machinists, maintenance workers, manufacturing representatives, medical assistants, merchant seamen, meter readers, military officers, miners, ministers, musicians, newspaper reporters, nuns, nurses, occupational therapists, oil-field roughnecks, optometrists, painters, paramedics, personnel directors, pharmacists, photographers, piano tuners, pilots, plumbers, police officers, porters, postmasters, printers, proofreaders, psychotherapists, purchasing agents, railroad carmen, ranchers, real estate agents, receptionists, registrars, researchers, restaurant owners, retail buyers, sales clerks, sanitation workers, sculptors, secretaries, securities traders, shipping clerks, shopkeepers, silversmiths, small-business owners, social workers, soil testers, supervisors, tax consultants, tax representatives, taxidermists, teachers, telephone operators, tennis instructors, traffic monitors, travel agents, travelling salesmen, truck drivers, typists, USDA food inspectors, veterinarians, waitresses, welders, welfare investigators, and writers.

Our participants come from every one of the fifty states. While most of them live in the large population centres – California, New York, Florida, and Texas – the Arthritis Survey reached Myrtle Creek, Oregon; Boonville, Missouri; Blue Diamond, Washington; Horse Cave, Kentucky; Iron River, Wisconsin; Hepzibah, Georgia; Ceresco, Nebraska; and Eagle, Alaska. We also had a total of nineteen participants from the Bahamas, Puerto Rico, and Canada. We drew the line there, however, and denied the survey requests we received from residents of Spain, England, Chile, the Philippines, and other foreign countries, because we wanted to focus on practitioners and treatments that would be accessible to North American readers.

The characteristics of the survey group match the national portrait of people with rheumatoid arthritis and osteoarthritis in terms of age and sex. In all, 68 percent of them are in their forties, fifties, or sixties, and 67 percent are women. We counted 216 participants with rheumatoid arthritis, 139 with osteoarthritis, and 71 with a combination of both. (You'll find a summary of the demographics, including age of onset, in Appendix B.)

The participants who answered our ads are 'self-selected' volunteers, as opposed to subjects picked at random. A few researchers contend that self-selected participants are somehow special or atypical – that they answer a call for volunteers because they have 'an axe to grind,' and that this invalidates their responses. However, our earlier survey research project, which was described in our book *Backache Relief* (Times Books, 1985; NAL/Signet, 1986, and a Book-of-the-Month Club Alternate Selection), brought in very few people who had nothing but an axe to grind. Most of the participants in that survey responded because they had found an effective approach to back pain, after years of searching for one, and wanted to share what they had learned. In the Arthritis Survey, too, the respondents wrote in to share their experiences, not air their grievances.

In the hospitals where clinical trials are conducted, research subjects are also self-selected, to a degree. Even though potential subjects literally arrive on the doorstep because illness drives them to seek treatment, their participation in trials is by no means automatic. Researchers must solicit volunteers by approaching each patient who has the disease of interest, explaining the nature of the study and the risks involved, and then getting the patient's consent in writing. Ethical concerns have put an end, thank goodness, to the only truly random selection process in human studies: that of experimenting upon the unwitting or unwilling inmates of asylums, state hospitals, and penitentiaries, or on soldiers, prisoners of war, or the poor.

Advertising for subjects as we did is a well-established research practice. Health scientists looking for appropriate outpatient volunteers to serve as research subjects have used all imaginable approaches to attract them, including newspaper ads, radio spots, posters, press releases, and by making appearances at civic-group meetings. Paying research subjects is likewise standard procedure. Volunteers typically receive free medical care or a direct cash payment for their participation.

Tabulating and analyzing the data from the Arthritis Survey questionnaires was a massive job that took more than six months. It was further complicated, and *greatly* enriched, by those participants who not only wrote all over the printed form but then tacked on a page or two – or eight or nine – of extra details. This was not the kind of material that could be fed into a computer or turned over to research assistants. We read every questionnaire at least three times and began keeping tallies by hand. These eventually filled some four hundred spreadsheets, which we had to tailor-make to our purposes. On several of the popular drug treatments, for example, we often needed as many as thirty to forty columns for the side effects alone.

In addition to the wealth of information from our participants, we also used online medical literature services to give us monthly updates on relevant current research reported in the medical journals. We took each month's list to the medical-school library at the State University of New York's Stony Brook campus, where we read the original articles in their entirety. This helped us explain and augment the information from our participants with the latest research findings from professionals in nutrition, rheumatology, orthopaedics, and related fields.

Appendix A
Arthritis Survey Questionnaire*

Dear Survey Participant,

Thank you for agreeing to take part in our nationwide Arthritis Survey.

We will use the information you provide as the basis for a new book we are writing about *osteoarthritis* and *rheumatoid arthritis*. In the hope of helping others, we ask you to tell us your experiences, opinions about the treatments you have tried, and tips on how to live with arthritis.

Our first book, *Backache Relief* (Times Books, 1985; NAL/Signet, 1986), based on a similar nationwide survey, was chosen as a Book-of-the-Month Club alternate selection. The arthritis book will be published by St. Martin's Press in 1989.

You have our word that we will treat your personal information with respect and keep it *confidential*. Your name will not be used in the book or put on any kind of mailing list.

Please try to answer the questions with as much *detail* as you can give. If you need more space, feel free to attach extra pages; we are interested in *everything* you have to say about arthritis.

As a token of our thanks for the time you spend sharing your knowledge, we will be happy to send you a check for $8 within 7 to 10 days of receiving your *fully completed* questionnaire.

Name/Address/Age/Sex/Occupation

Check which arthritis you have: osteoarthritis–rheumatoid– (Other forms of arthritis are *not* included in this survey.)

What parts of your body are arthritic?

How long have you had arthritis? (If less than 6 months, please do not fill out the questionnaire.)

On a scale of 0 to 10, where 0 means pain-free and 10 means intense pain that keeps you from doing anything, how would you

---

* To save space, the survey questions are printed here in list form without the blank areas where participants wrote their responses.

rate your condition on average? Circle one number: 0 1 2 3 4 5 6 7 8 9 10

[pain-free]   [intense pain]

Professional Care

Please list all the *kinds* of practitioners who have treated you. (For example, rheumatologist, internist, physiatrist, chiropractor, osteopath, physical therapist, nurse, Yoga instructor, etc.)

Please look at the list you just wrote and put three plus signs (+ + +) after those who gave you a *great deal of help* that lasted *a year or more.*

Put two plus signs (+ +) after those who gave you *a little help* that lasted *a year or more.*

Put one plus sign (+) after those who gave you *only temporary relief.*

Put a zero (0) after those who *didn't help at all.*

Put a minus sign (−) after those who *made you feel worse.*

In the space below, please comment about the practitioners you have seen. (For example, tell *how* they helped you or made you worse.)

Are you satisfied with the care you are receiving now? If not, what are you planning to do?

What kinds of arthritis diagnostic *tests* have you taken? (For example, X rays, blood tests, arthroscopy, joint aspiration, etc.)

What would you say about these tests to someone who needed to take them? (Are they expensive, painful, useful, etc.?)

Do you take *aspirin?*

If yes, how much each day? Check one: plain buffered coated What does it do for you (pain relief, side effects, etc.)?

Treatments

What prescription drugs do you take? (Some examples are Deltasone, Dolobid, Feldene, Indocin, Motrin, Naprosyn, Oraflex, Orudis, Ridaura, Tolectin, etc.)

Now give (+ + +) to pills that helped you *a great deal* for *a year or longer.*

Put (+ +) after any that helped you *a little bit* for *a year or longer.*

Put (+) after those that gave *only temporary relief.*

Put (0) after the ones that *did no good.*

Please give as many details as you can about your reaction to these pills, including any side effects (dizziness, nausea, etc.).

Please list any *injection* treatments you have had (gold, methotrexate, cortisone, etc.) and tell what they did for you.

Please list other professional treatments you've tried (acupuncture, physical therapy, splints, biofeedback, manipulation, massage, etc.).

Of these, what helped the most? What made no difference? Did any treatment injure you?

Surgery

Have you had surgery for arthritis?

If no, skip to the section on Exercise.

If yes, please name the joint(s) involved and what was done (total knee replacement, partial hip replacement, wrist fusion, etc.), including the year you had the operation.

If you have an artificial joint and know its brand name (Zimmer knee, Techmedica hip, etc.) please give it:

How long did it take to fully recover from surgery?

What follow-up treatment (physical therapy, exercise advice, etc.) did you receive after your operation(s)?

Please tell the outcome (pain relief, greater mobility, infection, etc.) of your operation(s).

What advice would you offer someone considering arthritis surgery?

Exercise

Do you exercise (stretch, swim, walk, etc.) for arthritis? If no, please skip to Other Treatments.

If yes, please tell *what you do* and *how much time* each day you devote to exercise:

How did you learn exercises? (Doctor, book, class, etc.)

What benefit(s) do you get from exercise?

If you have ever been harmed by exercise, please tell what happened:

What exercise advice can you offer other arthritis sufferers?

Other Treatments

Please list any over-the-counter remedies (liniments, pills other than aspirin, etc.) you've used for arthritis, and tell what they did for you.

If you have tried any arthritis treatments that most doctors reject (copper bracelet, insect venom, hormone, etc.) please list them and describe what they did for you.

Please give any helpful information (danger, cost, etc.) you can for others thinking of trying the treatment(s) you just named.

Nutrition

Have you changed the way you eat (avoid some foods, eat more of others, etc.) because of arthritis? If yes, please give details:

What has your doctor told you about nutrition and arthritis?

Does arthritis affect your food shopping and cooking? If yes, in what way?

What vitamins/minerals, if any, do you take, and what do they do for you?

Please give *comments* or *questions* you have about nutrition and arthritis:

Self-Help

What things do you do for yourself (rest, warm baths, ice bags, etc.) that give you pain relief?

What do you do to lift your spirits?

Does *stress* make your pain worse?

If yes, what techniques (deep breathing, imagery, etc.) help you reduce stress?

Have you changed your *home* or *workplace* and the things in it (raised toilet seat, bed board, etc.) because of arthritis? Please list the changes:

Please name the most *useful items* you've discovered (homemade, store-bought or mail-order) for arthritis sufferers, and where to get them.

What are some of the ways you've found for doing *common activities* (from cleaning house to making love) without increasing pain or injury?

We are *not* affiliated with the Arthritis Foundation, but we would like to know if that group has helped you in any way (information, support, etc.):

If you would be willing to discuss exercise or practical tips in depth with us, please give your area code and phone number:

Best time to call: AM − − PM − −

If you know another arthritis sufferer who might be willing to participate in our survey, please give his or her name and address:

Thanks Again!

Appendix B
Survey Demographics

The 1,051 participants in our Arthritis Survey are a diverse group of 352 men and 699 women. We knew even before we began soliciting volunteers that we would have more women than men in our survey population, since rheumatoid arthritis affects about three times as many women as men, and osteoarthritis is also more common among women.

	Number of Participants with Rheumatoid Arthritis	Number of Participants with Osteoarthritis	Number of Participants with Both Forms
Men	153	188	11
Women	263	376	60
Total	416	564	71

Our participants range in age from twelve to ninety-three, but more than two-thirds of them are now in their forties, fifties, and sixties.

Age Range	Number of Participants in This Age Range	Percent of Total
10–19	7	1%
20–29	44	4%
30–39	117	11%
40–49	165	16%
50–59	224	21%
60–69	325	31%
70–79	144	14%
80–89	21	2%
90–99	1	–
Age not stated	3	–

Arthritis is frequently called a disease of old age, despite the fact that hundreds of thousands of children suffer from juvenile rheumatoid arthritis. Even the two forms of arthritis covered in our survey – osteoarthritis and rheumatoid arthritis – take their toll among the young and middle-aged. More than half of our participants, or 557 individuals, are under the age of sixty *now*, and 450 of them had arthritis before they reached age forty.

Age at Onset	Number of Participants	Percent of Total
0–9	26	2%
10–19	71	7%
20–29	140	13%
30–39	213	20%
40–49	247	24%
50–59	209	20%
60–69	95	9%
70–79	25	2%
80–89	2	–
Unstated	23	2%

Although most of our participants have found relief in a combination of professional treatments and self-help strategies, they have endured their share of pain. Here's how they rate themselves, on average, on our pain scale, where 0 means pain-free at present, and 10 signifies intense pain that keeps them from doing anything.

Pain Rating	Number of Participants	Percent of Total
0	10	1%
1	25	2%
2	53	5%
3	102	10%
4	133	13%
5	209	20%
6	150	14%
7	139	13%
8	111	11%
9	53	5%
10	45	4%
No answer	21	2%

We had to pool and average the answers of those who gave themselves a range-type rating, such as '2 to 4,' or more than one answer, such as '4, except during flare-ups, when it jumps to about 9½.' Several participants who gave no answer to this question went to some lengths explaining how hard it was to put a number rating on pain. It was simpler, by far, to say which joints were, or had been, painful.

Affected Joint(s)	Number of Participants Affected There
Knees/Legs	634
Hands/Fingers	590
Spine	416
Shoulders	284
Feet/Toes	274
Hips/Pelvis	274
Neck	245
Elbows/Arms	232
Ankles	160
Wrists	150
'Most' or 'All' joints	125
Jaw	37
Ribs/Breastbone/Chest	18

We have more survey participants from California than from any other state, followed by New York, Florida, and Texas.

State	Number of Participants
Alabama	16
Alaska	4
Arizona	18
Arkansas	17
California	117
Colorado	15
Connecticut	9
Delaware	4
District of Columbia	1
Florida	64
Georgia	14
Hawaii	3

Idaho	7
Illinois	33
Indiana	29
Iowa	12
Kansas	11
Kentucky	13
Louisiana	15
Maine	5
Maryland	12
Tennessee	23
Texas	62
Utah	5
Vermont	1
Virginia	21
Massachusetts	15
Michigan	37
Minnesota	23
Mississippi	4
Missouri	21
Montana	4
Nebraska	10
Nevada	6
New Hampshire	5
New Jersey	30
New Mexico	6
New York	87
North Carolina	20
North Dakota	1
Ohio	52
Oklahoma	12
Oregon	19
Pennsylvania	45
Rhode Island	4
South Carolina	7
South Dakota	13
Washington	32
West Virginia	8
Wisconsin	37
Wyoming	3

Other Homes	Number of Participants
Alberta	1
British Columbia	3
Manitoba	1
Nova Scotia	1
Ontario	8
Saskatchewan	1
Bahamas	1
Puerto Rico	3

Appendix C
Drug Interactions

Medications used to treat arthritis, whether they are prescription drugs or over-the-counter products, can cause serious trouble when mixed with other medicines. This reference chart is a convenient guide that may alert you to potential problems, which you should discuss with your doctor.

The drugs are listed in alphabetical order. The information is based on the *Physicians' Desk Reference* and *The People's Pharmacy*.

Prescription Drugs		
Name	Type	Bad Matches and Their Possible Dangers
Azulfidine (sulfasalazine)	Anti-inflammatory	Digoxin (for heart trouble) – reduced absorption of digoxin
Butazolidin (phenylbutazone)	NSAID (Non-steroidal Anti-Inflammatory Drug)	Anticoagulants – bleeding
		Methotrexate (for cancer or rheumatoid arthritis) – increased toxic effects of methotrexate.
		Anticonvulsants (for seizures)– increased toxic effects of these drugs, including loss of balance
		Aspirin or other NSAIDs – gastrointestinal problems, including ulcers
		Oral diabetes drugs – extremely low blood sugar
		Penicillamine – blood and kidney disorders
Clinoril (sulindac)	NSAID	DMSO – reduced efficacy of Clinoril; peripheral neuropathy

		Aspirin – reduced efficacy of Clinoril Aspirin or other NSAIDs – gastrointestinal problems, including ulcers Dolobid (diflunisal) – reduced efficacy of Clinoril
Cortone (cortisone acetate)	See Deltasone	
Cuprimine (penicillamine)	Chelating agent/ Antirheumatic	Gold – serious blood and kidney disorders Antimalarial – blood and kidney disorders Cytotoxic drugs – blood, kidney disorders Butazolidin – blood and kidney disorders
Decadron (dexamethasone)		See Deltasone
Deltasone (prednisone)	Steroid	Anticonvulsants – reduced efficacy of Deltasone Antituberculosis drugs – reduced efficacy of both Deltasone and these drugs Aspirin and other salicylates – reduced efficacy of aspirin or other salicylate Barbiturates (certain sedatives) – reduced efficacy of Deltasone Diuretics – depleted potassium stores Oral contraceptives – Increased toxic effects of Deltasone Live vaccines – failure of vaccine to take effect; onset of illness it's meant to prevent
Depen (penicillamine)		See Cuprimine
Disalcid (salsalate)	NSAID	Gout medications – reduced efficacy of these drugs

		Anticoagulants – bleeding
		Aspirin and other salicylates – toxic levels of active ingredient, as the drugs are so closely related
		Oral diabetes drugs – extremely low blood sugar
Dolobid (diflunisal)	NSAID	Anticoagulants – bleeding
		Antacids (taken regularly) – reduced efficacy of Dolobid
		Acetaminophen – elevated blood levels of acetaminophen, posing threat to liver.
		Indocin (indomethacin) – fatal gastrointestinal hemorrhage
		Clinoril (sulindac) – reduced efficacy of Clinoril
		Naprosyn (naproxen) – decreased urinary excretion of Naprosyn
		Aspirin or other NSAIDs – gastrointestinal problems, including ulcers
Easprin (aspirin)	Salicylate (NSAID)	Anticoagulants – hemorrhage
		Oral diabetes drugs – extremely low blood sugar
		Insulin – extremely low blood sugar
		Gout medications – small doses of aspirin reduce efficacy of these drugs
		Alcohol – gastrointestinal bleeding
		Steroids – increased risk of ulcers
		Butazolidin – increased risk of ulcers

		Phenobarbital – reduced efficacy of aspirin
		Beta blockers – reduced anti-inflammatory effect of aspirin
		Antacids – changes in Easprin's enteric coating
		Methotrexate – increased toxicity of methotrexate
		Other NSAIDs – Gastrointestinal problems, including ulcers
Feldene (piroxicam)	NSAID	Anticogulants – bleeding
		Aspirin – reduced efficacy of Feldene
		Aspirin or other NSAIDs – gastrointestinal problems, including ulcers
Imuran (azathioprine)	Immuno-suppressive	Allopurinol (for gout) – increased toxicity of Imuran
		Alkylating agents such as cyclophosphamide and chlorambucil – cancer
Indocin (indomethacin)	NSAID	Dolobid (diffunisal) – fatal gastrointestinal hemorrhage
		Aspirin – reduced efficacy of Indocin
		Aspirin or other NSAIDs – gastrointestinal problems, including ulcers
		Probenecid (for gout) – increased blood levels of Indocin
		Lithium (for depression) – elevated lithium levels and possible lithium toxicity
		Diuretics (for hypertension) – reduced efficacy of the diuretic; kidney problems
		Beta blockers – reduced efficacy of beta blocker

Meclomen (meclofenamate sodium)	NSAID	Anticoagulants – bleeding
		Aspirin – greater blood loss in the stool than from either drug alone
Medrol (methylprednisolone)		See Deltasone
Methotrexate (methotrexate)	Antimetabolite	Butazolidin – increased toxicity of Methotrexate Aspirin and other salicylates – increased toxicity of Methotrexate
Motrin (ibuprofen)	NSAID	Anticoagulants – bleeding Aspirin – reduced efficacy of Motrin Aspirin or other NSAIDs – gastrointestinal problems, including ulcers
Nalfon (fenoprofen calcium)	NSAID	Aspirin – reduced efficacy of Nalfon Phenobarbital – reduced efficacy of Nalfon Anticoagulants – bleeding Anticonvulsants (for seizures) – increased toxicity of these drugs
Naprosyn (naproxen)	NSAID	Anaprox (naproxen sodium) – elevated blood levels of the active ingredient, as the drugs are very closely related Diuretics – kidney trouble Anticoagulants – bleeding Beta blockers – reduced efficacy of beta blocker Probenecid – increased Naprosyn potency Methotrexate – increased toxicity of methotrexate

Orudis (ketoprofen)	NSAID	Aspirin – reduced efficacy of Orudis
		Diuretics – kidney failure
		Probenecid – inhibited excretion of Orudis
Plaquenil (hydroxychloroquine sulfate)	Antimalarial	Penicillamine – bone-marrow depression; kidney trouble
Prednisone		See Deltasone
Rheumatrex (methotrexate)		See Methotrexate
Ridaura (auranofin)	Gold (Antirheumatic)	Dilantin (for epilepsy) – increased blood levels of Dilantin
Rufen (ibuprofen)		See Motrin
Sulfasalazine		See Azulfidine
Tolectin (tolmetin sodium)	NSAID	Anticoagulants – bleeding
		Diuretics – kidney trouble
		Aspirin and other NSAIDs – gastrointestinal problems, including ulcers
Zorprin (aspirin)		See Easprin
Advil (ibuprofen)		See Motrin
Anacin (aspirin)		See Easprin
Anacin-3 (acetaminophen)	Analgesic	Dolobid – elevated levels of acetaminophen, posing threat to the liver
Arthritis Pain Formula (aspirin)		See Easprin
Arthritis Strength Bufferin (aspirin)	See Easprin	
Ascriptin (aspirin)		See Easprin
Bufferin (aspirin)		See Easprin
Datril (acetaminophen)	See Anacin-3	
Medipren (ibuprofen)		See Motrin
Nuprin (ibuprofen)		See Motrin
Panadol (acetaminophen)		See Anacin-3
Tylenol (acetaminophen)		See Anacin-3
Tylenol Extra Strength (acetaminophen)		See Anacin-3

Selected Bibliography

The following list of books has been supplied by Arthritis Care, which has carefully selected those from among the many published on the subject that have been found to be popular and useful. The publishers are grateful to Arthritis Care for permission to reproduce it here.

General

The Arthritis Helpbook: A tested self-management program for coping with your arthritis.

Authors: K. Lorig and J. F. Fries.

Description: The basis of education-in-arthritis programmes in many countries, this shows what can be achieved by understanding, exercise and self-management.

Publisher: Addison-Wesley, 3rd edition, 1990 (ISBN 0201524031)

Price: £11.45 including p&p

Available from: Projectlink, Old Vicarage, 84 Hampton Rd, Twickenham, Mddx TW2 5PX

Arthritis at Your Age?

Author: Jill Holroyd

Description: Written by, for and about people with arthritis, especially younger people.

Mini-review: Combines the author's chattiness with the authority of a well-sourced, comprehensive, academic work.

Publisher: Grindle Press, 1992 (ISBN 0951881604)

Available from: Grindle Press, PO Box 222, Ipswich, Suffolk, IP9 1HE

Price: £7.95 + £1.65 p&p

Arthritis: Dr Smith's Postbag

Authors: Mike Smith & Sharon Kerr

Description: Advice, information and reassurance in an approachable style. Based on the letters he receives, with many quotations from them.

Publisher: Kyle Cathie, 1993 (ISBN 1856260852)

Price: £3.99

Living with Arthritis: People with arthritis talk about coping from day to day

Author: M. Leitch

Description: A series of personal accounts of day-to-day experiences.

Mini-review: A very positive and encouraging book, but the information about sources of advice is becoming dated.

Publisher: Collins, 1987 (ISBN 0002182440) (Pbk)

Available from: Arthritis Care, 18 Stephenson Way, London NW1 2HD

Price: Free

Living with Arthritis

Author: J. Shenkman

Description: For children of 10 years upwards, explaining about arthritis, its treatment and coping with disability.

Mini-review: This well presented and illustrated book is the only layperson's book to describe the different kinds of joints. Designed for children, it is suitable for everyone.

Publisher: F. Watts, 1990 (ISBN 0749601000)

Price: £6.95

Research

All About Arthritis, Past, Present and Future

Author: Derrick Brewerton

Description: Explains the scientific aspects of arthritis research and treatment to general readers.

Publisher: Harvard University Press, 1992 (ISBN 0674016157)

Price: £15.95

Types of Arthritis

Ankylosing Spondylitis

A Guidebook for Patients

Author: National Ankylosing Spondylitis Society

Description: Practical information about diagnosis, treatments, especially exercise.

Publisher: NASS

Available from: NASS, 5 Grosvenor Crescent, London SW1X 7ER

Price: Free

Rheumatism and Arthritis: What they are and what you should know about them

Author: M. I. V. Jayson and A. St J. Dixon

Description: Describes all the main forms of arthritis, devoting a major section to Ankylosing Spondylitis.

Mini-review: The book does not live up to its claims except for Ankylosing Spondylitis.

Publisher: Pan Books, rev. ed., 1991 (ISBN 033031842X) (Pbk)
Price: £4.99

Rheumatoid Arthritis
Coping with Rheumatoid Arthritis
Author: R. H. Phillips
Description: Practical advice from a psychologist.
Publisher: Avery, 1989 (ISBN 0895293714)
Price: £8.95

Lupus
Coping with Lupus: A guide to living with lupus
Author: R. H. Phillips
Description: Covers positive strategies to cope with emotional reactions, stress, fatigue, relationships and especially depression.
Publisher: Avery, 1987 (ISBN 0895292521)
Price: £8.95
Lupus: A guide for parents
Author: G. R. V. Hughes
Description: An introductory booklet for people with lupus.
Publisher: G. R. V. Hughes, no date.
Available from: Arthritis Care
Price: £1.28 incl. p&p.

Osteoarthritis
Coping with Osteoarthritis
Author: Robert Phillips
Description: Teaches management and coping strategies.
Publisher: Avery, 1990 (ISBN 0895293935)
Price: £8.95

Osteoporosis
Avoiding Osteoporosis
Authors: Dr A. Dixon and Dr A. Woolf
Description: Includes causes, symptoms, preventative measures, treatments, etc.
Mini-review: Thorough and helpful, but unnecessarily alarming about spinal osteoporosis.
Publisher: Optima, 1989 (ISBN 0356154459)
Price: £5.99
Bone-loading: The new way to prevent and combat the thinning bones of osteoporosis
Authors: A. Simkin and J. Ayalon

Description: What can be done by exercise.

Mini-review: The exercise programmes need to be closely related to the medical condition being managed.

Publisher: Multimedia Books, 1990 (ISBN 1853750379) (Pbk)

Price: £7.50

Understanding Osteoporosis: Every woman's guide to preventing brittle bones

Author: W. Cooper

Description: Explains the causes and effects of osteoporosis. Includes hormone replacement therapy and statements from women on living with osteoporosis.

Publisher: Arrow, 1990 (ISBN 0099706202)

Price: £3.99

Living with Arthritis

Carers

Caring at Home: A handbook for people looking after someone at home – someone young or old, handicapped or disabled, ill or frail

Author: N. Kohner

Description: Provides basic information, sources of further information, and ways of coping with problems.

Publisher: National Extension College, rev. ed., 1993 (ISBN 1853560049)

Available from: BEBC, PO Box 1496, Poole, Dorset BH1 3YD

Price: £6.95

Diet

Some of the general books already listed have good chapters on diet, e.g. *Arthritis at Your Age?* and *The Arthritis Helpbook.*

Food for Thought

Author: Arthritis Care

Description: Leaflet on eating a balanced diet, supplements and food intolerance.

Publisher: Arthritis Care

Price: Free

The Complete Guide to Food Allergy and Intolerance

Authors: Dr J. Brostoff and L. Gamlin

Description: A popular book about a controversial subject, distinguishing types of reaction to food and elimination diets.

Publisher: Bloomsbury, 2nd ed, 1992 (ISBN 0747512604) (Pbk)

Price: £9.99

Arthritis: The allergy connection

Author: Dr J. Mansfield

Description: A controversial book about how arthritis might be helped by treatment for allergies.

Publisher: Thorsons, 1990 (ISBN 0722519036) (Pbk)

Publisher: Lansdowne Large Print Books, new ed, 1991 (ISBN 0745155286) (Pbk)

Price: £6.95

Exercise

The following books on arthritis relate specifically to exercise. For a full list of titles see *Arthritis: What Really Works* by Dava Sobel and Arthur Klein (Robinson 1994).

Baum, G. *Aquarobics* (Arrow Books, 1991). Step-by-step exercises in water devised by a physiotherapist.

Cooper Clinic, Dallas, USA *Arthritis – Your Complete Exercise Guide* (Human Kinetic Publishers). This is a proactive exercise program for the enthusiast. Rarely is the label 'complete' appropriate, but in this case it may be.

Hills, M. *The Curing Arthritis Exercise Book* (Sheldon Press). Illustrated exercises, with advice on diet.

Sayce, V. and Fraser, I. *Exercise Beats Arthritis* (Thorsons, 1992). A well-illustrated book of straightforward, simple exercises.

Disability

Directory for Disabled People: A handbook of information and opportunities for disabled and handicapped people

Authors: A. Darnborough and Derek Kinrade

Description: A comprehensive guide to the services and opportunities available.

Mini-review: Too comprehensive for most individual needs, this is a vital tool for groups.

Publisher: Woodhead Faulkner with RADAR, 6th ed, 1991 (ISBN 0859417018)

Price: £19.95

Aquarobics: Getting fit and keeping fit in the swimming pool

Author: G. Baum

Description: A well-illustrated book of step-by-step exercises in water devised by a physiotherapist, with sections on problem backs, hips, and knees and for people who are older, overweight or pregnant.

Publisher: Arrow Books, new ed, 1991 (ISBN 0099875101) (Pbk)

Price: £9.99

Exercise Beats Arthritis: An easy-to-follow programme of exercises

Authors: V. Sayce and I. Fraser

Description: This Australian book provides exercises for every joint for people with arthritis.

Mini-review: An excellent book of straightforward, simple exercises, well illustrated. There are useful tips on the different forms of arthritis and good instructions on the overall nature of diet in arthritis.

Publisher: Thorsons, 1992 (ISBN 0722527160) (Pbk)

Price: £9.00

Pain and stress management

Back Pain: The facts

Author: Malcolm Jayson

Description: Non-technical information on the causes of back pain and its effects, medical and surgical treatments, complementary therapies and self-help.

Publisher: Oxford University Press, 3rd ed, 1992 (ISBN 019262248X)

Price: £6.99

Beating Back Pain

Author: Dr J. Tanner

Description: A comprehensive introduction to preventing, treating and overcoming back and neck pain. Includes descriptions of orthodox and complementary medical approaches as well as on self-management techniques and pain management.

Publisher: Dorling Kindersley with the British Holistic Medical Association, 1987 (ISBN 0863181635) (Pbk)

Price: £6.99

Coping Successfully with Pain

Author: Neville Shone

Description: A practical guide to learning about pain, exercise and relaxation.

Publisher: Sheldon, 1992 (ISBN 0859696405) (Pbk)

Price: £4.99

Overcoming Stress

Author: Dr V. Coleman

Description: A practical, easy-to-understand book to help the general reader understand stress. It explains its causes and how to cope with it.

Publisher: Sheldon, 1988 (ISBN 0859695603)

Price: £5.95

A Self-Help Pain Management Programme
Author: R. Everatt
Description: For people with intractable pain, including pacing and relaxation.
Publisher: SHIP (Self Help In Pain, Whitstable)
Available from: SHIP, 33 Kingsdown Park, Tankerton, Kent CT5 2DT. Tel: (0227) 264677
Price: £2.50

Personal Relationships
Our Relationships, Our Sexuality: A guide for younger people with arthritis
Author: Young Arthritis Care/Kata Kolbert
Description: Explores myths and images concerning disability and sexuality and seeks to answer some common questions. Written by people with arthritis.
Publisher: Arthritis Care, 1992 (ISBN 0952030322)
Price: £3 or free to Arthritis Care members
Living, Loving & Ageing: Sexual and personal relationships in later life
Authors: W. Greengross and S. Greengross
Description: Tackles sexual issues in a straightforward fashion.
Publisher: Age Concern England, 1989 (ISBN 0862420709) (Pbk)
Price: £4.95
Publisher: ISIS Large Print Books, new ed, 1992 (ISBN 1856950409)
Price: £11.95

Pregnancy
Baby Challenge: Handbook on pregnancy for women with physical disability
Author: M. J. Campion
Description: Includes a chapter about women with arthritis.
Mini-review: An excellent chapter with straightforward advice on problems likely to be encountered by patients suffering from inflammatory arthritis who become pregnant and care for a young child.
Publisher: Routledge, 1990 (ISBN 0415048591) (Pbk)
Price: £10.99

Useful UK Addresses

The Arthritis and Rheumatism Council for Research
Copeman House
St Mary's Court
St Mary's Gate
Chesterfield
Derbyshire S41 7TD
Tel: 0870 850 5000 or
01246 558033
www.arc.org.uk

Arthritis Care
18 Stephenson Way
London NW1 2HD
Tel: 020 7380 6555
www.arthritiscare.org.uk

Arthritis Care is a registered charity and is the largest voluntary organization working with people with arthritis. A publications list and membership details are available from the address above. Arthritis Care publishes a quarterly magazine, *Arthritis News*, free to members, and has branches and local contacts throughout the UK. Contact them for information about self-help groups for particular forms of arthritis.

The following list of arthritis-related organizations has been supplied by Arthritis Care.

Behçet's Syndrome Society
3 Church Close
Lambourn
Hungerford RG17 8PU
Tel: 01488 71116
www.behcets-society.fsnet.co.uk

Bone Dysplasia Group
Child Growth Foundation
2 Mayfield Avenue
Chiswick
London W4 1PW
Tel: 0181 995 0257

British Sjögren's Syndrome Association
20 Kingston Way
Nailsea
Bristol BS19 2RA
Tel: 01275 854215

Children's Chronic Arthritis Association
Ground Floor
Amber Gate
City Wall Road
Worcester WR1 2AH
Tel: 01905 745595
www.ccaa.org.uk

**Dermatomyositis &
Polymyositis Support**
146 Newtown Road
Woolston
Southampton
Hants SO19 9HR
Tel: 023 80 449708
www.myositis.org.uk

Ehlers-Danlos Support Group
PO Box 337
Aldershot GU12 6WZ
Tel: 01252 690940
www.ehlers-danlos.org

Ekbom Support Group
(Restless Leg Syndrome)
18 Rodbridge Drive
Thorpe Bay
Essex SS1 3DF
Tel: 01702 582 002
www.ekbom.org.uk

Fibromyalgia Support Group:
PO Box 26, Stourbridge,
West Midlands DY9 8YL.
Tel: 01384 820052.
(Enclose SAE if writing. Arthritis
Care can supply details of local
fibromyalgia support groups.)

General Osteopathic Council
176 Tower Bridge Road
London
SE1 3LU
Tel: 020 7357 6655
www.osteopathy.org.uk

Lupus UK
St James House
Eastern Road
Romford
Essex RM1 3NH
Tel: 01708 731251
www.lupusuk.com

Marfan Association UK
Rochester House
5 Aldershot Road
Fleet
Hampshire GU51 3NG
Tel: 01252 810472
www.marfan.org.uk

**National Ankylosing
Spondylitis Society (NASS)**
PO Box 179
Mayfield
East Sussex TN20 6ZL
Tel: 01435 873527
www.nass.co.uk

**National Association for the
Relief of Paget's Disease**
323 Manchester Road
Walkden
Worsley
Manchester M28 3HH
Tel: 0161 799 4646
www.paget.org.uk

**National Osteoporosis
Society**
Camerton
Bath BA2 0PJ
Tel: 0845 4500230
www.nos.org.uk

Perthes Association
PO Box 773
Guildford
Surrey GU1 1XN
Tel: 01483 306637
www.perthes.org.uk

Psoriatic Arthropathy Alliance
PO Box 111
St Albans
Herts AL2 3JQ
Tel: 0870 7703212
www.paalliance.org

Raynaud's and Scleroderma Association
112 Crewe Road
Alsager
Cheshire ST7 2JA
Tel: 01270 872776
www.raynauds.org.uk

Restricted Growth Association
(includes children)
PO Box 4744
Dorchester DT2 9FA
Tel: 01308 898445
www.restrictedgrowth.co.uk

Sarcoidosis Association (UK)
(also British Association of
Sarcoidosis Patients):
19 Ashurst Close, Blackbrook,
St Helens, WA11 9DN
Tel: 01744 28020

Scleroderma Society
3 Caple Road
London NW10 8AB
Tel: 020 8961 4912
www.sclerodermasociety.co.uk

Scoliosis Association (UK)
2 Ivebury Court
323–327 Latimer Road
London W10 6RA
Tel: 020 8964 5343
www.sauk.org.uk

Useful UK Addresses (Exercise)

The following organizations work with people with arthritis. With the exception of the Arthritis and Rheumatism Council for Research and Arthritis Care (a charity, and the largest voluntary group for arthritis sufferers) these groups should be helpful specifically for guidance on exercise.

The Arthritis and Rheumatism Council for Research
Copeman House
St Mary's Court, St Mary's Gate
Chesterfield, Derbyshire
S41 7TD

Arthritis Care
18 Stephenson Way
London NW1 2HD
Tel: 0171 916 1500
(10a.m. – 4p.m., Mon. – Fri.);
freephone helpline 0800 289170
(12p.m. – 4p.m. Mon. – Fri.)

Northern Ireland
Arthritis Care Northern Ireland Manager
31 New Forge Lane
Belfast BT9 5NW
Will be able to supply you with a list of branches throughout the region.

Scotland
Arthritis Care Scotland Manager
68 Woodvale Avenue
Bearsden, Glasgow G61 2NZ
Will be able to supply you with a list of branches throughout Scotland.

Children's Chronic Arthritis Association
47 Battenhall Avenue, Worcester
WR5 2HN. Tel: 01905 763556

Disabled Living Foundation:
380–384 Harrow Road, London
W9 2HU. Tel: 0171 289 6111

National Back Pain Association
16 Elmtree Road, Teddington
Middlesex TW11 8ST
Tel: 0181 977 5474

National Osteoporosis Society
PO Box 10, Radstock
Bath, Avon BA3 3YB
Tel: 01761 471771

The Pain Society
9 Bedford Square
London WCIB 3RA
Tel: 0171 636 2750

Index

Page numbers given in italic refer to illustrations